Pediatric Tumors of the
Genitourinary Tract

Pediatric Tumors of the Genitourinary Tract

Editors

Bruce H. Broecker, M.D.
Departments of Surgery and Pediatrics
Medical College of Virginia
Richmond, Virginia

Frederick A. Klein, M.D.
Department of Surgery
Division of Urology
University of Tennessee Medical Center
Knoxville, Tennessee

Alan R. Liss, Inc., New York

Address all Inquiries to the Publisher
Alan R. Liss, Inc., 41 East 11th Street, New York, NY 10003

While the authors, editors, and publisher believe that drug selection and dosage and the specifications and usage of equipment and devices, as set forth in this book, are in accord with current recommendations and practice at the time of publication, they accept no legal responsibility for any errors or omissions, and make no warranty, express or implied, with respect to material contained herein. In view of ongoing research, equipment modifications, changes in governmental regulations and the constant flow of information relating to drug therapy, drug reactions and the use of equipment and devices, the reader is urged to review and evaluate the information provided in the package insert or instructions for each drug, piece of equipment or device for, among other things, any changes in the instructions or indications of dosage or usage and for added warnings and precautions.

Library of Congress Cataloging in Publication Data

Pediatric tumors of the genitourinary tract.

Includes bibliographies and index.
1. Genitourinary organs—Cancer. 2. Tumors in children. I. Broecker, Bruce H. II. Klein, Frederick A.
[DNLM: 1. Urogenital Neoplasms—in infancy & childhood.
WJ 160 P371]
RC280.G4P43   1988   618.92'9946   87-33898
ISBN 0-8451-4244-5

Contents

Contributors

John C. Adkins, Department of Surgery, Children's Hospital of Pittsburgh, Pittsburgh, PA 15213 [207]

J. Bruce Beckwith, Department of Pathology, The Children's Hospital, Denver, CO 80218 [25]

Mark F. Bellinger, Department of Pediatric Urology, Children's Hospital of Pittsburgh, Pittsburgh, PA 15213 [229]

William A. Brock, Department of Pediatric Urology, Schneider Children's Hospital, Long Island Jewish Medical Center, New Hyde Park, NY 11042 [49]

Bruce H. Broecker, Departments of Surgery and Pediatrics, Medical College of Virginia, Richmond, VA 23298; present address: Department of Surgery, Emory University School of Medicine, Atlanta, GA 30322 [ix,87,153]

Rebecca L. Byrd, Department of Pediatric Hematology—Oncology, Eastern Virginia Medical School, Norfolk, VA 23507 [61]

Richard H. Byrne, Department of Surgery, Georgetown University Medical Center, Chevy Chase, MD 20815 [113]

M. David Gibbons, Departments of Surgery and Pediatrics, Georgetown University Children's Medical Center, Washington, DC 20007 [113]

Martha Blechar Gibbons, Department of Human Development, University of Maryland, Washington, DC 20015 [299]

I. Gordon, Department of Pediatric Radiology, Hospital for Sick Children, London WC1 3JN, England [1]

Ronald Jaffe, Department of Pathology, Children's Hospital of Pittsburgh, Pittsburgh, PA 15213 [207]

Frederick A. Klein, Department of Surgery, Division of Urology, University of Tennessee Medical Center, Knoxville, TN 37920 [ix,177,283]

Thomas M. Krummel, Department of Pediatric Surgery, Medical College of Virginia, Richmond, VA 23298 [75]

The number in brackets is the opening page number of the contributor's article.

Walter Lawrence, Jr., Department of Surgery, Medical College of Virginia, Richmond, VA 23298 **[153]**

Gian Antonio M. Manzoni, Divisione Chirurgia Pediatrica, Ospedale Niguarda Ca'Granda, 20145 Milan, Italy **[113]**

Harold M. Maurer, Department of Pediatrics, Children's Medical Center, Medical College of Virginia, Richmond, VA 23298 **[139]**

C.D. Mitchell, Department of Hematology and Oncology, Hospital for Sick Children, London WC1 3JN, England **[187]**

James P. Neifeld, Department of Surgical Oncology, Medical College of Virginia, Richmond, VA 23298 **[95]**

P.N. Plowman, Department of Radiotherapy, St. Bartholomew's Hospital, London EC1A 7BE, England **[263]**

J. Pritchard, Department of Hematology and Oncology, Hospital for Sick Children, London WC1 3JN, England, **[187]**

Vincent M. Riccardi, Cytogenetics Research Laboratory, Baylor College of Medicine, Houston, TX 77030 **[241]**

Preface

The past two decades have witnessed a logarithmic increase in our knowledge and understanding of all aspects of cancer. Mysteries surrounding its origin and development are being unraveled at the same time as tremendous strides are occurring in diagnosis and management. Nowhere have these advances been more fruitful than in pediatric oncology. This volume brings together contributions from experts in various disciplines for a comprehensive discussion of the clinical management of children with genitourinary tumors.

Tumors of the genitourinary tract are responsible for between 25–30% of cancer occurring during childhood. The most common of these—neuroblastoma, Wilms' tumor, and rhabdomyosarcoma—are emphasized throughout the text in chapters on pathology, imaging, and genetics as well as in their respective individual chapters. Neuroblastoma continues to challenge us to find more effective treatment and improve overall survival. A number of new and innovative treatment modalities may help achieve that goal. The prognosis for children with Wilms' tumor and rhabdomyosarcoma has improved tremendously due in large part to superb cooperative multidisciplinary, multi-institutional studies such as the National Wilms' Tumor Study (NWTS) and the Intergroup Rhabdomyosarcoma Study (IRS). Although NWTS and IRS receive particular attention in this book, equally excellent European studies are discussed by the European contributors and data is introduced from that continent with which American clinicians may be less familiar.

The less common tumors of the adrenal, kidney, testes, and ovary have also been thoroughly covered by individual authors and there are chapters specifically addressing the long-term complications of antineoplastic therapy as well as the emotional impact of cancer on patients and their families.

Pediatric Tumors of the Genitourinary Tract is intended to be a clinical reference text of the most current information available on management of children with these tumors. In this rapidly changing field it is anticipated that future volumes will document a continuing improvement in prognosis for these children. We are indebted to the authors for the excellence of their contributions and to the staff at Alan R. Liss, Inc., who have made this book possible.

Bruce H. Broecker, M.D.
Frederick A. Klein, M.D.

Chapter 1
Imaging in Pediatric Genitourinary Malignancy

I. Gordon

The child with a suspected malignancy demands rapid evaluation to establish a diagnosis and to stage the malignant process. The department of radiology may provide images that strongly suggest a diagnosis, but no image is yet able to preclude histological confirmation of malignancy. The brief of the radiologist presented with a child who may have a malignancy is to assess the extent of the disease at presentation and guide the clinician's thoughts towards a relevant differential diagnosis. Frequently this may involve a combination of radiological and non-radiological methods, e.g., bone marrow trephine/aspirate, biochemical markers, and immunologic cell surface markers. It is imperative to know the exact diagnosis before embarking on a series of images that are not clinically useful or relevant [1]. The natural history of each malignancy and the most appropriate method for detecting relapse/recurrence must be coupled with the knowledge of the limitation of each modality of imaging if the site of recurrence is to be found.

The various imaging techniques have different degrees of invasiveness and unpleasantness for the child and have staggeringly different financial implications. These factors must all be considered when the team of oncologist, surgeon, radiotherapist, and radiologist come together to plan the investigation of the individual patient. Children with malignant disease will be frequent visitors to the radiology department, and, therefore, it is our policy to explain fully to the child and parent what we are doing. Patient preparation is important to ensure that the child's apprehension is reduced to the minimum and, therefore, maximum cooperation occurs between the radiographer

Pediatric Tumors of the Genitourinary Tract, pages 1–23
© 1988 Alan R. Liss, Inc.

and the child/parent. The results of the examination are made available to the parents through the clinical team within 12 hours in almost all cases.

RADIOLOGIST'S STRATEGY

In suspected malignancy the aim is to suggest a diagnosis or differential diagnosis and then stage the malignancy at the appropriate time. Followup of these children, searching for recurrance/relapse and/or the complications of therapy, is the basis for later investigation.

Diagnosis

To suggest an accurate differential diagnosis, using the least invasive methods is the first aim [2,3]. When a child presents with a mass, hematuria, or any other sign/symptom suggestive of an abdominal malignancy the radiologist's objective is to support or refute this suggestion. The chest and plain abdominal radiographs together with an abdominal ultrasound examination will frequently allow this broad division to be made.

No radiographic image, no matter how fine the detail, can offer a histologic diagnosis. While this limit of all imaging must be stressed, it is true that certain abdominal malignancies have such characteristic features that the radiologist has a very high probability of suggesting the correct histologic diagnosis.

Staging

This should only begin once the diagnosis has been firmly established either histologically or biochemically. There is however a conflict since accurate staging is required in order to instigate the correct treatment. Certain malignancies will receive preliminary chemotherapy rather than surgery. There is therefore a great deal of pressure on the radiologist to suggest the histologic diagnosis from the images in order that further imaging can be undertaken as soon as possible. In staging various malignancies, it is now accepted that accurate assessment of the skeleton requires a 99m technetium (Tc) isotope bone scan. Similarly if a secondary deposit in the lungs must be absolutely excluded then a CT scan is required [4]. Assessment of bulk disease in the abdomen can be done using ultrasound unless the disease is so extensive that the ultrasound cannot define the cranial or caudal extent; then CT is required. The liver is best assessed by more than one modality of imaging, and a combination of ultrasound and 99m Tc colloid liver/spleen scan or CT is required.

Complications

The radiologist may be helpful in detecting complications of therapy, as well as recurrent disease. The presence of an occult infection must always be kept in mind in immune-compromised children, and, at times, a child may be subjected to numerous imaging techniques in order to discover the presence of pus. Included in these investigations is radiolabeling white blood cells (WBC), which is now available in many departments [5,6]. The detection of recurrence in certain malignancies, e.g., Wilms' tumor or rhabdomyosarcoma, is heavily dependent on ultrasound and/or CT. Other malignancies tend to show up clinically with such rapidity that routine extensive imaging in the followup period is of little clinical help. This is common for neuroblastoma.

ULTRASOUND

This examination is non-invasive and does not expose the child to any radiation. Real-time equipment now available in most diagnostic departments provides high quality images of the liver, inferior vena cava (IVC), aorta, paraaortic nodes, and pancreas. The kidneys can be well visualized both in the supine and prone positions. The full bladder provides a good acoustic window for images for both the bladder base and remaining pelvic structures [7]. The ultrasound examination requires a quiet environment. The aim of the ultrasound examination is to identify a mass, define its full extent and echo characteristics, as well as identify the organ of origin. Information about the kidneys, liver, aorta, and IVC complete the examination. Whenever an abdominal mass is seen both kidneys must be identified. If a kidney cannot be seen, generally the mass arises from that organ. The echo characteristics allow a broad classification of the mass. If it is solid on ultrasound, then it must be considered malignant until proven otherwise. Rarely a hyperechogenic mass may be benign [8]. The characteristic appearances of a Wilms' tumor is that of hypoechogenic areas interspersed with echo-dense areas (Fig. 1-1A). A mass that is transonic may well be benign, but certain renal malignancies may have a cystic component and, therefore, the ultrasonographer must carefully look for any hyperechogenic area in the cystic renal mass (Fig. 1-3A). The so-called cystic Wilms' tumor is well recognized and must not be mistaken for a multilocular cyst. This tumor, if large, usually displaces adjacent structures. Neuroblastoma, the other common pediatric abdominal tumor, frequently has a homogeneously dense appearance, often with evidence of calcification (Fig. 1-5B). This tumor invades adjacent structures and may surround and encase vessels. Nevertheless, at times it may be

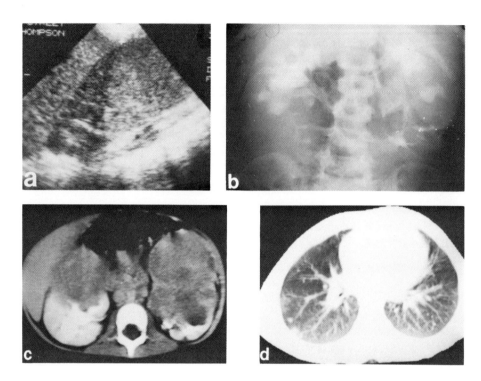

Fig. 1-1. This 4-year-old girl had abdominal pain and was found to have a left-sided abdominal mass. **a:** Ultrasound examination of the right kidney revealed a solid echogenic mass. The mass palpated on the left was also shown on ultrasound to be a solid renal mass. **b:** IVU clearly shows the bilateral nature of the intrarenal masses. **c:** CT scan of the kidneys confirms bilateral masses. **d:** Chest CT at that time was shown to have deposits not seen on the chest radiograph. **e:** Following various courses of chemotherapy, surgery was planned. Preoperative CT scan shows the relationship of the left renal artery to the mass in the left kidney. **f:** Digital subtraction angiogram (DSA) reveals the exact arterial supply to the left kidney and also demonstrates that this tumor is "avascular," with no malignant vessels. **g:** DSA of the right kidney shows not only the arterial anatomy but also malignant vessels on this side. **h:** ^{99m}Tc DMSA scan reveals the functioning renal parenchyme that guides the surgeon in determining what is surgically feasible.

impossible to distinguish between a Wilms' in the upper pole of the kidney and an adrenal neuroblastoma [9]. There must be careful systematic examination of all the other abdominal organs with positive identification of the major vessels as well as the liver. Abdominal ultrasonography is widely used and is the first examination in the radiology department. The examination is highly operator-dependent, and a skilled ultrasonographer should carry out

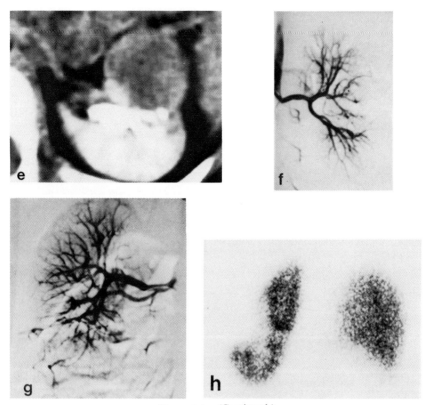

Figure 1-1. (Continued.)

the examination. The child may be unwell and in a strange environment with a great deal of equipment that he/she finds frightening. These factors add to the difficulty of getting the full cooperation of the child. The ultrasonographer might well need to repeat the examination the next morning after the child has not only had a night's rest but is a little more accustomed to the procedure.

It is important to realize the limitations of this examination. The areas that are difficult to evalute completely with the ultrasound include masses close to the hemidiaphragm where the superior extent of the mass cannot be seen. Masses in the pelvis, especially close to the pelvic side walls, cannot be completely seen. If there is a great deal of bowel gas then adequate images of the aorta, IVC, and adjacent areas may not be seen. Since the abdominal ultrasound examination may be the first imaging procedure, one must be

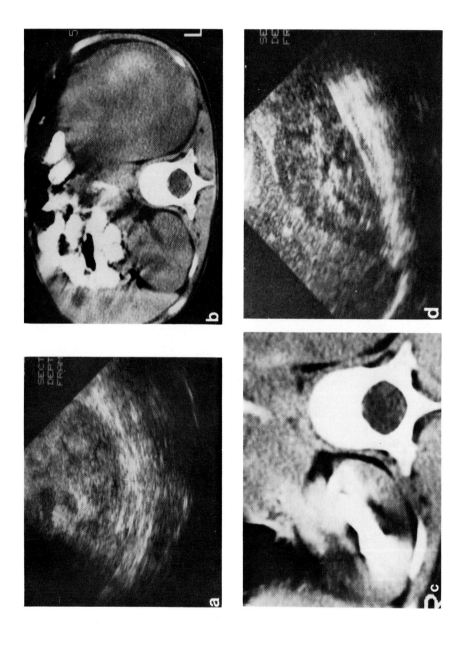

careful to ensure that an adequate examination has been carried out before attempting to draw conclusions about a mass and its extent and possible pathology.

RADIOLOGY

Chest Radiograph

Every child with a solid abdominal mass requires a frontal and lateral chest radiograph. If metastases are seen, then one has not only established the stage but has also confirmed the suspicion of malignancy from the ultrasound. A normal radiograph does not exclude the presence of metastasis and by itself is inadequate to accurately stage tumors that commonly metastasize to the lungs. Tomography also is relatively insensitive when compared to computed tomography (CT) and should no longer be undertaken if CT is available. The presence of a paravertebral mass, especially if adjacent to the lower dorsal spine, strongly suggests a neuroblastoma.

Plain Abdominal Radiograph

This film is helpful if calcification is present. Curvilinear calcification sugggests Wilms' tumor, while speckled calcification suggests a neuroblastoma (Fig. 1-6A). A tooth may be seen to suggest a dermoid/teratoma. Displacement of the bowel may be seen. Calcification may also represent renal calculi as seen in xanthogranulomatous pyelonephritis [8].

Intravenous Urogram (IVU)

This examination has been substantially replaced by the newer modalities of ultrasound and CT. It is difficult to list the appropriate indications for an IVU since many clinicians continue to be most comfortable with radiographic interpretations drawn from this more familiar examination. In addition, some

---

Fig. 1-2. This 2-year-old girl was noted to have hematuria. A left-sided abdominal mass was found on examination. **a:** Abdominal ultrasound examination shows that the mass arises from the left kidney and is solid. **b:** CT scan precontrast shows the left renal mass and raises suspicion about the normality of the right kidney. **c:** CT scan postcontrast of the right kidney shows that both the anterior and posterior aspects of this kidney are abnormal. **d:** Repeat ultrasound examination of the right kidney preoperatively failed to show the mass even though the ultrasonographer was aware of the results of the CT scan done 24 h previously. At surgery, a biopsy from the right kidney revealed unfavorable histology of Wilms' tumor. The same histology was obtained from the left kidney.

tumor protocols continue to require an IVU prior to randomization and treatment. It is easier to define when an IVU is not required. If the ultrasound examination has identified two normal kidneys with no evidence of any dilatation of the collecting systems, then the mass is neither arising from nor affecting the renal tract (Fig. 1-8C). If the mass is solid on ultrasound examination and completely contained within the kidney, then it is almost certainly a renal malignancy, probably a Wilms' tumor and an IVU is of no particular aid. Since contrast-enhanced CT scans are frequently carried out, an abdominal radiograph at the end of the CT scan may well satisfy radiologist, clinician, and protocol. An IVU may still be helpful when one is attempting to distinguish between a Wilms' tumor of the upper pole and a neuroblastoma.

Skeletal Survey

When searching for skeletal metastasis, a radiological survey is inappropriate. An isotope bone scan is required.

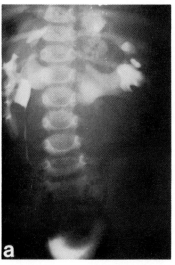

Fig. I-3. A 2-year-old boy with an abdominal mass noted by his grandmother. The boy was well. **a:** Ultrasound examination reveals a mass of mixed echogenicity. This mass with a partial echogenic character must be regarded as malignant. **b:** IVU shows a normal right kidney. The calyces of the left kidney are distorted by an intrarenal mass. Some calyces are displaced over the midline. **c:** CT scan after contrast shows how the kidney has been split by the intrarenal mass and the attenuation of the mass is mixed. This mass was a Wilms' tumor with favorable histology, a so-called cystic Wilms' tumor.

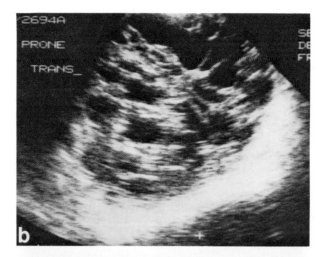

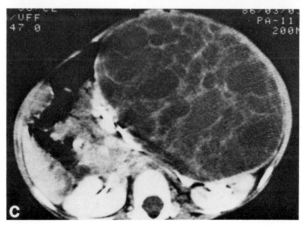

Figure 1-3. (Continued.)

Angiography

There are some indications for vascular studies in malignancy. The surgeon may request a renal arteriogram to aid with conservative surgery when Wilms' tumors are either bilateral (Fig. 1-1F,G), arise in a child with a solitary kidney, or occur in those children who are predisposed to further malignancy (e.g., hemihypertrophy, Beckwith-Weidemann syndrome, aniridia). Hepatic arteriography is requested by certain surgeons prior to partial hepatectomy in order to define the origin of the right hepatic artery and also to look at the hepatic venous drainage. Inferior vena cavography has largely

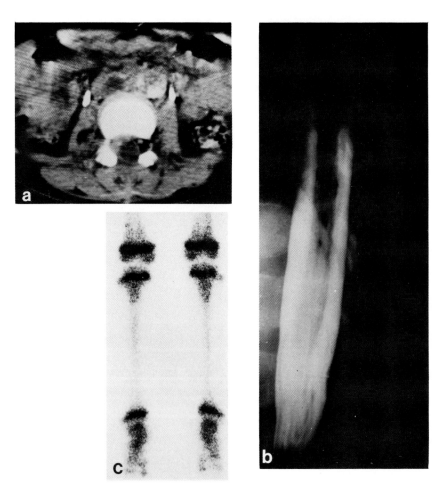

Fig. 1-4. This 1-year-old boy was noted to have stopped moving his legs and was unwell. **a:** CT scan shows a paravertebral mass and the spinal cord displaced laterally by a mass. **b:** Myelogram shows that contrast stops at the level of L4 due to the presence of a mass. **c:** ^{99m}Tc MDP bone scan shows that both knees are abnormal with loss of the normally clear hot epiphyseal plate. There is increased uptake of the isotope in the diaphysis. This was due to a stage IV neuroblastoma. **d:** Following six courses of chemotherapy, the repeat ^{99m}Tc MDP bone scan was normal. **e:** ^{123}I MIGB scan shows uptake of isotope in the midline at the site of the original tumor.

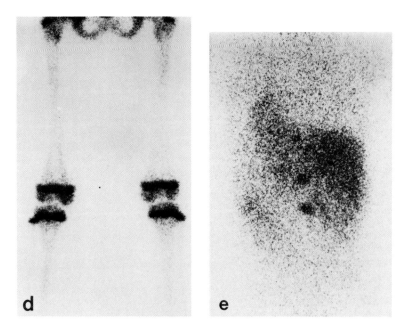

Figure 1-4. (Continued.)

been replaced by the combination of ultrasound and CT. It remains difficult to distinguish between an obstructed or flattened IVC due to tumor within the IVC or external compression by the tumor, respectively.

CT

The use of CT in both the chest and abdomen has, together with ultrasound, allowed complete delineation of most genitourinary malignancies.

Chest

This is the definitive examination for the detection of pulmonary metastasis. The increased sensitivity compared to tomography has been established. All children with a rhabdomyosarcoma or a Wilms' tumor require a chest CT. Even stage I Wilms' tumor may have micronodular metastasis. It is important to establish whether there is any difference between stage I with and without micronodular deposits in long-term followup. This has not yet been established.

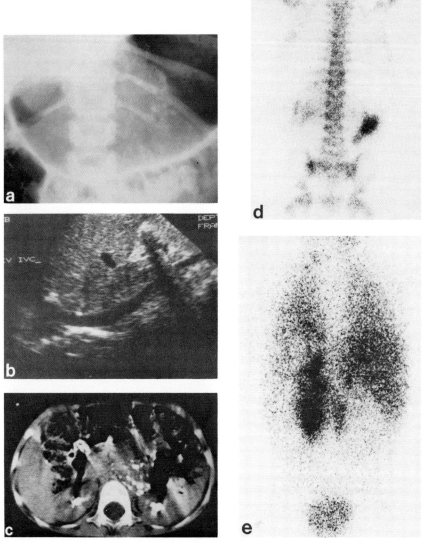

Fig. I-5. This 2-year-old boy presented unwell with anemia and anorexia, and was found to be hypertensive. **a:** Plain abdominal radiograph shows calcification in the left renal area strongly supporting the diagnosis of neuroblastoma. **b:** Ultrasound examination reveals that the calcified mass crosses the midline. The liver and IVC are clearly seen. The mass is elevating the IVC. **c:** CT scan shows contrast in both kidneys, the mass is again noted to cross the midline, and calcification is seen. **d:** ^{99m}Tc MDP bone scan of the spine shows that the right kidney is displaced and the left kidney is poorly seen. The mass takes up the isotope and is clearly seen as a hot area. **e:** ^{123}I MIBG scan shows the tumor to be taking up the isotope. The normal distribution of the isotope in the heart and right adrenal are also clearly seen.

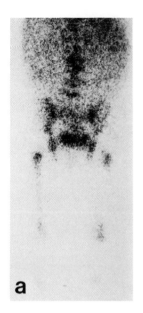
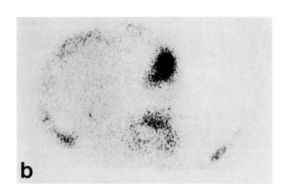

Fig. 1-6. This 1-year-old girl presented acutely unwell and had proptosis. She was found to have a neuroblastoma. **a:** [123]I MIBG scan shows abnormal accumulation of the isotope in the spine, pelvis, and both femurs. Normally the bone does not take up the isotope. **b:** Lateral view of the skull of the ^{123}I MIBG scan shows that there is increased uptake of the isotope in the region of the proptosis. The protosis was confirmed to be due to the tumor as judged from the response to chemotherapy.

Abdomen

The images should provide full visualization of the liver, spleen, pancreas, paraaortic nodes, IVC, and aorta, as well as the kidneys, ureters, and bladder. All children should be given oral as well as IV contrast (via a foot vein) and dynamic scans obtained. The renal veins are difficult to visualize. Indications for abdominal CT scan include all pelvic and abdominal masses that have a high probability of malignancy. The advantages of CT over ultrasound is the ability to assess local invasion more precisely, more accurate exclusion of stage V Wilms' tumor (bilateral disease), and assessment of lymph nodes. IVC involvement is also better demonstrated on CT [10]. Whenever there is a suspicion of intracaval tumor and the ultrasound has failed to outline the IVC, a CT should be done. In neuroblastoma; the cranial extent is often only seen using CT. Pelvic tumors, especially if they extend to the bony side walls, may only be fully visualized on CT. Tumors in the

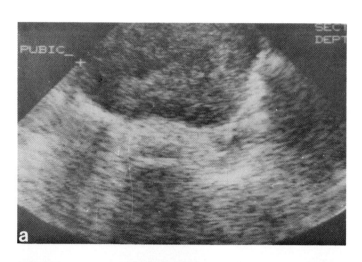

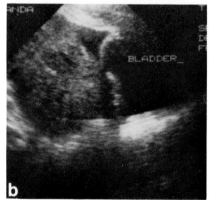

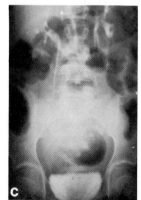

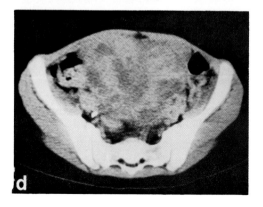

bladder base are well seen on ultrasound, and the results of CT (in my experience) have suggested that CT has nothing to offer in the followup of polypoid bladder tumors. Those arising in the prostate can only be accurately followed by CT. The suggestion of spinal cord involvement in neuroblastoma is another indication [11].

RADIOISOTOPES

The images provided are functional images in that the accumulation of the specific radiosotope is dependent on the function of the cells to which the isotope has been directed. Successful examinations require not only a dedicated technologist who is sympathetic to children, but also a great deal of patient cooperation. In a sick, miserable child this is a great deal to ask for, but a full explanation to both child and parent often removes the need for sedation. Long examinations, i,e., bone scans, are frequently done with the room lights dim and the mother reading a story. The environment in the room should be kept peaceful. The most frequently used isotope is ^{99m}Tc, which has a short half-life of 6.5 h and is a pure gamma energy emitter. The radiation dose is small, and the image quality is high. This isotope can be labeled to one of many specific compounds so that the labeled isotope will be taken up by only one cell type in the body. Iodine is also used labeled to metaiodobenzylguanidine (MIBG). This compound is specifically taken up by the adrenal glands and has also been shown to accumulate in both neuroblastoma and pheochromocytoma. Iodine has also been labeled to a monoclonal antibody (UJ13A) specific to neuroectodermally derived tissue and is useful in neuroblastoma [12].

^{99m}Tc Methyl Diphosphonate (MDP) Bone Scan

This isotope is absorbed onto the hydroxyapatite in the bone, and, therefore, the image represents areas of bone turnover. In the child, the growing

---

Fig. 1-7. This 12-year-old girl presented with a 4-day history of lower abdominal pain associated with pain in the left thigh. Examination revealed a large lower abdominal mass. **a:** Transverse abdominal ultrasound examination showed a "solid" mass independent from the bladder. **b:** Longitudinal ultrasound showed that the mass could not be separated from the uterus but was anterior to the rectum. Neither ovary could be identified. There were two normal kidneys. **c:** IVU shows a normal urinary tract with a mass above the bladder. **d:** CT scan confirms the mass and shows a mixed attenuation within the mass. This particular case shows how the ultrasound may be comprehensive for certain masses and that the IVU and CT did not add to the definition of the mass, which was rhabdomyosarcoma of the uterus. CT of the lungs and the ^{99m}Tc bone scan were normal (not illustrated).

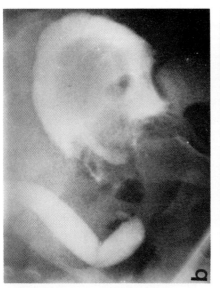

a

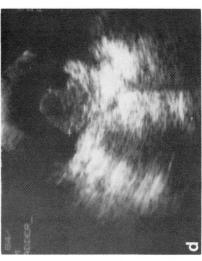

b

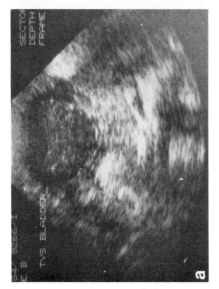

c

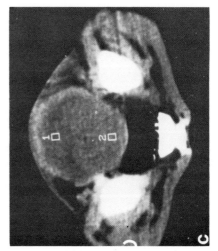

d

ends of the bones therefore show up as hot areas, but it must be remembered that the appearances of these areas change with the maturity of the skeleton. This is most obvious in the knee. In neuroblastoma, the malignancy permeates the skeleton rather than growing as discrete masses of malignancy. This causes a typical appearance with ill-defined areas of increased uptake most obvious around the knees (Fig. 1-5C,D) and also seen in the cranial vault. Almost any site can be involved. The isotope also accumulates in the primary tumor in over 65% of neuroblastoma. It is possible on a ^{99m}Tc MDP scan to strongly suggest the diagnosis of neuroblastoma when one sees the typical infiltration of the bones and the mass taking up the isotope. In Wilms' tumor, it is only the bone metastasizing tumor that requires regular bone scans both at diagnosis and followup. There is no role for bone scans in the regular followup of pelvic rhabdomyosarcoma.

^{99m}Tc Colloid Scans

These small particles are taken up by the reticuloendothelial cells, and, therefore depending on which particle is used, either a liver/speen scan or a combination of a liver/spleen scan and bone marrow scan is obtained. Although this bone marrow scan has been attempted in many institutions, it has found little use in clinical practice. The liver/spleen scan on the other hand has been found useful in helping to establish the involvement of the liver by the malignancy. The most accurate assessment of the liver requires at least two different techniques, yet even using a combination of liver/spleen scan, ultrasound, and CT it may be impossible to differentiate between a tumor that is compressing the liver from one that is infiltrating the liver.

^{99m}Tc Dimercaptosuccinic acid (DMSA)

This isotope fixes in the proximal tubules of the kidney. It may be useful if renal-sparing surgery is being planned in those children with bilateral Wilms' tumors or a Wilms' tumor arising in a child with a predisposition to malignancy, e.g., hemihypertrophy (Fig. 1-1H).

Fig. 1-8. This 10-month-old boy presented with hematuria and acute urinary retention. **a:** Abdominal ultrasound examination shows an echogenic mass within the bladder. **b:** Cystogram confirms the presence of the intravesical mass. **c:** CT scan again shows the mass; the paraaortic lymph nodes were normal. This was a rhabdomyosarcoma. **d:** Followup ultrasound examination clearly shows how well the tumor is responding to chemotherapy.

^{99m}Tc Hexamethylpropylene-amine Oxine (HMPAO)

This isotope may be used to label WBCs. The scan is a highly sensitive technique for the localization of an occult infection [6].

MIBG Labeled to Iodine 131 or 123

This isotope is taken up by the adrenergic nerve endings in the body and was first used clinically for the diagnosis of pheochromocytoma. The normal distribution of ^{131}I MIBG is into the salivary glands, heart, and liver. ^{123}I MIBG is also seen in the normal adrenal glands. This isotope provides good visualization of the primary neuroblastoma as well as secondary deposits (Figs. 1-5E,6).

The value in evaluating an abdominal mass is limited since biopsy of the mass is generally feasible. It may be useful however when the mass is not easily accessible for biopsy. The more important use may be in staging of neuroblastoma both at presentation and after chemotherapy. This applies to children with stage IV disease clinically in remission at the end of chemotherapy since these children frequently relapse. Another use may be to monitor therapy, including the response to chemotherapy, as well as distinguishing neuroblastoma from other causes of an abnormal ^{99m}Tc MDP bone scan. This is still a new technique, and its sensitivity and specificity have not been established. Therapeutic applications of MIBG labeled to 131 or 125 iodine are yet to be established.

UJI3A

This is a monoclonal antibody labeled with iodine. The antibody is specific for neuroectodermally derived tissue. Both animal and human studies using this isotope in vivo and in vitro have shown good results in neuroblastoma. The limited availability and high degree of skill required to make and label this isotope have limited its use [12].

MAGNETIC RESONANCE IMAGING

Magnetic resonance imaging (MRI) involves the use of a high, stable magnetic field into which the patient is placed. A radio frequency impulse of known short duration is applied to the magnetic field and sensitive radio frequency detectors then pick up the emitted radio frequency from the patient. The stable high magnetic field forces all the atoms to align according to the field force; the application of a short radio frequency pulse causes these cells to change their alignment rapidly. It is the process of realignment that is carefully measured and transformed into an image. The advantages of this technique are that no radiation is used, no known side effects have yet been demonstrated, the resolution is better than 1 mm, and bone does not cause an image problem. This enables visualization of the spinal cord without contrast. The disadvantage is the high cost of the equipment and the length of each examination (approximately 1 h per patient). The noise of the machine and claustrophobia are other recognized drawbacks to this technique. The use of MRI in genitourinary malignancy has yet to be established, since ultrasound and CT provide a great deal of anatomical information. The potential of this technique in the evaluation of the spinal cord in neuroblastoma is interesting. The development of tracers coupled to MRI may increase the potential usefulness of this technique in imaging of malignancies.

Magnetic Resonance Spectroscopy

Although this technique is not new, the possibility of in vivo spectroscopy with high quality images may open new horizons.

SPECIFIC TUMORS

The child may present clinically in a number of ways. It is the intention of this chapter to help the clinician handle any child in whom the diagnosis of a malignancy is suspected. One must emphasize the inability of any image to give a histological diagnosis, yet it is imaging that may point one to the correct diagnosis. Since radiation is not a major issue in this particular group of children, most of these children will undergo comprehensive staging and followup using what is regarded as the most sensitive technique. Virtually all the children will have an abdominal ultrasound examination and many will also have a CT scan early on in their investigation. It is, however, worthwhile trying to define various subgroups of patients so that the best use is made of the resources available and that the children are not subjected to unnecessary investigations.

Wilms' Tumor (Figs. 1-1–1-3)

If the ultrasound shows a solid renal or possible renal mass, then both a PA and lateral chest radiograph, as well as a CT scan, are required. The CT scan should include both the chest and abdomen pre- and postcontrast, as well as dynamic IVC imaging with contrast [10]. When ultrasound shows bilateral tumors, abdominal CT scan may be omitted. If lung metastases are seen on chest radiograph, then similarly, CT is not required.

Children who have inoperable tumors should be biopsied and treated with chemotherapy. This is followed by surgery if the tumor becomes operable.

Immediately preceding surgery, further imaging includes repeat ultrasound, CT scan, and ^{99m}Tc DMSA.

As regards operable tumors, if the histology is favorable, there is no further staging, only followup. If the histology is unfavorable, the procedure is as follows: anaplastic, no further staging; rhabdoid, brain CT scan; bone metastasizing, ^{99m}Tc bone scan, with chest radiograph and abdominal ultrasound followup.

Mesoblastic Nephroma

The imaging investigations for the diagnosis, staging, and followup are chest radiograph and abdominal ultrasound. These tumors usually present in early infancy [13], rarely metastasize, but may spread by local recurrence when the original surgery was associated with incomplete removal or spillage [14].

Neuroblastoma (Figs. 1-4–1-6)

The imaging should be done while the urinary biochemical analysis and even bone marrow aspiration and trephine biopsy are being undertaken [11]. Appropriate evaluation should include ultrasound, chest radiograph, abdominal radiograph, CT scan of abdomen pre- and postcontrast, ^{99m}Tc MDP bone scan and I MIBG scan.

Restaging should occur when the child has come to the end of chemotherapy. All the above investigations need to be repeated.

For stages I and II, no followup imaging is required. For stages III and IV, the role of routine followup is controversial; this center has found it to be of limited value. Over 40 children with stage IV disease underwent 240 ultrasound examinations and more than 120 ^{99m}Tc MDP bone scans, yet no child relapsed without clinical evidence of disease, and the imaging played no role in predicting either which children would relapse or when the relapse would occur. The role of I MIBG needs to be fully assessed since either this agent or I UJ13A (a monoclonal antibody) might change this situation.

Pheochromocytoma

When this diagnosis is suspected then evaluation should include ultrasound, I MIBG scan, and CT pre- and postcontrast. Most institutions still carry out venous sampling in the IVC and renal veins as well as arteriography. The child must be on adequate alpha and beta blockers prior to these investigations. The major aim of these studies is to accurately localize the tumors, but one must question their place in the light of recent advances using I MIBG.

Rhabdomyosarcoma (Figs. 1-7, 1-8)

All genitourinary rhabdomyosarcomas should have ultrasound, chest radiograph, CT scan of abdomen pre- and postcontrast, and ^{99m}Tc MDP bone scans. Followup should include ultrasound, CT scan, and chest radiograph.

The polypoidal bladder rhabdomyosarcoma is comprehensively imaged by ultrasound alone. The other rhabdomyosarcomata, especially those arising in the prostate, require both ultrasound and CT for adequate visualization of the mass, both for diagnosis and followup.

Lymphoma/Leukemia (Fig. 1-9)

Imaging plays a very small role in diagnosis and staging of both non-Hodgkin's lymphoma and leukemia [15]. The routine is for a chest radiograph and ultrasound examination to be done at the time of diagnosis. The demonstration of renal involvement allows the clinician to anticipate renal failure during induction chemotherapy.

CONCLUSIONS

The possible ways of creating an image are so wide that either the oncologist/surgeon is required to become a fully trained radiologist or the clinician must work closely with the radiologist. The various images created are based on different principles so that few clinicians could become proficient in these new imaging modalities while remaining deeply involved in clinical medicine. It is difficult even for the radiologist to remain fully proficient given the speed of current development. The radiologist is part of the team, and, at times, important decisions about patient management will be heavily influenced by his decision. This situation has altered the role of the radiologist who must be prepared to enter into this team philosophy.

Throughout this chapter, the title radiologist refers to ultrasonographer or radiologist or nuclear medicine physician. It is also assumed that there is easy access to all types of imaging equipment. There are, however, many clinical problems that can be solved in a number of different ways, and no one specific technique is always correct.

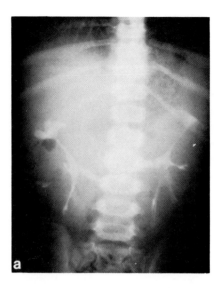

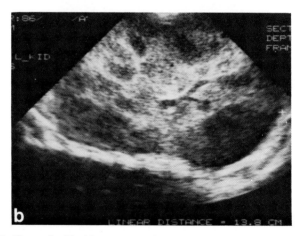

Fig. 1-9. This 18-month-old girl was not eating, irritable, and had bruising of the skin. Examination shows a protruberant abdomen due to a large mass. The diagnosis of leukemia was made on blood and bone marrow analysis. **a:** IVU shows two large kidneys with the calyces distorted and stretched by the "swollen" kidneys. **b:** Longitudinal section of the left kidney on ultrasound showing the enlarged kidney with masses within the kidney. **c:** Transverse scan of the right kidney shows a similar appearance, with the collecting system squashed by the leukemic deposits.

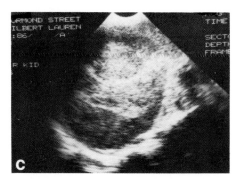

Figure 1-9. (Continued.)

REFERENCES

1. Schweisguth O: Solid Tumors in Children. New York: John Wiley, 1982.
2. Miller JH (ed): Imaging in Pediatric Oncology. Baltimore: Williams and Wilkins, 1985.
3. Parker BR, Castellino RA (eds): Pediatric Oncologic Radiology. St. Louis: Mosby, 1977.
4. Damgaard-Pederson K: The capabilities and limitations of CT. In Husband JE, Hobday PA (eds): Pediatric Oncology in Computerized Axial Tomography. Edinburgh: Churchill Livingstone, 1981.
5. Gordon I, Vivian G: Radiolabeled leukocytes: A new diagnostic tool in occult infection. Arch Dis Child 59:62–66, 1984.
6. Peters AM, Danpure HJ, Osman S et al.: Clinical experience with ^{99m}Tc hexamethylpropylene-amine oxine for labeling leucocytes and imaging inflammation. Lancet 2:946–949, 1986.
7. Garel L, Devred P, Leclere J: Retroperitoneal tumors. In Kalifa G. (ed.): Pediatric Ultrasonography. Berlin: Springer Verlag, 1986, pp 190–199.
8. Sweeney LE, Gordon I: A miserable child with an abdominal mass and more. Br J Radiol 59:707–708, 1986.
9. Hartman D, Sanders R: Wilms' tumor versus neuroblastoma. Usefulness of ultrasound in differentiation. J Ultrasound Med 1:117–122, 1982.
10. Reiman AH, Siefel MJ, Shakelford GD: Wilms' tumor in children: Abdominal ultrasound and CT evaluation. Radiology 160:501–505, 1986.
11. Resjo M, Harwood-Nash DC, Fitz CR, et al: CT metrizamide myelography for intraspinal and paraspinal neoplasms in infants and children. AJR 132:367–372, 1979.
12. Gordon I, Goldman A: A critical approach to imaging in neuroblastoma. In Pochedly C (ed): Pediatric Hem/Oncology Reviews. New York, Philadelphia: Praeger, 1985, pp 81–103.
13. Snyder H, et al.: Congenital mesoblastic nephroma: Relationship to other renal tumors in infancy. J Urol 126:513–516, 1981.
14. Hartman DS, Lesar MSL, Madewell JE, et al.: Mesoblastic nephroma: Radiologic-pathologic correlation of 20 cases. AJR 136:69–74, 1981.
15. Gore RM, Shkolinik A: Abdominal manifestations of pediatric leukemias: Sonographic assessment. Radiology 143:207–210, 1982.

Chapter 2
Pathological Aspects of Renal Tumors in Childhood

J. Bruce Beckwith

A number of recent advances in our understanding of the pathology of childhood renal neoplasia have major implications for clinicians. These advances form the basis of this chapter, which does not attempt to review completely all aspects of this complex subject. Material for this presentation is drawn largely from the files of the National Wilms' Tumor Study (NWTS) Pathology Center, for which the author has been responsible since the inception of the First NWTS (NWTS-1) in 1969.

Not all neoplasms of the kidney in childhood are Wilms' tumors. Several neoplastic entities formerly thought to be Wilms' tumors have been identified in recent years on the basis of distinctive structural and clinicopathological features [1]. Table 2-1 lists their estimated relative frequencies, extrapolated in part from the experience of NWTS-1 [2]. That study included routine registration of all cases thought preoperatively to represent Wilms' tumor. It is essential for clinicians and pathologists dealing with presumed Wilms' tumors to be alert to the possibility of these alternative diagnoses, since they have important implications with respect to therapy. These data also provide an approximation of the potential error rate to be anticipated when treating a presumptive case of Wilms' tumor prior to pathological confirmation of the diagnosis.

WILMS' TUMOR
Gross Appearance

Though usually unicentric, bilateral and multicentric tumors are often seen. At the time of this writing, 155 of 2,165 cases of confirmed Wilms' tumor

Pediatric Tumors of the Genitourinary Tract, pages 25–47
© 1988 Alan R. Liss, Inc.

TABLE 2-1. Relative Incidence of Renal Tumors in Childhood[1]

Tumor Type	Percentage
Wilms' tumor (favorable histology)	82.0
Wilms' tumor (anaplastic)	5.0
Clear cell sarcoma of kidney	6.0
Rhabdoid tumor	2.0
Mesoblastic nephroma	2.0
Renal neurogenic tumors	1.5
Adenocarcinoma	0.5
Renal lymphoma	0.5
Miscellaneous	0.5

[1]Cystic lesions or tumor-like conditions such as perirenal hemorrhage are not considered.

entered on NWTS-3 (7.2%) were bilateral at presentation. Bilaterality is the most obvious manifestation of multicentricity, though multicentric unilateral tumors are not uncommon. The frequency with which this occurs is difficult to establish, but in a report of 1,802 unilateral Wilms' tumors, we were able to confirm multicentricity in 133 (7.4%) [3]. These figures underscore the necessity for careful exploration of any renal parenchyma remaining in the patient after resection of the tumor. It is worthy of note that the presence of bilateral renal masses strongly favors the diagnosis of Wilms' tumor, since of the other neoplastic entities listed in Table 2-1, only renal lymphomas are likely to involve both kidneys. The presence of multicentric tumors suggests the presence of multifocal precursor lesions, as will be discussed below in the section on nephroblastomatosis. This suggests a constitutional predisposition to Wilms' tumor, either hereditary or acquired, and the presence of multicentric tumors should therefore alert the surgeon to an increased risk of either simultaneous or metachronous tumor development in the remaining kidney.

Localized tumors tend to be enclosed within a dense capsule, but on section, they characteristically present a soft, bulging appearance (Fig. 2-1), with a consistency and color often resembling that of brain tissue. It was this appearance that led to a number of 19th century reports of "encephaloid tumors" of kidney, now thought to have represented Wilms' tumor. In the event of preoperative or intraoperative disruption of the capsule, this consistency predisposes to spillage of tumor cells. Foci of hemorrhage, necrosis, or cyst formation may be present, but calcification is detectable in only about 1% of cases. The presence of stippled calcification and a diffusely hemorrhagic appearance should alert the surgeon or pathologist to the possibility of

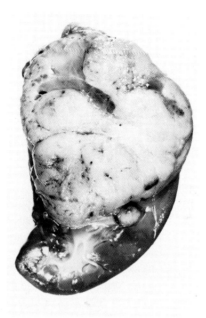

Fig. 2-1. Gross photograph of Wilms' tumor. Note bulging, pale surface and sharp demarcation from renal parenchyma.

intrarenal neuroblastoma, which may occur as a primary renal neoplasm, though more often it invades the kidney from an adjacent primary site.

Adhesions to adjacent structures may result from direct tumor invasion, but we have found that more frequently they result from an "inflammatory pseudocapsule" composed of reactive granulation tissue, which is usually seen in association with necrosis or hemorrhage in peripheral regions of the tumor. The significance of inflammatory pseudocapsule formation as a prognostic factor is under current study in the NWTS Pathology Center. Currently, inflammatory pseudocapsule formation is not a basis for upstaging on the NWTS. This is why surgeons are often surprised to learn that a tumor with prominent surface adhesions is considered a stage I tumor by the pathologist.

Histopathology

Wilms' tumor is notorious for a histological diversity that is exceeded in extent only by teratomas. A wide spectrum of cell types and stages of maturation produce an almost infinite variety of appearances, some of which replicate stages of normal nephrogenesis, while others represent cell types foreign to the kidney, such as skeletal muscle and mucinous epithelium. In addition to the classical triphasic admixture of blastemal, epithelial, and stromal elements, one may see tumors that are more or less monomorphous, being composed principally or exclusively of one of these elements. Such tumors often lead to controversy as to nomenclature. We have discussed elsewhere the practical and theoretical difficulties that may occur in attempting to distinguish some Wilms' tumors from renal adenocarcinomas, teratomas, and other tumor types [1].

Relationship of Wilms' Tumor Histology to Prognosis

In the context of modern therapy, most of the patterns of Wilms' tumor seem to bear little relationship to outcome. It has been suggested that tumors with a predominance of skeletal muscle, sometimes termed "fetal rhabdomyomatous nephroblastoma" [4], or those with abundant tubular differentiation [5,6] may be associated with a favorable outcome. Our experience suggests that these appearances are closely linked to younger patient age, with a majority of such tumors occurring in the first 2 years of life. It is not clear whether the tendency for good outcome is attributable to histopathology or is simply a reflection of the high cure rate generally observed when Wilms' tumor is diagnosed in the first 2 years of life. We have observed these allegedly favorable histological patterns to be associated with aggressive behavior on occasion, especially in older children.

It is important to recognize that the remarkable success that has been experienced in the treatment of Wilms' tumors has had the effect of obscuring patterns that might be inherently of low aggressiveness. As the effectiveness of therapy for a given tumor increases, the ability to recognize less aggressive variants of that tumor becomes diminished. It becomes essential, in this situation, to distinguish aggressive behavior of a given tumor in a "state of nature" from its behavior in the context of modern therapy. For example, we have observed that Wilms' tumors composed of sheets of blastemal cells tend to present with metastases and, hence, seem very aggressive prior to diagnosis. However, these same tumors usually respond well to therapy. Therefore the term "unfavorable histology" as used by the NWTS could more properly be termed "unresponsive histology." A tumor currently in the unfavorable category could become favorable when effective therapy for that particular pattern becomes available.

Significance of Anaplasia in Wilms' Tumor

Studies from the NWTS Pathology Center [1,7,8] have shown that the most important histopathological indicator of adverse prognosis of Wilms' tumor is the presence of large, hyperchromatic nuclei associated with multi-polar mitotic figures (Fig. 2-2). This change, termed "anaplasia," indicates the presence of a population of cells with polyploid DNA content. A recent study suggests that flow cytometry is an efficient and sensitive way to detect this change [9]. The incidence of anaplasia increases between 2 and 6 years of age and is rare before 2 years (Table 2-2). The significance of anaplasia in the first two NWTS trials is shown in Table 2-3.

The importance of anaplasia as a marker of adverse prognosis places responsibility on pathologists to ensure adequate sampling of the tumor. Even

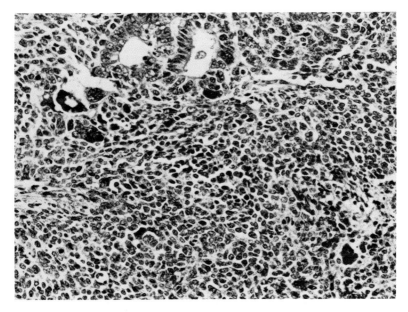

Fig. 2-2. Anaplastic Wilms' tumor. Multiple, obviously enlarged, hyperchromatic nuclei are visible.

TABLE 2-2. Age Incidence of Anaplastic Wilms' Tumor[1]

Age (yr)	No. patients	Anaplasia	Percentage
< 2	362	8	2
2–3	189	8	4
3–5	321	30	10
5–7	171	25	15
> 7	113	13	12

[1]Data modified from [8].

TABLE 2-3. Significance of Anaplasia in Wilms' Tumor[1]

	Anaplasia	No anaplasia
Total cases	49	720
Relapses	27 (55%)	101 (14%)
Tumor deaths	23 (47%)	39 (5%)

[1]NWTS-1 and 2, stages I–III.

when this cytological abnormality is present in one small focus, its prognostic significance remains. Criteria for adequacy of sampling are arbitrary, but NWTS protocols suggest that at least one generous section of tumor be obtained for every centimeter of tumor diameter. Excellent histological technique is necessary in order to accurately identify this change. Poorly fixed or stained specimens can lead to false positive or false negative results. For this reason, the surgeon should be certain the pathologist receives the specimen promptly and processes it expeditiously.

In a review of NWTS-2, a study in which anaplastic Wilms' tumors were treated the same as non-anaplastic lesions, only one relapse occurred among nine stage I anaplastic tumors. This finding suggests that early "micrometastases" do not occur in anaplastic Wilms' tumors. For this reason, the NWTS Committee currently recommends treating stage I anaplastic tumors in the same way as favorable histology tumors of the same stage. This emphasizes the importance of careful documentation of margins in presumed stage I anaplastic Wilms' tumors.

In our original paper defining histological criteria for unfavorable outcome, the tumors now termed rhabdoid tumor and clear cell sarcoma of kidney were recognized as distinctive lesions that possibly were variants of Wilms' tumor [7]. These are now thought to be distinctive clinical and pathological entities rather than variants of Wilms' tumor. These entities are discussed below, but are mentioned here because of the frequent confusion about the significance of so-called "sarcomatous stroma" in true Wilms' tumors. This should not be construed as a sign of adverse prognosis. In a true Wilms' tumor, the only criterion of "unfavorable histology" currently accepted by the NWTS is the presence of anaplasia.

NEPHROBLASTOMATOSIS

One of the most fascinating features of the natural history of Wilms' tumor is its frequent association with lesions thought to represent precursors of the tumor [10–15]. These precursor lesions are usually multiple and bilateral. They may be of microscopic size, may form grossly visible nodules, or appear as a diffuse "rind" of abnormal tissue around the surface of the kidney, causing massive uniform enlargement of one or both organs. The term "nephroblastomatosis" has been applied in different ways by different authors, but in this discussion it applies to any lesion of the kidney thought to be a precursor of Wilms' tumor, whether microscopic or macroscopic, multicentric or diffuse.

The literature on this subject is burdened by confusing systems of terminology and by controversy with respect to management. With two former NWTS fellows, I have reviewed this subject in a series of papers, upon which the present discussion is based [12–14]. We have proposed a considerable revision and simplification of existing schemes of classification and nomenclature, along with the description of an important subtype of nephroblastomatosis, "intralobar nephroblastomatosis" (ILN). ILN, as the name implies, occurs anywhere within the renal lobe, in contrast to "perilobar nephroblastomatosis" (PLN), which is found only at the lobar periphery, where the blastemal activity of the developing metanephros is concentrated during the latter part of gestation. These subtypes are illustrated in Figures 2-3 and 2-4. Our proposed classification of the major categories of nephroblastomatosis is presented in Table 2-4, and a new subclassification of the many recognized subtypes of PLN is given in Table 2-5.

Nephroblastomatosis is a frequent finding in kidneys bearing Wilms' tumors. We found PLN or ILN in 104 of 404 cases on NWTS-2 (25.7%) [14]. The frequency of finding these lesions is increased with more generous sampling of grossly uninvolved renal parenchyma [10]. In a series of unselected infant autopsies, we found PLN in nine of 1,035 cases, or approximately 1% [15]. Since it is estimated that only 1 in 10,000 infants will eventually develop a Wilms' tumor, it is apparent that most infants with these lesions never develop Wilms' tumors. This is important because of the occasional presence of PLN in renal tissue removed surgically for a reason other than Wilms' tumor [16,17]. We know of no evidence that this finding confers a markedly increased risk of tumor development, though the risk may be about that for the general population. The management of patients with this finding remains controversial. In a child with incidentally discovered PLN, who is not in a high risk group for developing Wilms' tumor (aniridia, hemihypertrophy, Beckwith-Wiedemann syndrome, Drash familial Wilms' tumor, etc.), we know of no evidence that the risk of tumor development exceeds 1%. Thus, the cost-effectiveness of intensive followup of such patients would seem to be low. On the other hand, when the patient is in a high risk category or has already developed one or more Wilms' tumors, the significance of finding nephroblastomatosis is considerable. In a recently

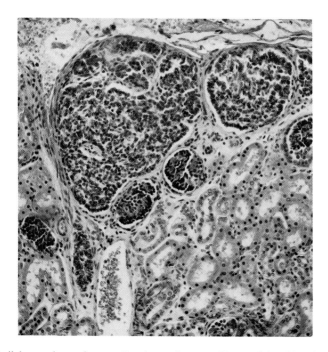

Fig. 2-3. Perilobar nephrogenic rests. Renal capsule at top. Note peripheral location in renal lobe and sharp demarcation from parenchyma.

completed study [14], we found that nephroblastomatosis in kidneys removed for Wilms' tumor was strongly correlated with the risk for subsequent tumor development in the remaining kidney. Among 404 patients studied on NWTS-2 for whom adequate tissue was available, there were no contralateral renal relapses among 300 patients without nephroblastomatosis. In patients with PLN alone, 5% later developed tumor in the remaining kidney. When ILN alone was present, the risk was approximately 17%, and when both types of lesion were present, it rose to 33%. These results suggest that careful followup by good imaging techniques is indicated for Wilms' tumor patients found to have nephroblastomatosis in addition to tumor, but is probably not necessary for the rest. Again, as with the search for anaplasia in Wilms' tumors, significant responsibility is placed on the pathologist to sample the specimen with care and to recognize precursor lesions in the grossly uninvolved renal parenchyma.

The surgeon operating for Wilms' tumor may be confronted with the problem of one or many small nodules of apparent tumor in the remaining

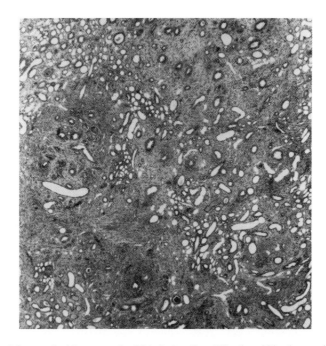

Fig. 2-4. Intralobar nephroblastomatosis. This lesion lies diffusely within the renal paren-chyma, without sharp margins. Medullary tubules are interspersed throughout the involved region.

TABLE 2-4. Proposed Classification of Major Categories of Nephroblastomatosis

	Comment
Perilobar (PLN)	Most common type. Occurs at lobar surface.
Intralobar (ILN)	Less frequent than PLN. Occurs anywhere in cortex or medulla.
Combined (PLN + ILN)	Discrete foci of ILN and PLN, with uninvolved renal tissue between lesions.
Panlobar	Extremely rare. No normal cortex or medulla is seen. Differs from diffuse PLN.

TABLE 2-5. Proposed Subclassification of Perilobar Nephroblastomatosis

Subtype	Macroscopic features	Histological subtypes
A. Nephrogenic rests	Not grossly visible.	Blastemal; epithelial; (glomerular, tubular, both present); sclerosing; adenomatous; mixed.
B. Hyperplastic rests	Multifocal oval or elongated, sharply demarcated lesions (see subtype D below).	Same as above.
C. Diffuse PLN	Resembles B, but more confluent, covering most cortical surfaces. May cause marked nephromegaly.	Same as above.
D. Multifocal perilobar Wilms' tumor	Same distribution as other subtypes of PLN. Differs from B in having spherical, compressive appearance.	Wilms' tumors. Epithelial or blastemal patterns predominate. Often has remnants of precursor lesion at edge of smaller tumors.

renal parenchyma. These may range in size from barely perceptible up to several centimeters. Some of these are early Wilms' tumors, while others may be enlarged precursor lesions that have not yet become true neoplasms. How should these be managed? My approach is quite conservative [18] and is based on the observation that small, early lesions are almost always well encapsulated and rarely exhibit invasive features. Therefore it is usually safe to perform limited local resection with a narrow margin of adjacent renal parenchyma. If the number or location of these lesions is such that their removal would endanger the entire kidney, it is worthwhile to attempt tumor reduction by chemotherapy. We have often seen complete ablation of viable tumor cells by a short course of preoperative chemotherapy.

In those cases where chemotherapy has achieved an apparently complete disappearance of tumor, "second look" procedures more often confuse than help clarify the situation. Nephroblastomatosis often remains following chemotherapy, presumably because of a longer cell cycle. Since the distinction between nephroblastomatosis and Wilms' tumor often cannot be made under the microscope, the finding of incompletely differentiated cells inevitably leads to a therapeutic dilemma. As an alternative to second look surgery, it is worth considering closely spaced imaging studies, reserving operative intervention for those situations where a new or enlarging nodule has appeared.

The objective of management of the various forms of nephroblastomatosis is to detect newly formed Wilms' tumors while they are still amenable to local resection, with maximal sparing of renal parenchyma. Since the patient with multiple precursor lesions may develop new Wilms' tumors over a considerable span of years, it is fortunate that modern imaging techniques are capable of extremely sensitive detection of small lesions and at the same time pose relatively little hazard to the long-term health of the patient.

There is no established standard concerning the frequency with which high-risk patients should be followed by appropriate imaging studies, but in several cases we have seen tumors progress over the course of 6 months from a size that was inapparent on an adequate study to a very large and even metastatic tumor that eventually led to death. These experiences have led us to suggest no more than a 3-month interval between examinations. If a suspicious or equivocal abnormality is apparent on one study, it may be safe to repeat the procedure at a shorter interval rather than proceeding immediately to surgical exploration.

MULTILOCULAR CYSTS (MLC) OF KIDNEY AND OTHER CYSTIC RENAL TUMORS

Solitary, multicystic nodular masses in the renal parenchyma of children have engendered lively debate. Prior to the advent of imaging techniques capable of demonstrating their cystic nature, such lesions were usually thought to be solid tumors until the specimen was incised following nephrectomy. Now that they are recognizable preoperatively in a majority of instances, it has become popular to consider partial nephrectomy for such cases [19]. Before undertaking such a procedure, the surgeon should be aware of the spectrum of neoplastic entities that can mimic the multilocular cyst of kidney, since some of these are locally aggressive or frankly malignant and, hence, cannot safely be managed by partial nephrectomy [20].

Multilocular Cysts

The multilocular cyst is classically defined as a solitary, oval to spherical mass within the renal parenchyma, composed of numerous non-communicating spaces separated by delicate septa composed of mature connective tissues. The spaces are lined by flattened or cuboidal epithelium. No nephronic elements, either mature or immature, are found within the lesion, and the cysts are not connected to the renal collecting system. Most definitions include unilaterality as a criterion for MLC, but bilateral specimens have been described [21]. The typical gross appearance of MLC is shown in Figure 2-5.

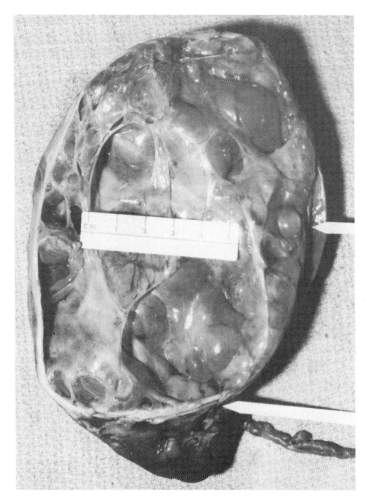

Fig. 2-5. Multilocular cyst of kidney. Gross specimen, opened. Note thin-walled septa. Two white arrows mark the sharply defined junction between lesion and uninvolved portions of kidney.

Relationship of MLC to other Cystic Renal Tumors

Lesions that can be confused with MLC are listed in Table 2-6. This or any other proposed classification of the principal cystic tumors of the child's kidney is certain to generate controversy. There is a lack of agreement as to the relationship of MLC to Wilms' tumor, and this has given rise to diverse

TABLE 2-6. Cystic Renal Tumors of Childhood

Multilocular cyst (MLC)
Cystic, partially differentiated nephroblastoma (CPDN)
MLC or CPDN with mural nodule(s) of Wilms' tumor
Wilms' tumor with focal or multifocal cystic change
Cystic congenital mesoblastic nephroma (CMN)
MLC with superimposed adenocarcinoma
Localized cystic dysplasia of kidney

schemes of classification and nomenclature. Joshi's review [22] contains a good discussion of this controversial subject. He has defined an entity known as "cystic, partially differentiated nephroblastoma" (CPDN), which grossly resembles MLC, but in which the septa are found to contain the incompletely differentiated elements seen in conventional Wilms' tumor. None of the cases of CPDN that he was able to identify metastasized, suggesting that these lesions might safely be treated by nephrectomy alone. Our experience corroborates Joshi's view, but it is important to distinguish typical CPDN, with immature elements conforming to the septa separating cysts, from cystic lesions with expanding, solid nodules of tumor, as such lesions may behave aggressively.

It is convenient to consider Wilms' tumor, MLC, and CPDN as forming a spectrum similar to that for the neuroblastoma series, with solid Wilms' tumor forming the most malignant end, MLC representing the benign end of the spectrum, and CPDN being an intermediate category analogous to the diffuse ganglioneuroblastoma. Some authors [23–25] have preferred the term "cystic nephroma" to MLC. This term has the advantage of conveying the neoplastic nature of the lesion and is perhaps less likely to lead to confusion with cystic malformations of the kidney.

It is important for the surgeon to be aware that congenital mesoblastic nephroma, a lesion with aggressive infiltrative borders and the capacity for recurrence and metastasis, and clear cell sarcoma of kidney may present with gross and imaging features identical to those of MLC [18,26]. These lesions will be discussed in more detail below, but are mentioned here because it would be inappropriate to treat them with partial nephrectomy. Therefore, when a partial nephrectomy for presumed MLC has been performed, it would seem prudent that the specimen be examined by a pathologist prior to closing the operative site. If the lesion is found to be one of these other entities, the nephrectomy could be completed expeditiously.

In adults, a few cases of adenocarcinoma arising in MLC have been reported [27], but at least some of these may have been incorrectly interpreted. The difficulties inherent in making this diagnosis are discussed by Taxy and Marshall [28].

CLEAR CELL SARCOMA OF KIDNEY (CCSK)

This unique renal tumor of childhood was first reported in abstract form by Kidd in 1970 [29]. It was separately identified by ourselves [7] and by Marsden et al. [30] in 1978 as a distinctive neoplasm with a particularly aggressive and unresponsive clinical behavior, including a propensity for skeletal metastases, which are almost never seen with conventional Wilms' tumor. This behavior led the latter authors to propose the term "bone-metastasizing renal tumor of childhood" for this tumor. These workers noted bone metastasis in 76% of 38 cases [31], as compared to 17% of 75 cases in our NWTS series [32]. This discrepancy may reflect an element of selection bias in the British series. CCSK comprised 4% of renal tumors of childhood entered on the NWTS prior to 1982 [32], but on NWTS-3 it comprises nearly 6% of cases, thus comprising the most commonly seen form of "unfavorable histology" renal tumor on NWTS-3. This apparently increased incidence is most likely attributable to increased recent awareness of the histological variants of CCSK.

Clinical Features

CCSK has an age distribution similar to that of Wilms' tumor, with relatively few cases diagnosed in the first year, and a peak incidence between 3 and 5 years of age. There is a distinct male preponderance, though this has been more prominent in the British series than in our own [32]. We are aware of no case occurring in the context of a Wilms' tumor-associated condition such as sporadic aniridia or hemihypertrophy.

Pathological Features

Grossly, there are no distinctive features that would permit the clinician to suspect this diagnosis in the absence of bony metastases. We are aware of no case of bilateral CCSK, so the finding of bilateral renal tumors would make this an unlikely diagnosis. CCSK often contains cysts, and we have illustrated a specimen [18] in which the cystic change was so prominent a feature as to invite confusion with multilocular cyst. The color is more often pale tan than gray, the latter being more typical of Wilms' tumor.

The classical histological appearances of CCSK are shown in Figure 2-6. The tumor is composed of very uniform cells with small nuclei having fine, evenly dispersed chromatin and inconspicuous nucleoli. The cytoplasm is

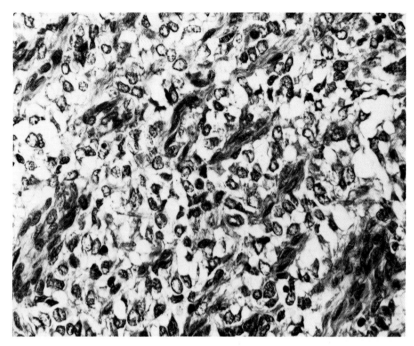

Fig. 2-6. Clear cell sarcoma of kidney. Columns of pale-stained tumor cells are separated by fine septa.

usually indistinct, being palely stained and with irregular, indistinct outlines. The cytoplasm is seen with the electron microscope to form delicate processes that enclose pools of intercellular matrix. This pale, vacuolated appearance led to our suggestion of the term CCSK, but occasionally there is moderate cytoplasmic eosinophilia, in which cases this term can be somewhat misleading. Tubules lined by basophilic cuboidal cells are often found dispersed singly through the tumor, especially near its periphery. It can be shown that these are preexistent renal tubules that have undergone metaplasia after having been surrounded and separated by tumor growth. Transitions between these tubules and tumor cells are not seen, in contrast to the transitions often seen in Wilms' tumor between blastemal and tubular elements. A distinctive feature is the presence of an evenly spaced fibrovascular network that subdivides the tumor into columns or bands of uniform size, typically five to ten cells wide.

In addition to the classic pattern of CCSK, many other variants have now been recognized. Sometimes the tumor cells become aligned along the vascular septa in a fashion resembling epithelial tubules, and in other cases they may form a diffuse myxoid matrix. In such cases the true diagnosis may only be recognized when foci of the classic pattern are seen. We have illustrated these variant forms elsewhere [1]. It is essential that the pathologist examining renal tumors of children be able to recognize CCSK including its variant forms, because of the prognostic significance of this diagnosis. This is potentially one of the most worrisome aspects of the use of fine needle aspiration in the diagnosis of pediatric renal tumors, as the presence of variant patterns can easily mimic Wilms' tumor.

The cell of origin of CCSK remains elusive. This subject has been reviewed recently and will not be discussed here [33].

Therapeutic Considerations

Unpublished results from NWTS-3 suggest that the intensified therapy used for unfavorable histology tumors in that study has produced a substantial improvement in outcome of CCSK patients. Therefore, the correct diagnosis of this entity is of urgent importance.

Another important point to be made is that CCSK, in contrast to anaplastic Wilms' tumor, is associated with a poor outcome even when the resected lesion appears to be limited to the kidney and completely removed (stage I). Of seven stage I CCSK patients entered on NWTS-2, all of which were treated the same as favorable histology Wilms' tumor, five died with metastatic disease. Thus, it appears that early microdissemination is the rule in this tumor, and it is not possible to be complacent about the therapy of seemingly localized primary tumors of this type.

RHABDOID TUMOR OF KIDNEY (RTK)

This tumor was first recognized as a distinctive entity in our 1978 review of the pathology of tumors entered on NWTS-1 [7]. It is the least common of the three entities considered in the unfavorable histology category of the NWTS, comprising only 2% of cases entered in the study. It is also the most malignant of the three tumor types. In a recently published review [34], it was found that only five of 45 reported patients of RTK for whom the initial tumor stage was known were alive and free of tumor at the time of reporting, and 37 (82%) had died of tumor, 34 within 1 year of diagnosis. Preliminary, unpublished results from NWTS-3 suggest that the intensified therapeutic protocols of that study have effected only a minor improvement in outlook for the patient with RTK.

Clinical Considerations

This tumor has several distinctive and unusual clinical features. Of 21 cases entered on NWTS-1 and 2, the age range was 3 months to 4.5 years, with a mean of 18 months and a median of 13 months [35]. The fact that nearly half of the patients were diagnosed in the first year of life contrasts sharply with Wilms' tumor and CCSK. Another distinctive feature is the occurrence of an apparently separate primary tumor of the midline posterior intracranial fossa, often producing hydrocephalus [34,36]. The intracranial tumor may appear substantially earlier than the renal tumor, or it may not present until several years later. There is an approximately 2:1 male: female ratio. Finally, hypercalcemia has been observed at presentation in a substantial number of reported cases [37], though this finding may also be present in another infantile renal tumor, the congenital mesoblastic nephroma [38].

Pathological Features

The gross features of RTK are not sufficiently distinctive to be helpful. Extrarenal extension or metastases is often present at the time of diagnosis, which may involve hematogenous or lymphatic routes. In addition to the apparently separate primary brain tumors mentioned above, metastases to the brain are often seen. Skeletal metastases are not uncommonly observed, so this finding is not specific for CCSK.

The microscopic appearances are distinctive. The tumor is monomorphous, being composed of rather large cells with abundant, usually acidophilic cytoplasm (Fig. 2-7). This lesion tends to infiltrate the renal parenchyma, isolating and separating glomeruli and tubules in a fashion similar to that of CCSK. This contrasts with the usual "pushing" border seen with Wilms' tumor. The tumor cells are characterized by huge, single nucleoli and usually by a hyaline acidophilic cytoplasmic inclusion that is seen ultrastructurally to consist of a whorled mass of intermediate filaments. It should be emphasized, however, that these inclusions are often difficult to find, and similar inclusions may occur in other tumor types, so their demonstration is not by itself proof of the diagnosis.

While RTK has an appearance that is quite distinctive and less likely to be mistaken for other renal tumors, an occasional specimen shows a somewhat tubular arrangement of tumor cells that can mimic Wilms' tumor, and on a few occasions we have seen spindling regions in RTK that led to a mistaken impression of congential mesoblastic nephroma. Confusion between meso-blastic nephroma and RTK is made more likely by the overlapping age ranges and by the occasional occurrence of hypercalcemia with both entitites, as mentioned above. This is one of those potentially disastrous situations where

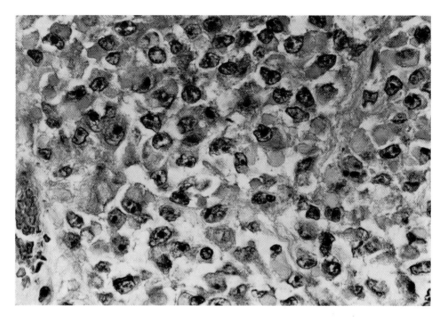

Fig. 2-7. Rhabdoid tumor of kidney. Large nuclei with prominent nucleoli are apparent. Rounded glassy areas in cytoplasm are filamentous inclusion bodies ultrastructurally.

an outspokenly malignant tumor can be confused with one that usually behaves in a benign fashion.

Other renal tumors can mimic RTK [39]. We have seen several blastemal Wilms' tumors with some tumor cells containing hyaline cytoplasmic inclusions. However, in these the nucleoli were not as large as in RTK. In adults, other tumors such as renal cell carcinomas, urothelial carcinomas, leiomyosarcomas, and metastatic melanomas have all been mistaken for RTK. One should be dubious about the diagnosis of RTK in patients over the age of 5 years.

The question of extrarenal rhabdoid tumors has recently generated considerable interest [34,40]. While some of these may eventually prove to be identical to RTK, we are becoming increasingly aware of the spectrum of "pseudo-rhabdoid" lesions [39] and suspect that the light microscopic and ultrastructural features of rhabdoid tumors may comprise a morphological phenotype that is not by itself specific for a single neoplastic entity. There seems no doubt that RTK is a clear-cut clinicopathological entity, but one that can be closely mimicked by other renal and extrarenal tumor types.

CONGENITAL MESOBLASTIC NEPHROMA (CMN)

This distinctive tumor of the infantile kidney has generated lively controversy and is an entity with which the surgeon operating on pediatric renal neoplasms must be familiar. Bolande and his colleagues, who originally defined and named this entity [41,42], emphasized its characteristically benign outcome. By so doing, they have rendered a valuable service to many hundreds of infants who have been spared the substantial dangers inherent in cancer chemotherapy and radiotherapy of the very young patient.

Pathological Appearance

The appearance of CMN is to a large extent related to the age of the patient. In newborns, the lesion is usually of modest cellularity (Fig. 3-8) and has strikingly irregular borders, with tongues of spindled cells extending a long distance into the renal parenchyma and into the perirenal soft tissues. It is this latter tendency that is of particular importance to the operating surgeon. CMN tends to extend beyond the renal capsule and is especially

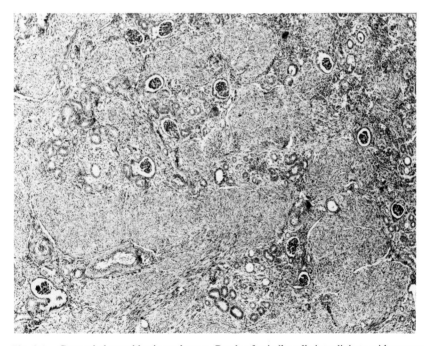

Fig. 2-8. Congenital mesoblastic nephroma. Bands of spindle cells interdigitate with uncompressed renal parenchyma.

likely to involve tissues in and beyond the renal sinus, sometimes going a considerable distance along the ureter. The surgeon should attempt to remove tissue well beyond the grossly apparent tumor margins. Despite its generally benign behavior, CMN often requires a more radical surgical removal than does Wilms' tumor, in which the margins are usually sharply defined, with a well-developed tumor capsule.

The spindle cells of a classic neonatal CMN are similar to those of fibromatosis, and most workers have characterized them as myofibroblasts. As the infant passes beyond the immediate perinatal period, one observes with increasing frequency the emergence of one or more regions of dense cellularity. Presumably because of a higher proliferative rate, these foci of "cellular CMN" progressively overgrow the original lesion. As this occurs, the tumor tends to develop a defined border with a pseudocapsule of compressed connective tissue, in which the remnants of the originally less cellular portions of the lesion may be apparent. CMN may invade vessels of the capsule or renal parenchyma and may even extend into the vena cava via the renal vein. Presumably this is the basis of their occasional metastasizing potential.

Prognostic Significance of Cellular CMN

Following the initially optimistic papers on CMN, there appeared a few case reports of local recurrences and metastases, as well as the recognition that some cases of CMN had worrisome histological features such as high cell density and numerous mitotic figures. This led us to sound a note of caution concerning these lesions in 1974 [43]. Since then, other examples of aggressive behavior have been reported. These have recently been summarized [44]. Based on these experiences, considerable concern and confusion has been generated concerning the so-called "cellular mesoblastic nephroma." We have been fortunate in having been able to review sections from all but one case of recurrent or metastatic CMN in the literature, plus five unreported cases [45]. It is noteworthy that only one documented case of recurrence was under 3 months of age at diagnosis, and in that case it is clear that tumor extended to the margin of ureteral extension and was transected during the nephrectomy. At this time the lesion was not unusually cellular, though its recurrence was densely cellular with moderate atypia.

It has been our observation that at least one-third of cases of CMN diagnosed in the first 3 months of life are of the cellular variety, yet none of these has subsequently recurred. The CMN recurrences other than the case cited above were all associated with lesions of the cellular type, and all were diagnosed beyond 3 months of age. This experience suggests that dense cellularity and numerous mitotic figures are not of ominous prognostic significance in infants under 3 months of age, but are occasionally associated with local recurrence or metastasis beyond that age. These findings become increasingly worrisome with each month of life beyond that point.

Necrosis and hemorrhage are frequently cited as adverse prognostic features in CMN, but this contrasts with our experience. Tumor rupture, on the other hand, has been associated with recurrence of several tumors, all of which were of the densely cellular variety.

We are concerned about any CMN that seems to have been incompletely removed and about the hypercellular lesion in infants older than 3 months. Vascular invasion is also of potentially ominous significance. Fortunately, most of these tumors are recognized in the early weeks of life, when the chances of recurrence are minuscule if an adequate margin of uninvolved tissue is secured.

MISCELLANEOUS RENAL TUMORS OF CHILDREN

Renal adenocarcinomas of children appear to be similar in biological behavior to the same lesions in adults [46]. On rare occasions, a composite tumor consisting of an admixture of typical Wilms' tumor with foci of renal adenocarcinoma may be observed [1]. The number of reported cases is too small to establish which tumor type is the major determinant of outcome in this circumstance. Urothelial malignancies of children are extremely rare [47]. Neuroblastomas of the kidney may occur as intrarenal primary lesions, but more commonly they appear to involve the kidney secondarily. Lymphomas, particularly of the Burkitt variety, may present in a fashion resembling either unilateral or bilateral Wilms' tumor. Each of these tumors seems, on the basis of small numbers of observed cases, to behave no differently than would be expected in an extrarenal primary site.

REFERENCES

1. Beckwith JB: Renal tumors and other renal tumors of childhood: A selective review from the National Wilms' Study Pathology Center. Hum Pathol 14:481, 1983.
2. Ehrlich RM, Blumberg SD, Gyepes MT, et al.: Wilms' tumor misdiagnosed preoperatively: A review of 19 National Wilms' Tumor Study-1 cases. J Urol 122:790, 1979.
3. Breslow NE, Beckwith JB: Epidemiological features of Wilms' tumor: Results of the National Wilms' Tumor Study. JNCI 68:429, 1982.
4. Wigger HJ: Fetal rhabdomyomatous nephroblastoma—a variant of Wilms' tumor. Hum Pathol 7:613, 1976.
5. Chatten J: Epithelial differentiation in Wilms tumor: A clinicopathologic appraisal. Perspect Pediatr Pathol 3:225, 1976.

6. Lawler W, Marsden HB, Palmer ML: Wilms tumor—histologic variation and prognosis. Cancer 40:1122, 1975.
7. Beckwith JB, Palmer NF: Histopathology and prognosis of Wilms tumor. Cancer 41:1937, 1978.
8. Bonadio JF, Storer B, Norkool P, et al.: Anaplastic Wilms tumor: Clinical and pathologic studies. J Clin Oncol 3:513, 1985.
9. Douglass EC, Look AT, Webber B, et al.: Hyperdiploidy and chromosomal rearrangements define the anaplastic variant of Wilms tumor. J Clin Oncol 4:975, 1986.
10. Bove KE, McAdams AJ: The neophroblastomatosis complex and its relationship to Wilms tumor: A clinicopathologic treatise. Perspect Pediatr Pathol 3:185, 1976.
11. Machin GA: Persistent renal blastema (nephroblastomatosis) as a frequent precursor of Wilms tumor: A pathological and clinical review. Am J Pediatr Hematol Oncol 2:165, 253, 353, 1980.
12. Beckwith JB, Kiviat NB, Bonadio JF: Studies of nephroblastomatosis. I. Introduction and classification (submitted for publication).
13. Kiviat NB, Beckwith JB: Studies of nephroblastomatosis. II. Intralobar nephroblastomatosis and related Wilms tumors. A report of the National Wilms Tumor Study (NWTS) (submitted for publication).
14. Bonadio JF, Beckwith JB, Kiviat NB, Sim DA: Studies of nephroblastomatosis. III. Clinical significance of nephrogenic rests associated with unilateral Wilms tumor (submitted for publication).
15. Bennington JL, Beckwith JB: Tumors of the kidney, renal pelvis and ureter. In Atlas of Tumor Pathology, 2nd series. Washington D.C.: Armed Forces Institute of Pathology, 1975.
16. Gaddy CD, Gibbons MD, Gonzales ET Jr., et al.: Obstructive uropathy, renal dysplasia and nodular renal blastema: Is there a relationship to Wilms tumor? J Urol 134:330, 1985.
17. Craver R, Dimmick J, Johnson H, et al.: Congenital obstructive uropathy and nodular renal blastema. J Urol 136:305, 1986.
18. Beckwith JB: The John Lattimer Lecture. Wilms tumor and other renal tumors of childhood: An update. J Urol 136:320, 1986.
19. Banner MP, Pollack HM, Chatten J, et al.: Multilocular renal cysts: Radiologic-pathologic correlation. Am J Roentgenol 136:239, 1980.
20. Beckwith JB, Kiviat NB: Multilocular renal cysts and cystic renal tumors. Am J Roentgenol 136:435, 1980.
21. Chatten J, Bishop HC: Bilateral multilocular cysts of the kidney. J Pediatr Surg 12:749, 1977.
22. Joshi VV: Cystic, partially differentiated nephroblastoma: An entity in the spectrum of infantile renal neoplasia. Perspect Pediatr Pathol 5:217, 1979.
23. Boggs L, Kimmelstiel P: Benign multilocular cystic nephroma: Report of two cases of so-called multilocular cyst of the kidney. J Urol 76:530, 1966.
24. Gallo G, Penchansky L: Cystic nephroma. Cancer 39:1322, 1977.
25. Abt AB, Demers LM, Schochat SJ: Cystic nephroma: An ultrastructural and biochemical study. J Urol 122:539, 1977.
26. Ganick DJ, Gilbert EF, Beckwith JB, et al.: Congenital cystic mesoblastic nephroma. Hum Pathol 12:1039, 1981.
27. Sadlowski RW, Smey P, Williams J, et al.: Adenocarcinoma in a multilocular renal cyst. Urology 14:512, 1979.
28. Taxy JB, Marshall FF: Multilocular renal cysts in adults. Possible relationship to renal adenocarcinoma. Arch Pathol Lab Med 107:633, 1983.

29. Kidd JM: Exclusion of certain renal neoplasms from the category of Wilms tumor. Am J Pathol 59:16a, 1970.
30. Marsden HB, Lawler W, Kumar PM: Bone metastasizing renal tumor of childhood. Morphological and clinical characteristics from Wilms tumor. Cancer 42:1916, 1978.
31. Marsden HB, Lawler W: Bone metastasizing renal tumour of childhood. Histopathological and clinical review of 38 cases. Virchows Arch [A] 387:341, 1980.
32. Haas JE, Bonadio JF, Beckwith JB: Clear cell sarcoma of the kidney with emphasis on ultrastructural studies. Cancer 54:2978, 1984.
33. Sotelo-Avila C, Gonzalez-Crussi F, Sadowinski S, et al: Clear cell sarcoma of the kidney: A clinicopathologic study of 21 patients with long-term follow-up evaluation. Hum Pathol 16:1219, 1986.
34. Sotelo-Avila C, Gonzalez-Crussi F, deMello D, et al.: Renal and extrarenal rhabdoid tumors in children: A clinicopathologic study of 14 patients. Seminars Diagn Pathol 3:151, 1986.
35. Palmer NF, Sutow W: Clinical aspects of the rhabdoid tumor of the kidney: A report of the National Wilms' Tumor Study group. Med Pediatr Oncol 11:242, 1983.
36. Bonnin JM, Rubinstein LJ, Palmer NF, et al.: The association of embryonal tumors originating in the kidney and in the brain. A report of seven cases. Cancer 54:2137, 1984.
37. Rousseau-Merck MF, Nogues C, Nezelof C, et al.: Infantile renal tumors associated with hypercalcemia. Characterization of intermediate filament clusters. Arch Pathol Lab Med 107:311 1983.
38. Vido L, Carli M, Rizzoni G, et al.: Congenital mesoblastic nephroma with hypercalcemia. Pathogenetic role of prostaglandins. Am J Pediatr Hematol Oncol 8:149, 1986.
39. Weeks DA, Beckwith JB, Mierau GW: "Pseudo-rhabdoid" tumors of the kidney. Lab Invest 54:10P, 1986.
40. Tsuneyoshi M, Daimaru Y, Hashimoto H, et al.: Malignant soft tissue neoplasms with the histologic features of renal rhabdoid tumors: An ultrastructural and immunohistochemical study. Hum Pathol 16:1235, 1985.
41. Bolande RP, Brough AJ, Izant RJ: Congenital mesoblastic nephroma of infancy. Pediatrics 40:272, 1967.
42. Bolande RP: Congenital mesoblastic nephroma of infancy. Perspect Pediatr Pathol 1:237, 1973.
43. Beckwith JB: Mesenchymal renal neoplasms of infancy revisited. J Pediatr Surg 9:803, 1974.
44. Joshi VV, Kaznicka J, Walters TR: Atypical mesoblastic nephroma: Pathologic characterization of a potentially aggressive variant of conventional congenital mesoblastic nephroma. Arch Pathol Lab Med 110:100, 1986.
45. Beckwith JB, Weeks DA: Congenital mesoblasic nephroma. When should we worry? Arch Pathol Lab Med 110:98, 1986.
46. Raney RB, Palmer N, Sutow WW, et al.: Renal cell carcinoma in children. Med Pediatr Oncol 11:91, 1983.
47. Karmi S, Averill R, Young JD: Malignant urothelial tumors in childhood. Urology 21:178, 1983.

Chapter 3
Congenital Mesoblastic Nephroma and Nephroblastomatosis

William A. Brock

The remarkable advances made in the treatment of Wilms' tumor over the last few decades, coupled with an explosion of knowledge in the field of genetics has enabled us to better characterize renal tumors of childhood and thus provide more specific and successful treatment for each child.

Two pathologic entities have been identified which are related to Wilms' tumor in very different ways. Congenital mesoblastic nephroma (CMN), previously felt to be an infantile Wilms' tumor, has now been shown to be a separate entity requiring decidedly different management. Lesions of the nephroblastomatosis complex, on the other hand, are felt to represent a subset of Wilms' tumor "precursors," some of which are genetically determined. Together CMN and NBT may represent two points on the continuous line between normal embryologic development of the kidney and the disordered embryology which can manifest as frank Wilms' tumor.

CONGENITAL MESOBLASTIC NEPHROMA

Congenital mesoblastic nephroma (CMN) is the most common renal neoplasm encountered in the newborn period and the second most common malignancy seen in neonates after sacrococcygeal teratoma [1–4]. Kastner first described the histology of CMN in 1921 and characterized it as a sarcomatous lesion [1,5]. Prior to Bolande's review in 1967, tumors characteristic of CMN were considered to be congenital Wilms' tumors or were

Pediatric Tumors of the Genitourinary Tract, pages 49–60

grouped with renal hamartomas as leiomyomatous hamartomas, fetal renal hamartomas, and mesenchymal hamartomas [1,6–8]. Bolande recognized that CMN was a unique lesion that could be distinguished clinically and pathologically from true congenital Wilms' tumor by its benign clinical behavior, a preponderance of mesenchymal derivatives, and lack of the malignant epithelial components typical of Wilms' tumor [6]. A definite infiltrative tendency distinguishes CMN from hamartomas with more limited growth potential. Since Bolande's initial report and later review of 48 cases the majority of these other lesions have been reclassified as CMN [9]. Bolande's description allows a more precise prognosis, avoiding the tendency to overtreat infants utilizing a Wilms' tumor chemotherapy protocol, while recognizing a greater potential for local recurrence and spread than seen with simple hamartomas.

There have been more than 100 cases of CMN reported in the English literature to date [3,10]. A review of 3,340 patients entered into the National Wilms' Tumor Study (NWTS) from 1969 to 1984 revealed only 24 renal malignancies in children under 30 days of age. Eighteen of these (75%) were congenital mesoblastic nephromas and only four were considered true congenital Wilms' tumor [4]. In the earlier NWTS report, congenital mesoblastic nephroma was the final diagnosis in 54 of 1,905 (2.8%) patients entered, irrespective of age [2].

Pathology and Pathogenesis

The involved kidney is often markedly enlarged, attaining weights over 50 grams [6]. On cut section, the majority of parenchyma is diffusely replaced by tumor, which exhibits a uniformly pale, yellow-gray, rubbery whorled surface reminiscent of a uterine fibroid or leiomyosarcoma. The pseudocapsule seen in Wilms' tumor is absent, and the margin between the tumor and adjacent compressed renal parenchyma is indistinct. The tumor may extend into the perinephric connective tissue, especially near the hilum. Areas of hemorrhage, necrosis, or cyst formation are uncommon.

Histologically, the tumor is composed of broad, interlacing bands or sheets of immature connective tissue cells that are predominantly fibroblasts [6,9,11,12]. Mitotic figures may be seen but are not prominent. The tumor is devoid of the epithelial elements seen in Wilms' tumor, though glomeruli and tubules may appear as nests trapped within the invading sheets of tumor. Islets of hematopoiesis or bars of immature cartilage are occasionally seen [3,6,13]. The tumor cells are elongated and spindle-shaped and may contain "cigar-shaped" nuclei; nuclear pleomorphism is not prominent. The cytoplasm is pale pink and finely fibrillar, and cell borders are indistinct [6,12].

A cellular variant of CMN that contains hyperchromatic nuclei and more prominent mitotic activity has been described [14–16]. This sarcomatous-appearing variant is associated with a higher risk of recurrence and aggressive biologic behavior when seen in children older than 3 months of age and may be a precursor of the clear cell sarcoma variant of Wilms' tumor [1,17,18].

Several histologic characteristics of CMN are basic to the various theories of its origin and include: 1) primarily mesenchymal composition of the tumor, 2) invasion and almost complete replacement of the involved kidney by the tumor, and 3) an aggressive cellular variant. Early fetal differentiation of the metanephric blastema is primarily stromagenic; glomeruli and outer cortical layers of the kidney develop later in nephrogenesis. A mutagenic event occurring early in nephrogenesis could lead to overgrowth of the mesenchymal elements. The later development of epithelial components would not be affected except by permeation and replacement with mesenchymal derivatives [1,2,6,12]. A second mutational event could then account for malignant transformation of a mesoblastic nephroma into the cellular variety and subsequently to clear cell sarcoma [19]. Bolande et al. have hypothesized that CMN represents a cytodifferentiated Wilms' tumor in which development of the mesenchymal components is associated with maturation or suppression of growth of neoplastic epithelial components [6].

Clinical Features

The mean age at diagnosis of CMN in the National Wilms' Tumor Study was 3.44 months [2]. There have been rare reports in older children [2,3,20]. There does not appear to be a race predilection. Males are affected 1.5 times more often than females [2,9,10,12]. The most common presentation is that of an asymptomatic, palpable mass noted during the newborn examination. The mass is solid, unilateral, and can attain a very large size. Hematuria (18%), renin-mediated hypertension (4%), congestive heart failure secondary to arteriovenous shunting in the tumor, and hypercalcemia may occur [21–23]. Maternal polyhydramnios and fetal prematurity have been noted frequently. [10,12,24–28]. The etiology of the polyhydramnios is unknown, and it is not certain whether prematurity is secondary to the polyhydramnios and premature rupture of the membranes. The incidence of associated congenital anomalies is similar to that seen with Wilms' tumor (14%), though hemihypertrophy has been reported only once [10].

The most common cause of an abdominal mass discovered in the newborn period is hydronephrosis or a multicystic kidney. These lesions are sonolucent and should be readily distinguished from CMN by ultrasound alone. A plain radiograph of the abdomen in a child with CMN shows a large flank mass that often crosses the midline; calcification is rarely seen [29]. Sonography will demonstrate the solid nature and renal origin of the mass and may show either a homogeneous or complex pattern, but cannot differentiate CMN from a Wilms' tumor [28,29]. Prenatal diagnosis is possible and should be considered whenever polyhydramnios is encountered during fetal ultrasonography [26,27,28]. An intravenous urogram commonly shows delayed contrast excretion on the side of the tumor. The collecting system, if visualized, is displaced and distorted by the intrarenal mass, which compresses rather than invades it; hydronephrosis is uncommon [29]. Radionuclide renal scans are of little help in the diagnosis of CMN, and computer assisted tomography is non-specific [10,20]. Angiography, in addition to being hazardous in the newborn, is also non-specific and of little assistance in differentiating CMN from other intrarenal tumors; non-homogeneous hypervascularity and neovascularity may be seen [3,21,29].

Treatment

Nephrectomy is the treatment of choice for CMN. There have been few reports of recurrence after nephrectomy seen primarily in the face of incomplete resection or in children treated after 3 months of age [2,15,30–32]. The tendency to finger-like perinephric extension of the tumor necessitates a more radical form of nephrectomy to ensure complete removal and avoid recurrence [17]. In addition, this tendency to extension has led to a 20% incidence of intraoperative rupture of the tumor [2]. The majority of deaths associated with CMN have been due to postoperative complications or the effects of radiation or chemotherapy [2,3,15]. Adjuvant therapy is unnecessary in the vast majority of cases of CMN and should be reserved for any tumor that was incompletely resected or in which intraoperative rupture occurred. Children older than 3 months of age at the time of diagnosis, with highly mitotic, cellular variants should also be considered for chemotherapy with reduced doses of actinomycin D and vincristine as currently utilized for favorable histology, stage 1 Wilms' tumor [2,15,17]. Multimodal adjuvant therapy with surgery, chemotherapy, and radiation should be reserved for the rare patient who develops metastatic disease [2,32]. The non-cellular form of the tumor does not appear to be a precursor of Wilms' tumor, and the prognosis of infants with CMN treated by wide nephrectomy alone is excellent. Even in the rare cases with recurrence or metastasis, salvage has generally been affected by chemotherapy with or without radiation [2,30–32].

NEPHROBLASTOMATOSIS

The definition of histologic features that differentiate subtypes of renal tumors in children has enabled more accurate prediction of biological behavior and allowed us to fine tune therapy so that maximun survival is achieved with minimal treatment-related toxicity. Central to our improved appreciation of the biology of Wilms' tumor is an understanding of the natural history of the nephroblastomatosis complex of lesions (NBT). Many pediatric tumors histologically resemble the embryonic stages of their tissue of origin; NBT represents an example of this relationship between disordered embryogenesis and oncogenesis [33]. The term nephroblastomatosis was first used in 1961 to describe a case of bilateral nephromegaly caused by diffuse persistence of fetal renal blastema, felt now to be an example of pannephric or pancortical NBT (34–36]. A number of related lesions that are considered to be part of the nephroblastomatosis complex have since been described.

The normal human kidney develops by inductive interaction between the ampullae of the dividing ureteric bud and the metanephric blastema. Nephrons and supporting tissue are induced to develop in a layered fashion by the continually bifurcating ureteric buds. The earliest nephrons formed tend to lie deepest within the kidney, while those formed later occupy a more peripheral, subcapsular position [17,36]. This sequence of nephrogenesis is complete by 36 weeks of gestation, at which time no further metanephric blastema remains. Nephrogenic blastemal tissue persisting beyond 36 weeks of gestation, blastema found in areas of the fetal kidney other than the cortical neogenic zone, or blastema found in quantities greater than that expected for the state of fetal nephron development are considered persistent renal blastema and part of the nephroblastomatosis complex [37]. Persistent renal blastema varies from microscopic foci of nodular renal blastema to a diffuse, confluent pannephric form, depending on the time during nephrogenesis at which it began. The persistence of fetal renal blastema may represent the first prezygotic or early embryologic stage in Knudson's two-stage theory of oncogenesis [19,38]. The nature of the second oncogenic event that allows development of Wilms' tumor in this persistent premalignant substrate is unknown.

NBT in its most severe, diffuse form is incompatible with extrauterine life. An appreciation of the more "benign" forms of NBT is also clinically important since several subtypes are considered to be precursors of Wilms' tumor, and when found in association with Wilms' tumor, imply a significant potential for synchronous or metachronous bilateral malignancy. A large body of circumstantial evidence for the premalignant nature of NBT has accumulated. The evidence revolves around the relative incidences of NBT and Wilms' tumor, the coexistence of NBT and Wilms' tumor in the same kidney, and, in cases of bilateral Wilms' tumor, the increased incidence of NBT in teratologic disorders known to be associated with Wilms' tumor and the structural and histological similarities found between subtypes of NBT and Wilms' tumor [19,38–43]. In addition, biopsy-proven progression of NBT to Wilms' tumor has been reported [41–45].

Lesions of the NBT complex are found incidentally at autopsy in one of every 200 to 400 infants less than 4 months of age but are rare in older children [35,39,47–49]. This age-related decreasing incidence may reflect a tendency for NBT to regress or mature or may reflect the fact that NBT is seen more frequently in association with other congenital anomalies, which themselves lead to perinatal mortality and a skewed autopsy population sample [39–41,48]. The incidence of NBT in the population of otherwise healthy children is unknown. Lesions of the NBT complex, however, accompany Wilms' tumor in approximately 40% of all cases, are present in 21% of uninvolved kidneys opposite a Wilms' tumor, in 60% of kidneys with multifocal Wilms' tumors, and in virtually 100% of cases of bilateral Wilms' tumor [35,38,39,48].

Classification

Machin and Beckwith have devised similar systems to classify the lesions of the NBT complex, according to the pattern of distribution of the persistent blastema in the renal lobule [17,37]. This pattern is related to the time when disordered embryogenesis occurred; more central, diffuse, or intralobar lesions develop earlier in embryogenesis than more superficial lesions. While up to 50% of Wilms' tumors are felt to arise in areas of NBT, not all subtypes of the nephroblastomatosis complex of lesions progress to the malignant state.

Diffuse pancortical, pannephric NBT. This is a very rare form of NBT that is incompatible with life. The disorder presents as diffuse, palpable, bilateral nephromegaly. All renal tissue is replaced by proliferative fetal blastema, and the infants succumb to pulmonary hypoplasia or neonatal renal failure. The potential for malignant degeneration is unknown.

Diffuse superficial NBT. This lesion is also uncommon, with only nine cases reported to 1984. Earlier reports of diffuse bilateral Wilms' tumor may have represented occurrences of diffuse superficial NBT rather than true malignancy. The diffuse nature of this peripherally located rind of blastemal tissue causes bilateral, palpable nephromegaly. The calyceal system is distorted on intravenous urography and may be mistaken for adult type polycystic kidney disease. Arteriography will show a characteristic lack of opacification of the peripheral, cortical rind of NBT, with increased opacification of the medullary tissue [40,41]. Renal sonography reveals nephromegaly and diffuse thickening of the renal cortex [50]; the rind of cortical nephroblastomatosis will not enhance on computed tomograms [51]. On gross examination the nephromegaly is diffuse rather than tumorous, and the jacket of blastemal tissue has a pink, uniform, fleshy appearance that is separated by a sharp margin from the uninvolved parenchyma. Histologically, diffuse superficial NBT is composed of confluent subcapsular masses of tightly packed nephrogenic epithelial cells that resemble the nephrogenic zone of the fetal kidney [40]. The tissue histology may resemble that of Wilms' tumor; two of the nine cases reported to date have gone on to develop frank Wilms' tumor [37,44–46].

Multifocal superficial, perilobar NBT. This is the most common type of NBT encountered. It is seen with increased frequency in the teratologic syndromes known to be associated with Wilms' tumor and is found in virtually 100% of cases of bilateral Wilms' tumor. The lesions are focal and appear in the grossly uninvolved cortex of kidneys containing Wilms' tumor as discontinuous collections of metanephric blastemal cells along with differentiated tubules and stromal elements [37]. The lesions are located in areas affected late in embryogenesis. Three subtypes are recognized. 1) Nodular renal blastema—microscopic, encapsulated, non-mitotic nodules that retain nephrogenic capacity. They are located in the subcapsular cortex (Fig. 3-1). 2) Metanephric hamartoma—larger lesions (up to 3 cm diameter) that are differentiated into tubular, or less commonly, stromal elements. They are

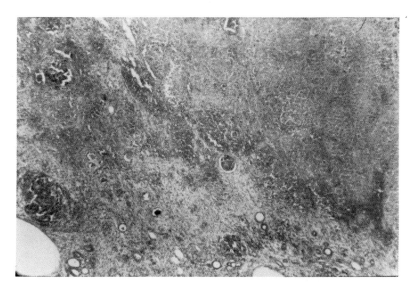

Fig. 3-1. Focus of subcapsular nodular renal blastema in patient with bilateral Wilms' tumor.

subcapsular and do not exhibit mitotic activity. The lesions will occasionally appear as sclerotic hamartomas composed of collagenous tissue. 3) Wilms' tumorlets—hamartomas greater than 1 cm in diameter with histologic features of Wilms' tumor and a high degree of mitotic activity. These lesions may represent the earliest stages in the development of Wilms' tumor (Fig. 3-2).

Larger lesions of multifocal perilobar NBT may appear as discrete masses on ultrasound and have a mixed echo pattern. The masses exhibit decreased attenuation levels and are non-enhancing on computed tomography [50]. All the subtypes of multifocal superficial perilobar NBT may coexist within the same kidney and appear to be the precursor substrate from which many Wilms' tumors develop [37].

Multifocal deep cortical, intralobar NBT. This form of NBT lies deeper within the kidney near the corticomedullary junction and is currently emerging as a separate entity [17]. The lesions may be mistaken for Wilms' tumor because the nodules vary in size, become confluent, and appear to invade

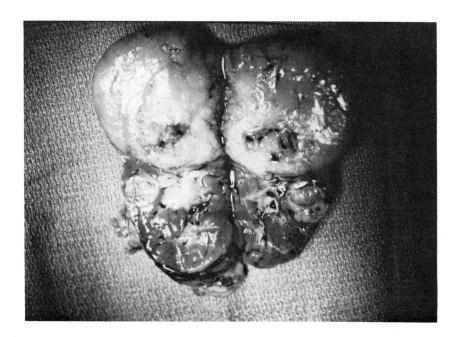

Fig. 3-2. Bisected surgical specimen from 1-yr-old girl with hemihypertrophy who developed Wilms' tumor in lower pole of left kidney. Tumor proved to be multifocal with grossly visible Wilms' tumorlets. Microscopic examination also revealed areas of nodular renal blastema.

adjacent tissue. A significant stromal component mimics triphasic Wilms' tumor, and some areas may exhibit a high mitotic rate. Wilms' tumors that develop from multifocal deep cortical NBT differ structurally from those arising in superficial, perilobar NBT. Sixteen percent of children in the NWTS II found to have intralobar NBT developed a metachronous contralateral Wilms' tumor [17].

Management

Because the presence of NBT in association with Wilms' tumor implies multifocal or bilateral disease, the preoperative, prenephrectomy appreciation of its presence would be advantageous in planning renal-conserving therapy. Nephroblastomatosis should be suspected and sought in children with Wilms' tumor presenting at an early age, those with other congenital or chromosomal abnormalities, cases of unilateral multifocal Wilms' tumor, and familial cases of Wilms' tumor [39–41].

Management of diffuse superficial NBT and nephromegaly is a dilemma since the relative risk of malignant escape of this form of NBT is unknown. Machin suggests a need for prolonged chemotherapy with vincristine and actinomycin D and long-term followup [52]. The lesions may progress to sclerosing metanephric hamartomas or escape to frank Wilms' tumor after apparent regression [44,45,47,52,53].

Beckwith feels that incidentally discovered microscopic foci of multifocal superficial NBT (nodular renal blastema) in a non-malignant multicystic, dysplastic, or obstructed kidney pose a low risk of malignant degeneration and require no therapy or followup [12,17,54,55].

The possibility of concomitant NBT must be considered in a Wilms' tumor kidney because of the implications regarding bilaterality. Aggressive contralateral exploration would seem to be indicated prior to examination of the tumor-bearing kidney in children at risk for NBT [17]. If frozen section biopsy of any suspicious areas in the "normal" kidney show NBT, a renal-preserving procedure may be indicated on the side of the frank Wilms' tumor since the risk of metachronous development of Wilms' tumor in the normal kidney is so high. In the child with Wilms' tumor and a normal contralateral kidney, frozen sections should be performed on the nephrectomy specimen looking for associated NBT; if NBT is present, a biopsy of the normal kidney should be performed [38,52]. There is a danger of overtreatment of NBT in these situations. Therapy based on the stage and histology of the frank Wilms' tumor should suffice for multifocal or contralateral NBT, though prolonged followup with quarterly renal sonography is necessary. The overall prognosis for children with Wilms' tumor that developed in a substrate of NBT is good, and therapy should be centered around the concept of preserving renal parenchyma and minimizing treatment-related toxicity.

REFERENCES

1. Wigger HJ: Fetal hamartoma of kidney. Am J Clin Pathol 51:323, 1969.
2. Howell CG, Othersen HB, Kiviat NE, et al.: Therapy and outcome in 51 children with mesoblastic nephroma: A report of the National Wilms' Tumor Study. J Pediatr Surg 17:826, 1982.
3. Biggers RD: Congenital mesonephric blastoma. Urology 21:302, 1983.
4. Hrabovsky EE, Othersen HB, Jr., de Lorimier A, et al.: Wilms' tumor in the neonate: A report from the National Wilms' Tumor Study. J Pediatr Surg 21:385, 1986.
5. Arensman RM, Belman AB: Ruptured congenital mesoblastic nephroma: Chemotherapy and irradiation as adjuvants to nephrectomy. Urology 15:394, 1980.
6. Bolande RP, Brough AJ, Izant RJ, Jr.: Congenital mesoblastic nephroma of infancy: A report of eight cases and the relationship to Wilms' tumor. Pediatrics 40:272, 1967.
7. Kay S, Pratt CB, Salzberg AM: Hamartoma (leiomyomatous type) of the kidney. Cancer 19:1825, 1966.
8. Bogdan R, Taylor DEM, Mostofi FK: Leiomyomatous hamartoma of the kidney. A clinical and pathological analysis of 20 cases from the kidney tumor registry. Cancer 31:462, 1973.
9. Bolande RP: Congenital mesoblastic nephroma of infancy. Perspect Pediatr Pathol 1:227, 1973.
10. Yazaki T, Kawai H, Akimoto M, et al.: Congenital mesoblastic nephroma. Urology 20:446, 1982.
11. Shen SC, Yunis EJ: A study of the cellularity and ultrastructure of congenital mesoblastic nephroma. Cancer 45:306, 1980.
12. Snyder HM, III, Lack EE, Chetty-Baktavizian A, et al.: Congenital mesoblastic nephroma: Relationship to other renal tumors of infancy. J Urol 126:513, 1981.
13. Gerber A, Gold JH, Bustamante S, et al.: Congenital mesoblastic nephroma. J Pediatr Surg 16:758, 1981.
14. Beckwith JB: Mesenchymal renal neoplasms of infancy revisited. J Pediatr Surg 9:803, 1974.
15. Beckwith JB, Weeks DA: Congenital mesoblastic nephroma: When should we worry? Arch Pathol Lab Med 110:98, 1986.
16. Joshi VV, Kasznicka J, Walters TR: Atypical mesoblastic nephroma: Pathologic characterization of a potentially aggressive variant of conventional congenital mesoblastic nephroma. Arch Pathol Lab Med 110:100, 1986.
17. Beckwith JB: Wilms tumor and other renal tumors of childhood: An update. J Urol 136:520, 1986.
18. D'Angio GJ, Duckett JW, Jr., Belasco JB: Tumors: Upper urinary tract. In Kelalis PP, King LR, Belman AB (eds): Clinical Pediatric Urology, 2nd ed. Philadelphia: W.B. Saunders, 1985.
19. Knudson AG, Jr., Strong LC: Mutation and cancer: A model for Wilms' tumor of the kidney. JNCI 48:313, 1972.
20. Bitter JJ, Harrison DA, Kaplan J, et al.: Case report: Mesoblastic nephroma. J Comput Assist Tomogr 6:180, 1982.

21. King DR, Buck D, Kleinman PB, et al.: Congenital mesoblastic nephroma. Am J Dis Child 132:1139, 1978.
22. Bauer JH, Durham J, Miles J, et al.: Congenital mesoblastic nephroma presenting with primary reninism. J Pediatr 95:268, 1979.
23. Shanbhogue LKR, Gray E, Miller SS: Congenital mesoblastic nephroma of infancy associated with hypercalcemia. J Urol 135:771, 1986.
24. Favara BE, Johnson W, Ito, J: Renal tumors in the neonatal period. Cancer 22:845, 1986.
25. Blank E, Neerhout RC, Burry KA: Congenital mesoblastic nephroma and polyhydramnios. JAMA 240:1504, 1978.
26. Geirsson RT, Ricketts NEM, Taylor DJ, et al.: Prenatal appearance of a mesoblastic nephroma associated with polyhydramnios. J Clin Ultrasound 13:488, 1985.
27. Walter JP, McGahan JP: Mesoblastic nephroma: Prenatal sonographic detection. J Clin Ultrasound 13:686, 1985.
28. Apuzzio JJ, Unwin W, Adhate A, et al.: Prenatal diagnosis of fetal renal mesoblastic nephroma. Am J Obstet Gynecol 154:636, 1986.
29. Hartman DS, Lesar MSL, Madewell JE, et al: Mesoblastic nephroma: Radiologic-pathologic correlation of 20 cases. AJR 136:69, 1981.
30. Walker D, Richard GA: Fetal hamartoma of the kidney: Recurrence and death of patient. J Urol 110:352, 1973.
31. Fu Y, Kay S: Congenital mesoblastic nephroma and its recurrence: An ultrastructural observation. Arch Pathol 96:66, 1973.
32. Crussi FG, Avila CS, Kidd JM: Malignant mesenchymal nephroma of infancy: Report of a case with pulmonary metastases. Am J Surg Pathol 4:185, 1980.
33. Machin GA: Persistent renal blastema (nephroblastomatosis) as a frequent precursor of Wilms' tumor; a pathological and clinical review. Part 1. Am J Pediatr Hematol Oncol 2:165, 1980.
34. Hou LT, Holman RL: Bilateral nephroblastomatosis in a premature infant. J Pathol Bacteriol 82:249, 1961.
35. Bove KE, McAdams AJ: The nephroblastomatosis complex and its relationships to Wilms' tumor; a clinicopathologic treatise. Perspect Pediatr Pathol 3:185, 1976.
36. Machin GA: Persistent renal blastema (nephroblastomatosis) as a frequent precursor of Wilms' tumor; a pathological and clinical review. Part 2. Am J Pediatr Hematol Oncol 2:253, 1980.
37. Machin GA: Persistent renal blastema as a precursor of Wilms' tumor. In Pochedly C, Baum ES (eds): Wilms' Tumor: Clinical and Biological Manifestations. New York: Elsevier, 1984.
38. Machin GA: Nephroblastomatosis and bilateral nephroblastomata. Arch Pathol Lab Med 102:639, 1978.
39. Bove KE, Koffler H, McAdams AJ: Nodular renal blastema: Definition and possible significance. Cancer 24:323, 1969.
40. Chadarevian JP, Fletcher BD, Chatten J, et al.: Massive infantile nephroblastomatosis: A clinical, radiological and pathological analysis of four cases. Cancer 39:2294, 1977.
41. Haddy TB: Nephroblastomatosis: Clinical manifestations and management. In Pochedly C, Baum ES (eds): Wilms' Tumor: Clinical and Biological Manifestations. Elsevier Publ., New York: Elsevier, 1984.
42. Pochedly C: Persistent renal blastema: A seed of Wilms' tumor? Hosp Practice, Vol. 16, May, 83, 1981.
43. Rous SW, Bailie MD, Kaufman DB, et al.: Nodular renal blastema, nephroblastomatosis, and Wilms' tumor: Different points on the same disease spectrum? Urology 8:599, 1976.

44. Haddy TB, Bailie MD, Bernstein J, et al.: Bilateral, diffuse nephroblastomatosis: Report of a case managed with chemotherapy. J Pediatr 90:784, 1977.
45. Kulkarni R, Bailie MD, Bernstein J, et al: Progression of nephroblastomatosis to Wilms' tumor. J Pediatr 96:178, 1980.
46. Haddy TB: Management of bilateral diffuse nephroblastomatosis. J Pediatr 97:501, 1980.
47. Rosenfield NS, Shimkin P, Berdon W, et al.: Wilms tumor arising from spontaneously regressing nephroblastomatosis. AJR 135:381, 1980.
48. Bove KE, McAdams AJ: Multifocal nephroblastic neoplasia. JNCI 61:285, 1978.
49. Breslow NE, Beckwith JB: Epidemiological features of Wilms' tumor: Results of the National Wilms' Tumor Study. JNCI 68:429, 1982.
50. Foley LL, Campbell JB, Heideman RL, et al.: Imaging of nephroblastomatosis. AJR 141:853, 1983.
51. Franken EA, Jr., Yiu-Chiu V, Smith WL, et al.: Nephroblastomatosis: Clinicopathologic significance and imaging characteristics. AJR 138:950, 1982.
52. Machin GA: Persistent renal blastema (nephroblastomatosis) as a frequent precursor of Wilms' tumor; a pathological and clinical review. Part 3. Am J Pediatr Hematol Oncol 2:353, 1980.
53. Heideman RL, Haase GM, Foley CL, et al.: Nephroblastomatosis and Wilms' tumor: Clinical experience and management of seven patients. Cancer 55:1446, 1985.
54. Gaddy CD, Gibbons MD, Gonzales ET, Jr., et al.: Obstructive uropathy, renal dysplasia and nodular renal blastema: Is there a relationship to Wilms tumor? J Urol 134:330, 1985.
55. Snyder HM, Duckett JW, Elder JS: Nodular renal blastema in a multicystic kidney. Soc Pediatr Urol Newsletter, April, p. 36, 1986.

Chapter 4
Wilms' Tumor—Medical Aspects

Rebecca L. Byrd

Wilms' tumor is the most common malignancy of the genitourinary tract in children and accounts for approximately 8% of all childhood malignancies [1]. Over the past two decades, there has been dramatic improvement in the survival of patients with Wilms' tumor. This improved survival is the result of a multidisciplinary approach that includes surgery, radiation therapy, and chemotherapy.

EPIDEMIOLOGY

Data from the Third National Cancer Survey indicates that the annual incidence for Wilms' tumor is 7.8 per million children under 15 years of age [2]. The risk of developing Wilms' tumor is one in 10,000 live births [3]. There are about 500 cases of Wilms' tumor in the United States annually. Wilms' tumor accounts for 8% of all pediatric malignancies and ranks fifth among solid tumors of children behind central nervous system tumors, lymphomas, neuroblastomas, and soft tissue sarcomas.

The tumor occurs with an equal frequency among boys and girls and has a peak age incidence during the third year of life. Three-fourths of the patients are less than 5 years of age at diagnosis and 90% occur in those under 7 years of age [4]. Wilms' tumor is rare in the newborn, adolescent, and adult.

Wilms' tumor occurs in either an hereditary or non-hereditary form [5–7]. The hereditary form is transmitted in an autosomal dominant manner. It develops at an earlier age, tends to be bilateral and/or multicentric. All

Pediatric Tumors of the Genitourinary Tract, pages 61–73
© 1988 Alan R. Liss, Inc.

bilateral cases and up to 20% of unilateral Wilms' tumors may be due to the hereditary form [6].

Patients with Wilms' tumor may have additional abnormalities [5,8–10]. The most frequently diagnosed are aniridia, hemihypertrophy, and genitourinary abnormalities. Of 547 children evaluated in the National Wilms' Tumor Study (NWTS), aniridia was noted in 1.1%, hemihypertrophy in 2.4%, and genitourinary abnormalities in 4.4%.

Aniridia may occur in both familial and sporadic forms. Approximately two-thirds of the cases are familial. Wilms' tumor occurs almost exclusively in the sporadic form of aniridia. The incidence of aniridia in the general population is 1 in 50,000. In contrast, Miller et al.'s survey reveals an incidence of 1 in 73 cases among children with Wilms' tumor [11]. Other abnormalities that may be seen when aniridia and Wilms' tumor are present include congenital eye lesions, mental retardation, and genitourinary abnormalities [11]. The cytogenetic analysis of multiple cases of Wilms' tumor with aniridia reveal a deletion in the short arm of chromosome 11 (−11p13) [12,13]. Children with sporadic aniridia should be evaluated frequently with physical examinations and ultrasonography as they have a 1 in 3 chance of developing a Wilms' tumor [14].

The frequency of hemihypertrophy in the general population is 0.003% [15]. Among the children with Wilms' tumor, the incidence is 2.4% [15]. Hemihypertrophy may not be apparent until after the diagnosis of Wilms' tumor and may be ipsilateral or contralateral to the involved kidney.

The most common abnormalities associated with Wilms' tumor are genitourinary [10,11]. These include hypospadias, cryptorcidism, ureteral duplication, and anomalies of the kidney (hypoplasia, horseshoe or fused or ectopic kidneys).

CLINICAL PRESENTATION AND DIAGNOSTIC EVALUATION

Most children with Wilms' tumor are otherwise healthy and receive medical attention because of an enlarged abdomen or mass that has been felt by a parent. Occasionally, a tumor may be discovered during routine examination. Other frequent presenting signs and symptoms include fever (23%), hematuria (25%), abdominal pain (37%), and hypertension (6.3%) [16–20]. Physical examination usually reveals a smooth, non-tender mass confined to one side of the abdomen.

Laboratory evaluation of a child suspected of having a Wilms' tumor should include a complete blood count and differential, platelet count, urinalysis, serum chemistries, and urinary catecholamines. Karyotyping should be obtained in patients with congenital abnormalities. A bone marrow examination is indicated to exclude stage IV neuroblastoma.

Preoperative radiographic evaluation should document the presence of an intrarenal mass, establish the normal function of the contralateral kidney, determine the patency of the inferior vena cava, and document the presence or absence of pulmonary metastases. The evaluation should begin with a plain radiograph of the abdomen. This will demonstrate a mass of homogeneous density that displaces the bowel gas pattern. Calcifications are unusual and, when present, are in the periphery of the tumor mass [21,22]. The common features on intravenous urography are displacement and distortion of the collecting system. Non-visualization of the kidney has been reported in between 5 and 33% of Wilms' tumors [21–25]. Ultrasonography and computerized tomography scanning (CT scan) will differentiate a non-functioning kidney due to a Wilms' tumor from renal agenesis, multicystic kidney, or hydronephrosis. The CT scan may also detect metastatic involvement of the liver or lymph nodes in the retroperitoneum and a thrombus in the inferior vena cava [26–29], as well as direct tumor extension into the liver and other adjacent organs. An inferior vena cavagram is indicated if caval assessment by ultrasound or CT scan is indeterminate. Arteriography is rarely indicated. A plain radiograph of the chest should be performed to evaluate the presence of pulmonary metastases. The value of whole lung tomography and computerized tomography of the lung is uncertain and has not been evaluated adequately in patients with Wilms' tumor.

Skeletal metastases are rare and only seen in the sarcomatous type of Wilms' tumor. A radionuclide bone scan and skeletal survey should be performed postoperatively in children with the clear cell sarcoma type. In those children with rhabdoid histology, a computerized tomography or radionuclear brain scan should be performed because of the possibility of brain metastases.

PROGNOSTIC FACTORS

The two most important prognostic factors for Wilms' tumor are the stage and histology of the tumor [30–33]. Several staging systems have been used for Wilms' tumor. The current staging system as used in the National Wilms' Tumor Study III (NWTS-III) (Table 4-1) was developed as prognostic factors from the two previous national studies were identified. Patients with positive lymph nodes are now assigned to stage III. Gross tumor spillage and peritoneal contamination also places the patient in stage III. When a tumor is biopsied or minor spillage is confined to the flank, the patient is staged as II.

TABLE 4-1. National Wilms' Tumor Study Treatment Groups

Stage I	Tumor limited to the kidney and was completely excised. The surface of the renal capsule was intact. The tumor was not ruptured before or during removal. There was no residual tumor apparent beyond the margins of resection.
Stage II	Tumor extends beyond the kidney but was completely excised. There was regional extension of the tumor. The renal vessels outside the kidney substance were infiltrated or contained tumor thrombus. The tumor may have been biopsied or there may have been local spillage of tumor confined to the flank. There was no residual tumor apparent beyond the margins of resection.
Stage III	Residual non-hematogenous tumor confined to the abdomen. One or more of the following occurred: 1) tumor extends beyond surgical margins either micro- or macroscopically, 2) diffuse peritoneal contamination by tumor spillage or peritoneal implants, 3) involved lymph nodes beyond the abdominal paraaortic chains, and/or 4) tumor was not completely resectable because of local infiltration into vital structure.
Stage IV	Hematogenous metastases. Deposits beyond stage III, e.g., lung, liver, bone, and/or brain.
Stage V	Bilateral renal involvement either initially or subsequently.

This stage is determined by the surgeon at the time of the operation and is confirmed by the pathologist. In the NWTS-II, 64% of the patients were in groups I and II, 19% in group III, 12% in group IV, and 5% in group V [4].

Various histological and pathological subtypes of Wilms' tumor are now recognized. Data from the NWTS reveals that patients can be separated on the basis of favorable or unfavorable histology [29–33]. Unfavorable histology includes anaplasia, clear cell sarcomas, and rhabdoid tumors. (Clear cell sarcomas and rhabdoid tumors, while considered unfavorable Wilms' tumor variants in early NWTS, are now each considered a separate entity, as noted by Beckwith in Chapter 2, this volume.) All other histologic features are considered favorable. The unfavorable histology group constitutes 12% of all the cases in the NWTS but includes 52% of all deaths [29]. The rhabdoid subtype has a high mortality rate and is associated with cerebral metastases. The clear cell subtype is characterized by a strong tendency to metastasize to bone.

TREATMENT

Although Wilms' tumor was first described in 1814 by Runce [34], Max Wilms reviewed the literature and added seven cases of his own in 1899 [35].

The outlook for a child with Wilms' tumor in the early years of the 20th century was poor [36,37]. By 1950, advances in anesthetic and surgical techniques improved sufficiently to reduce operative mortality from 20% to less than 5% [38]. At the same time the role of postoperative flank or whole abdominal radiation was defined by Gross and Newhauser [39]. The addition of radiotherapy to surgical resection increased 2-year survival rates to 50%. In 1956, dactinomycin was found to be effective in children with metastatic Wilms' tumor [40]. Similar results were observed with vincristine [41]. By 1965 with multimodal therapy, consisting of surgery, radiation therapy, and dactinomycin or vincristine, over 80% of children survived 2 years or longer [42]. The surgical treatment of Wilms' tumor will be discussed in Chapter 5.

Radiation Therapy

Since the first reported case by Friedlaender in 1916 of treatment of a malignant renal tumor in a child by radiation alone, radiation has become widely used as a supplement to the treatment of Wilms' tumor [43]. Silver first reported the beneficial effect of preoperative radiation [44]. Subsequently, an increase in cure rate from 19 to 47% was achieved by the addition of postoperative radiation therapy [44–47]. The addition of radiation therapy to surgery, whether given before or after, significantly increased the cure rate.

Preoperative radiation therapy can shrink large tumors, thereby facilitating surgery, and reduce tumor rupture [47,48]. Those who are reluctant to give preoperative radiation therapy cite the possibility of misdiagnosis prior to tissue confirmation. Further arguments against preoperative radiation are possible stage changes and difficulties with histological evaluation.

Marked improvement in survival has been noted with postoperative flank irradiation. The NWTS designed control trials to determine if all patients benefited from radiation. The results of the NWTS-II determined that patients of any age with a stage I tumor and favorable histology given actinomycin D plus vincristine did not require postoperative irradiation [49]. At present, the policy in the majority of cancer centers is to give no postoperative radiation therapy for stage I tumors with favorable histology. The necessity of radiation therapy in stage II with favorable histology is currently being evaluated in the NWTS-III. Radiation therapy is indicated for any patient with an unfavorable histology or a stage III tumor with favorable histology.

The technique of radiation therapy is rather uniform. Two parallel opposed fields are used that include the tumor bed, the ipsilateral renal vessels, and the immediate nodal drainage area [50]. The field is extended across the midline to include the entire width of the vertebral bodies to avoid asymmetrical growth and subsequent scoliosis [51]. The opposite kidney is outside the treated area. A high voltage linear accelerator is used.

A daily dose of 150–200 rad are delivered five times per week. The total dose recommended is 2,000 rad whether given just to the tumor bed or to the whole abdomen. High doses are used for older children with unfavorable histology or metastatic disease. The doses are based on estimates of normal tissue tolerance for children who are also receiving radiation-enhancing agents (dactinomycin, adriamycin).

Chemotherapy

In order to determine the most effective therapy for Wilms' tumor, three cooperative groups—Children's Cancer Study Group, Acute Leukemia Group B, and Southwest Oncology Group—formed the first National Wilms' Tumor Study Group. The first controlled trial, National Wilms' Tumor Study-I (NWTS-I) was launched in 1969.

In NWTS-I, double-agent chemotherapy using vincristine and dactinomycin was demonstrated to be superior to either agent alone [42]. Postoperative radiation therapy was not found to be necessary in younger patients with early stage disease. In this study, relapse-free survival improved from 55 to 80%.

The second study, NWTS-II, was begun in 1974 and was built on the results of NWTS-I. This study sought to determine whether postoperative radiation therapy was necessary in children with group I disease if dactinomycin and vincristine were both used and whether the addition of adriamycin to vincristine and dactinomycin would improve survival in children with groups II, III, and IV disease. The results showed that survival was approximately 90% in group I patients with postoperative chemotherapy alone whether given for 6 or 15 months [52]. The addition of adriamycin to vincristine and dactinomycin improved relapse-free survival for groups II and III disease of favorable histology from 72 to 90%.

The NWTS-III is currently in progress. The objectives of this study are to 1) decrease therapy and its toxicities for children at low risk (low stage, favorable histology), 2) intensify therapy in an attempt to improve survival for children at high risk (high stage, unfavorable histology), 3) identify late effects of treatment, and 4) identify genetic or other etiologic factors [4]. This study is now closed to patient entry and data is being evaluated.

Treatment of Bilateral Disease

Wilms' tumor present in both kidneys affects approximately 5% of all patients [17,42,52–56]. The treatment of children with bilateral Wilms' tumor must be individualized. Treatment should be directed at preserving as much renal tissue as possible [4,53–56]. More than one surgical procedure may be required. The degree of renal involvement is generally unequal, and the most common surgical procedure is nephrectomy on the more involved side and tumor excision or partial nephrectomy on the less involved side. Renal-sparing procedure should be employed bilaterally when technically possible. Presurgical treatment with drug therapy and radiotherapy is effective in reducing tumor bulk and should be employed in bilateral disease when it will make a renal-sparing procedure technically more feasible. Bilateral nephrectomy and renal transplantation has been performed for bilateral Wilms' tumor, but results are generally inferior to renal-sparing procedures [57–61].

Bilateral Wilms' tumor is usually of a favorable histologic pattern and has a good prognosis. Survival rates for bilateral Wilms' tumor range from 60 to 87% [54,56,61–63].

Treatment of Recurrent Disease

Children with Wilms' tumor who relapse may be salvaged with a multidisciplinary team approach. The most common site of relapse is the lung [55,64]. The NWTS committee has reviewed the cure rate for children who relapse [64]. Patients with group I disease were salvaged more easily than those with groups II and III disease. Children with metastatic tumor at diagnosis did worse than children with subsequent metastases. Prognosis was worse for those patients who relapsed early (less than 6 months from diagnosis), who had unfavorable histology, or had recurrent abdominal disease [64–66]. Since the relapsed patients were not treated in a controlled fashion, it is difficult to determine the most successful management. Vincrintine and dactinomycin (although used in patients prior to relapse) and adriamycin have been successfully employed with or without radiation therapy.

The prognosis for children who develop pulmonary metastases after adjuvant chemotherapy is approximately 50% [55,67–69]. The prognosis for children who develop recurrent disease at other sites is generally poor, but successes have been reported [55].

SURVIVAL

Overall survival rates for children with Wilms' tumor are excellent [33,42,52,70]. Two-year relapse-free survival rates for stages I, II, III, and IV are 95, 90, 84, and 54%, respectively. The 2-year survival rate for patients with unfavorable histology is 54% and 90% for those with favorable histology. The presence of nodal disease has a significant adverse effect on relapse-free survival rates. Fifty-four percent of patients with positive nodes and 82% of those with negative nodes survived relapse-free [42,52].

LATE EFFECTS

As more children are surviving Wilms' tumor, clinicians are identifying long-term effects of antineoplastic treatment [71–74]. Objectives of the NWTS-III are to reduce the length of treatment (and therefore presumably treatment complications) without sacrificing survival, to follow the children who survive and document the long-term effects, and, if possible, to identify the etiologies. Several of the more common late effects of treatment for Wilms' tumor will be discussed.

Wilms' tumor patients who undergo a nephrectomy followed by radiation therapy are at risk of developing radiation nephritis in the remaining kidney [73,75,76]. Radiation nephritis may occur months to years after treatment and is characterized by hypertension, proteinuria, anemia, and renal failure. The severity of renal dysfunction correlates directly with the dose of radiation. Once the symptoms of progressive renal failure develop, the treatment is supportive.

Musculoskeletal structures can be affected by radiotherapy. The first reported case of radiation-induced scoliosis was published by Arkin in 1950 in a child treated for Wilm's tumor. Oliver et al. studied 21 children who had been treated for Wilms' tumor [74]. Flank atrophy was present in all patients on the side treated with radiotherapy. Other noted abnormalities included asymmetry of vertebral bodies, vertebral end-plate irregularities, scoliosis, kyphosis, platyspondyly, and hypoplasia of the ileum. Riseborough et al. reported vertebral abnormalities in 70% of children previously treated for Wilms' tumor [77]. Changes in vertebral bodies usually occur within 5 years after radiation, while scoliosis and kyphosis may not occur until many years later [77–79].

Both radiation and chemotherapy may affect the gastrointestinal system. The major late effects seen in Wilms' tumor patients include hepatic injury and chronic enteritis [72,73]. Liver dysfunction is more common if the entire liver volume has received doses of more than 3,000 rads over an interval of 3 weeks. Adriamycin and dactinomycin may potentiate the reaction to radiation [80–82]. This enhancement has been postulated as the explanation for hepatic toxicity reported by Tefft. In this review, 15 patients developed liver abnormalities; all but three recovered [72].

Approximately 5% of patients who receive radiation therapy to the abdomen in doses of 4,000–5,000 rads will develop gastrointestinal complications. Patients who have had previous abdominal surgery or chemotherapeutic agents like adriamycin or dactinomycin are at greater risk for radiation enteritis. In the review of Cassady et al., the gastrointestinal tract was the most frequent site of complications. Sixteen Wilms' tumor patients had 21 episodes of small bowel obstruction, with 20 requiring surgical intervention [73].

The major effect of cancer therapy on the lung is interstitial pneumonitis and pulmonary fibrosis. The volume of lung irradiated and the dose of radiation are the most important predisposing factors. Symptoms generally do not occur for 9–12 months and are uncommon when doses of less than 3,000 rads are given. In general, children treated for lung metastases will tolerate up to 1,400 rad (with chemotherapy) [83]. Pulmonary complications are more common in patients who relapse and receive more than one course of radiation and chemotherapy [72,73].

Individuals treated for childhood cancer have an increased risk (up to 15%) for developing a second malignancy. Twenty-four cases of second neoplasms have been reported in 23 individuals previously treated for Wilms' tumor [71,84–93]. These tumors were diagnosed between 1 year and 26 years following treatment, with a median of 12 years. All but one patient received radiation and ten received a combination of chemotherapy and radiation therapy. All but three developed the second tumor in the irradiated field.

SUMMARY

Wilms' tumor has a high rate of cure even when metastic disease is present. The multidisciplinary approach to the tumor has been a model in the field of pediatric oncology. Over the past two decades, there has been improvement in treatment as a result of identification of histological subtypes, precise staging of the disease, and accurate assessment and followup of the patients' response to treatment.

In the future, patients with poor prognostic features and worse survival need more intense or innovative therapy, while those with more favorable features may receive less therapy. More attention needs to be focused on the toxic effect of therapy, the genetic aspects of the disease, and epidemiologic factors influencing the development of Wilms' tumor.

REFERENCES

1. Hanson MR, Mulvihill JJ: Epidemiology of cancer in the young. In Levine AS (ed): Cancer in the Young, 1st ed. New York: Masson Publishing, 1982, p 3.

2. Cutler SJ, Young JL: Third National Cancer Survey: Incidence Data. Nat Cancer Inst Monog 41, March, 1975.
3. Young JL, Miller RW: Incidence of malignant tumors in US children. J Pediatr 86:254, 1975.
4. Belasco JB, Chatten J, D'Angio GJ: Wilms' tumor. In Sutow WW, Fernbach DJ, Vietti TJ (eds): Clinical Pediatric Oncology, 3rd ed. St Louis: CV Mosby, 1984, p 588.
5. Breslow NE, Beckwith JB: Epidemiological features of Wilms' tumor: Result of the National Wilms' Tumor Study. JNCI 68:429, 1982.
6. Matsunaga E: Genetics of Wilms' tumor. Hum Genet 57:231, 1981.
7. Knudson AG, Strong LC: Mutation and cancer: A model for Wilms' tumor of the kidney. JNCI 48:313, 1972.
8. Fontana VJ, Ferrara A, Perciaccante R: Wilms' tumors and associated anomalies. Am J Dis Child 109:459, 1965.
9. Miller RW: Relationship between cancer and congenital defects: An epidemiologic evaluation. JNCI 40:1079, 1968.
10. Pendergrass TW: Congenital anomalies in children with Wilms' tumor. Cancer 37:403, 1976.
11. Miller RW, Fraumeni JF, Manning MD: Association of Wilms' tumor with aniridia, hemihypertrophy, and other congenital abnormalities. N Engl J Med 270:922, 1964.
12. Miller RW: Birth defects and cancer due to small chromosomal deletions. J Pediatr 96:1031, 1980.
13. Yunis JJ, Ramsay NKC: Familial occurrence of the aniridia: Wilms' tumor syndrome with deletion of 11p13-14.1. J Pediatr 96:1027, 1980.
14. Pilling GP: Wilms' tumor in seven children with congenital aniridia. J Pediatr Surg 10:87, 1975.
15. Green DM: The diagnosis and management of Wilms' tumor. Pediatr Clin North Am 32:735, 1985.
16. Aron BS: Wilms' tumor: A clinical study of eighty-one patients. Cancer 33:637, 1974.
17. Ledlie EM, Mynors LS, Draper GJ, et al.: Natural history and treatment of Wilms' tumors: An analysis of 335 cases occurring in England and Wales 1962–1966. Br Med J 4:195, 1970.
18. Pearson D, Duncan WB, Pointon RCS: Wilms' tumor—A review of 96 consecutive cases. Br J Radiol 37:154, 1964.
19. Perez CA, Kaiman HA, Keith J, et al.: Treatment of Wilms' tumor and factors affecting prognosis. Cancer 32:609, 1973.
20. Sukarochana K, Tolentlon W, Kiesewetter WB: Wilms' tumor and hypertension. J Pediatr Surg 7:573, 1972.
21. Guozhen Z: Intravenous urography in nephroblastoma. Chinese Med J 92:405, 1979.
22. Lalli AF, Ahstrom L, Ericsson NO, et al.: Nephroblastoma (Wilms' tumor): Urographic diagnosis and prognosis. Radiology 87:495, 1966.
23. Andersen J, Steenskor V: Radiologic and prognostic aspects of Wilms' tumor. Acta Radiol 22:353, 1981.
24. Canty TG, Nagaraj HS, Shearer LS: Nonvisualization of the intravenous pyelogram—A poor prognostic sign in Wilms' tumor. J Pediatr Surg 14:825, 1979.
25. Cremin BJ: Nonfunction in nephroblastoma (Wilms' tumor). Clin Radiol 30:197, 1979.
26. Hunig R, Kinser J: Ultrasonic diagnosis of Wilms' tumor. Am J Roentgenol Radium Ther Nucl Med 117:119, 1973.
27. Goldstein HM, Green B, Weaver RM: Ultrasonic detection of renal tumor extension into the inferior vena cava. AJR 130:1083, 1978.

28. Green B, Goldstein HM, Weaver RM: Abdominal pansonography in the evaluation of renal cancer. Radiology 132:421, 1979.
29. McArdle CR: Ultrasonic diagnosis of liver metastases. J Clin Ultrasound 4:265, 1976.
30. Beckwith JB: Wilms' tumor and other renal tumors of childhood: A selective review from the National Wilms' Tumor Study Pathology Center. Hum Pathol 14:481, 1983.
31. Beckwith JB, Palmer NF: Histopathology and prognosis of Wilms' tumor: Results from the First National Wilms' Tumor Study. Cancer 41:1937, 1978.
32. Beckwith NE, Palmer NF, Hill LR, et al.: Prognosis of Wilms' tumor patient without metastases at diagnosis—Results of the National Wilms' Tumor Study. Cancer 41:1577, 1978.
33. Breslow N, Churchill G, Beckwith JB, et al.: Prognosis for Wilms' tumor patients with nonmetastatic disease at diagnosis. Results of the Second National Wilms' Tumor Study. J Clin Oncol 3:521–531, 1985.
34. Runce TF: Case of fungus haematodes of the kidneys. Med Phys J 32:19, 1814.
35. Wilms M: Die Mischgeschwulste de Nieren. Leipzig: Arthur George, 1899, p 1–90.
36. Ladd WE: Embryoma of the kidney (Wilms' tumor). Ann Surg 108:885, 1938.
37. Ladd WE, White RR: Embryoma of the kidney (Wilms' tumor). JAMA 117:1858, 1941.
38. Harvey RM: Wilms' tumor: Evaluation of treatment methods. Radiology 43:689, 1950.
39. Gross RE, Newhauser EBD: Treatment of mixed tumors of the kidney in children. Pediatrics 6:843, 1950.
40. Farber S, Toch R, Sears EM, Pinkel D: Advances in chemotherapy of cancer in man. Adv Cancer Res 4:1, 1956.
41. Sutow WW, Sullivan MP: Vincristine in primary treatment of Wilms' tumor. Tex State J Med 61:794, 1965.
42. D'Angio GJ, Evans AE, Preslow JV, et al.: The treatment of Wilms' tumor: Results of the National Wilms' Tumor Study. Cancer 38:633, 1976.
43. Friedlaender A: Sarcoma of kidney treated by roentgen-ray. Am J Dis Child 12:328, 1916.
44. Silver HK: Wilms' tumour (embryoma of kidney). J Pediatr 31:643, 1947.
45. Gross RE, Neuhauser EBD: Treatment of mixed tumors of the kidney in childhood. Pediatrics 6:643, 1950.
46. Klapproth HJ: Wilms' tumor: A report of 45 cases and an analysis of 1351 cases reported in the world literature from 1940 to 1958. J Urol 81:633, 1959.
47. Jereb B, Eklund G: Factors influencing the cure rate in nephroblastoma. Acta Radiol Ther 12:84, 1973.
48. Lemerle J, Voute PA, Tournade MD, et al.: Preoperative versus postoperative radiotherapy, single versus multiple courses of actinomycin-D in the treatment of Wilms' tumor. Preliminary results of a controlled clinic trial conducted by the International Society of Pediatric Oncology (SIOP). Cancer 38:647, 1976.
49. D'Angio GJ, Evans AE, Breslow N, et al.: The treatment of Wilms' tumor. Cancer 38:633, 1976.
50. D'Angio GJ, Tefft M, Breslow N, Meyer JA: Radiation therapy of Wilms' tumor: Results according to dose, field, postoperative timing and histology. Int J Radiat Oncol Biol Phys 4:769, 1978.
51. Neuhauser EBD, Wittenborg MH, Berman CZ, et al.: Irradiation effects of roentgen therapy on the growing spine. Radiology 49:637, 1952.
52. D'Angio JG, Evans A, Breslow N, et al.: The treatment of Wilms' tumor: Results of the Second National Wilms' Tumor Study. Cancer 47:2302, 1981.

53. Bishop HC, Tefft M, Evans AE, et al.: Survival in bilateral Wilms' tumor: Review of 30 National Wilms' Tumor Study Cases. J Pediatr Surg 12:631, 1977.
54. Bond JV: Bilateral Wilms' tumor. Lancet 2:482, 1975.
55. Green DM, Jaffe N: Wilms' tumor—Model of a curable pediatric malignant solid tumor. Cancer Treat Rev 5:143, 1978.
56. Wasiljew BK, Bresser A, Raffensperger J: Treatment of bilateral Wilms' tumor—A 22 year experience. J Pediatr Surg 17:265, 1982.
57. Anderson KD, Altman RP: Selective resection of malignant tumors using bench surgical techniques. J Pediatr Surg 11:881, 1976.
58. DeLorimier AA, Belzer FO, Kountz SL, et al.: Simultaneous bilateral nephrectomy and renal allotransplantation for bilateral Wilms' tumor. Am J Surg 122:275, 1971.
59. Lilly JR, Pfister RR, Putmann Wc, et al.: Bench surgery and renal autotransplantation in the pediatric patient. J Pediatr Surg 10:623, 1975.
60. Penn I: Renal transplantation for Wilms' tumor: Report of 70 cases. J Urol 122:793, 1979.
61. Dimaria JE, Hardy BE, Brezinski A, et al.: Renal transplantation in patients with bilateral Wilms' tumor. J Pediatr Surg 14:577, 1979.
62. Asch MJ, Siegel S, White L, et al.: Prognostic factors and outcome in bilateral Wilms' tumor. Cancer 56:2524, 1985.
63. Bishop HC, Tefft M, Evans AE, et al.: Survival in bilateral Wilms' tumor—Review of 30 National Wilms' Tumor Study cases. J Pediatr Surg 12:631, 1977.
64. Sutow WW, Breslow NE, Palmer NP, et al.: Prognosis in children with Wilms' tumor metastases prior to or following primary treatment. Am J Clin Oncol 5:339, 1982.
65. Kim T, Zaatori GS, Baum ES, et al.: Recurrence of Wilms' tumor after apparent cure. J Pediatr 107:44, 1985.
66. D'Angio GJ, Evans AE, Breslow N, et al.: Biology and management of Wilms' tumor. In Levine AD (ed): Cancer in the Young. New York: Masson Publishing, 1982, pp 633–662.
67. Bellani FF, Gasparini M, Bonadonna G: Adriamycin in Wilms' tumor previously treated with chemotherapy. Eur J Cancer 11:593, 1975.
68. Sutow WW, Thurman WG, Windmiller J: Vincristine (leurocrinstine) sulfate in the treatment of children with metastatic Wilms' tumor. Pediatrics 12:880, 1963.
69. Vietti TJ, Sullivan MP, Haggard ME, et al.: Vincristine sulfate and radiation therapy in metastatic Wilms' tumor. Cancer 25:12, 1970.
70. Clouse JW, Thomas PRM, Griffith RC, et al.: The changing management of Wilms' tumor over a 30 year period 1949–1978. Cancer 56:1484, 1985.
71. Byrd RL, Levine AS: Late effects of treatment of Wilms' tumor. In Pochedley C, Baum ES (eds): Wilms' Tumor: Clinical and Biologic Manifestations. New York: Elsevier, 1984, pp 339–354.
72. Tefft M: Radiation related toxicities in National Wilms' Tumor Study I. Int J Radiat Oncol Biol Phys 2:455, 1977.
73. Cassady JR, Tefft M, Filler RM, et al.: Consideration of the radiation therapy of Wilms' tumor. Cancer 32:598, 1973.
74. Oliver JH, Gluck G, Gledhill RB, et al.: Musculoskeletal alterations following treatment for Wilms' tumor. J Bone Joint Surg 58:526, 1976.
75. Arneil GC, Emmanuel IG, Flatman GE: Nephritis in two children after irradiation for Wilms' tumor. Br Med J 285:996, 1982.
76. Mitus A, Tefft M, Feelers FX: Long-term follow-up of renal function of 108 children who underwent nephrectomy for malignant disease. Pediatrics 44:912, 1969.

77. Riseborough EJ, Grabias SL, Burton R, et al.: Skeletal abnormalities following the irradiation of Wilms' tumor. J Bone Joint Surg 58:526, 1976.
78. Arkin AM, Pack GT, Ranschoff NS, et al.: Radiation-induced scoliosis: A case report. J Bone Joint Surg 32:401, 1950.
79. Newhauser EDB, Kaplan HS: Growth retardation in children after megavoltage irradiation of the spine. Radiology 59:637, 1952.
80. McVeagh P, Ekart H: Hepatotoxicity of chemotherapy following nephrectomy and radiation therapy for right-sided Wilms' tumor. J Pediatr 87:627, 1975.
81. Jayabose S, Sherde A, Lanzkowsky P: Hepatotoxicity of chemotherapy following nephrectomy and radiation therapy for right-sided Wilms' tumor. J Pediatr 88:898, 1976.
82. Holcenberg JS, Kum LE, Ring BJ, et al.: Effect of hepatic irradiation of the toxicity and pharmacokinetics of adriamycin in children. Int J Radiol Oncol Biol Phys 7:953, 1981.
83. Littman P, Meadows AT, Polgar G: Pulmonary function in survivors of Wilms' tumor: Patterns of impairment. Cancer 37:2773, 1976.
84. Meadows AT, Strong LC, Li FP, et al.: Oncogenesis and other late effects of cancer treatment in children. Radiology 114:175, 1975.
85. Meadows AT, Jarrett P: Pigmented nevi, Wilms' tumor and second malignant neoplasms. J Pediatr 93:889, 1978.
86. Li FP, Cassady JR, Jaffe N: Risk of second tumors in survivors of childhood cancer. Cancer 35:1230, 1975.
87. Li FP: Second malignant tumors after cancer in children. Cancer 40:1899, 1977.
88. Schwartz AD, Lee H, Baum ES: Leukemia in children with Wilms' tumor. J Pediatr 87:374, 1975.
89. Banner MP, Bleshman MH, Novick DE: Renal cell carcinoma in a patient successfully treated for Wilms' tumor. J Roentgenol 128:77, 1977.
90. Reimer RR, Fraumeni JF, Reddick R, et al.: Breast carcinoma following radiotherapy of metastatic Wilms' tumor. Cancer 40:1450, 1977.
91. Sabio H, Teja K, Elkon D, et al.: Adenocarcinoma of the colon following the treatment of Wilms' tumor. J Pediatr 95:424, 1979.
92. Opitz JM: Adenocarcinoma of the colon following Wilms' tumor. J Pediatr 96:775, 1980.
93. Li FP: Colon cancer after Wilms' tumor. J Pediatr 96:954, 1980.

Chapter 5
Wilms' Tumor—Surgical Aspects

Thomas M. Krummel

Surgical resection remains the cornerstone of Wilms' tumor treatment and provides the information necessary for appropriate application of chemo- and radiation therapy. It is hoped that the surgical perspective in this chapter, in tandem with the medical view of Chapter 4, will provide a contemporary discussion of Wilms' tumor therapies.

HISTORICAL PERSPECTIVE

Jessop performed the first nephrectomy in a child with this tumor in 1877 [1]; Kocher reported a similar operation in 1878 [2].

A confusing plethora of pathologic terms accumulated, including fungus haematodes of the kidney embryonal sarcoma, adenomyosarcoma, mesoblastic sarcoma, congenital sarcoma of the kidney, sarcoma muscularis, until Max Wilms [3], a German surgeon, reviewed the existing literature on childhood renal tumors. He recognized common pathologic features in all of these descriptions, added seven cases of his own, and thus his name as the eponym.

Prior to the advent of adjuvant therapy, Gross and Neuhauser reviewed the results of purely operative treatment of Wilms' tumor during three "eras" at the Children's Hospital [4]. From 1914 to 1930, the survival rate was 14.9% with an operative mortality of 23%. Between 1931 and 1939, the cure rate rose to 32% and then to 47% between 1940 and 1947. No operative deaths were noted after 1932.

Pediatric Tumors of the Genitourinary Tract, pages 75–86
© 1988 Alan R. Liss, Inc.

The modern era of combined modalities began with Farber's report in 1954 [4].

PREOPERATIVE SURGICAL CONSIDERATIONS

Children with Wilms' tumor are typically well at initial presentation with a flank mass [6]. Atypical presentations of note include the occasional ruptured Wilms' tumor with evidence of peritonitis [7,8] and posttraumatic hematuria due to an occult Wilms' tumor.

Following the physical and laboratory examinations outlined in Chapter 4, a number of diagnostic x-ray studies are available. Intravenous pyelography (IVP), ultrasonography (US), or computerized tomography (CT) scan and contrast injection in the inferior vena cava (IVC) [9,10] all have some utility; on radiologic bases the surgeon must be able to identify the lesion and renal anatomy, confirm contralateral renal presence and function, screen for tumor embolus in the IVC, and document metastatic pulmonary disease.

Preoperative documentation of a Wilms' tumor in a unilateral kidney, a horseshoe kidney, or a pelvic kidney, or the existence of bilateral Wilms' tumors permits rational and orderly evaluation and treatment and obviates catastrophic blunders. Arteriography is not generally needed except if hemi-nephrectomy is contemplated [11] or rarely for angiographic embolization of large hemorrhagic tumors [12]. Should tumor embolus be identified in the IVC, additional studies including right heart catheterization [13,14] may be necessary to identify the extent of the embolus and thus extraction planned, as discussed below, since tumor embolization with subsequent cardiac arrest is well recognized [15,16]. Determination of urinary catecholamines aids in the discrimination of neuroblastoma; occasionally bone marrow examination may be helpful to exclude state IV neuroblastoma.

Following such documentation, the child is prepared for operation. Mechanical and intraluminal antibiotic bowel prep is administered as well as intravenous antibiotics; preoperative evaluation by the anesthesiologist, and provisions for postoperative care in a pediatric intensive care unit are indicated.

Preoperative errors in diagnosis will still occur. Thus, there is no substitute for intelligent intraoperative assessment with operative strategies based thereon.

GENERAL OPERATIVE TECHNIQUE

The technique of nephrectomy remains essentially unchanged from Ladd's description [17]. Following induction of general anesthesia, adequate supradiaphragmatic arterial and venous access is achieved. The involved side is elevated slightly (Fig. 5-1) and the chest and abdomen prepared as a single sterile field. The abdominal incision must provide wide transperitoneal exposure of both kidneys; a transverse, midline, or paramedian incision may be used. The specific choice is based on the surgeon's experience; despite claims to the contrary, there is no clear advantage to any of these incisions. Thoracic extension may occasionally prove necessary later but need not be incorporated prior to abdominal exploration.

Following incision, the small bowel is eviscerated, and the abdominal cavity is explored for metastases; the liver is palpated and the contralateral kidney is explored. Gerota's fascia must be incised allowing direct inspection and palpation of all surfaces with biopsy of any nodules. It would, of course, be remarkable to encounter gross lesions unrecognized from the preoperative radiologic studies but small ($\leqslant 1$ cm) lesions may exist undetected.

After exploration, preoperative strategies can be modified if necessary; curative resection remains the goal. The colon is elevated and its peritoneal reflection incised from its flexure to the pelvis (Fig. 5-2A). Involvement of the colon or mesocolon warrants en bloc resection.

Complete exposure of the IVC, the aorta and subsequent identification of all major vessels is next achieved (Fig. 5-2). Beginning in the pelvis, the ipsilateral iliac vessels are identified and traced cephalad. The gonadal vessels and ureter are identified, ligated, and divided. Dissection continues up the aorta and cava; on the left side the inferior mesenteric vein is mobilized to the right. Once the IVC is dissected and both renal veins are identified, the major arterial branches of the aorta are delineated. If preoperative studies document caval involvement or should palpation of the renal vein and IVC disclose tumor thrombus not recognized preoperatively, control of the cava above and below the renal vein is warranted to permit complete safe extraction. If intraluminal tumor is limited to the renal vein or should a right-sided bulky lesion preclude safe in continuity ligation of the vein, a side-biting vascular clamp is applied to the lateral wall of the cava, allowing a cuff resection with the renal vein. Closure with vascular suture techniques is then performed (Fig. 5-2E).

Minimal tumor thrombus in the cava can be locally extracted. If the IVC contains extensive tumor, more elaborate techniques discussed below are warranted.

The renal vein is divided following ligation and suture ligation. The arterial supply is then promptly divided to prevent renal engorgement.

Excision of the tumor is then accomplished by establishing a plane of dissection outside of Gerota's fascia inferiorly, sweeping up posteriorly to

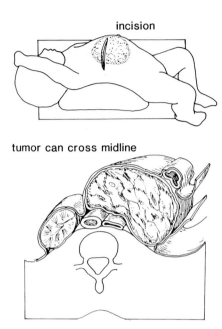

incision

tumor can cross midline

Fig. 5–1.   Generous transperitoneal incision. Transverse approach shown here. Retroperitoneal relationship to the aorta, vena cava, and contralateral kidney depicted.

the diaphragm. This is usually easy; however, care must be taken to avoid tumor rupture with attendant upstaging of the tumor. Though preoperative curative radiation and chemotherapy in the International Society of Pediatric Oncology (SIOP) have been shown to reduce the risks of tumor rupture [18], the lack of tissue diagnosis has made this approach unattractive.

The upper pole is then freed medially with careful ligation of all tumor vessels. The adrenal is commonly removed with the tumor; it may be spared in small, lower pole lesions.

Tumor locally invasive into lumbar muscles or diaphragm should be excised with a generous cuff of normal muscle. Paraaortic lymphadenectomy is clearly not therapeutic; however, excision allows histologic examination as gross inspection is notoriously inaccurate [19]. Bleeding is controlled, the National Wilms' Tumor Study (NWTS) surgical checklist completed, and the wound closed.

SPECIFIC OPERATIVE PROBLEMS
Bilateral Wilms' Tumor

At operation for bilateral disease, as for unilateral tumors, the surgeon's goal remains complete excision with adequate preservation of functional renal

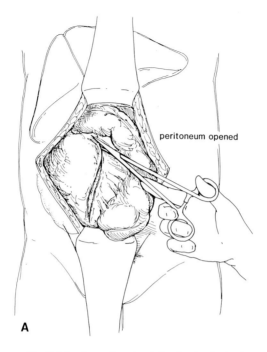

peritoneum opened

A

Fig. 5–2A. Lateral peritoneal reflection incised.

mass. When feasible, a unilateral nephrectomy of the larger tumor with excision by partial nephrectomy of the contralateral tumor has been performed [20,21]. Others have suggested unilateral nephrectomy of the larger tumor with contralateral radiation [22,23]. Such an approach is warranted only if complete excision is achieved with adequate residual kidney. Bilateral partial nephrectomies have also been employed [24]. If the surgeon's goal cannot be accomplished, then bilateral biopsy for staging is indicated. Bilateral nephrectomy followed by renal transplantation is recommended only when irradiation and chemotherapy have failed [25,26].

If resection is incomplete following chemotherapy and irradiation, a second laparotomy is planned if response is documented by CT scan. At reoperation, the priorities for resection remain unchanged.

Horseshoe Kidney

Wilms' tumor in a horseshoe kidney can present a perplexing problem [27]. However, surgical therapy is generally similar to unilateral or bilateral disease depending on tumor and fusion location [28], with resection of the involved side and the isthmus.

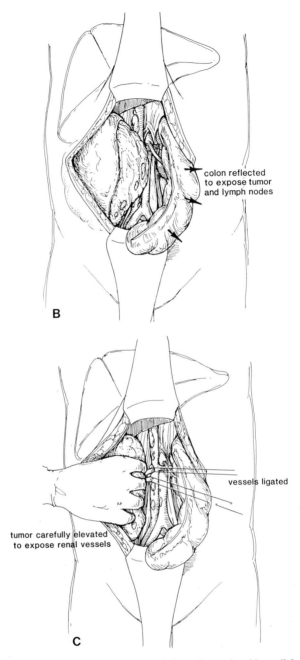

B

colon reflected
to expose tumor
and lymph nodes

vessels ligated

tumor carefully elevated
to expose renal vessels

C

Fig. 5–2B. Exposure of the aorta, vena cava, and visceral vessels with medial reflection of the colon.

Fig. 5–2C. Cephalad dissection of the vena cava completed with identification control and ligation of the renal artery and vein.

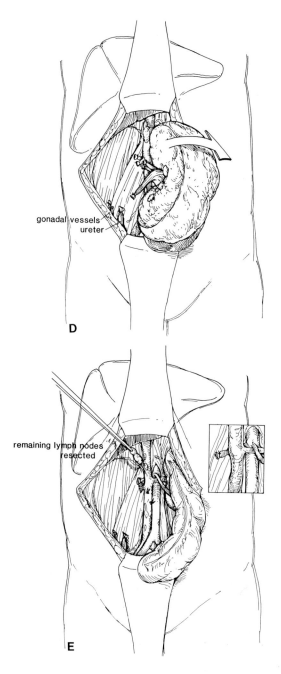

gonadal vessels
ureter

D

remaining lymph nodes
resected

E

Fig. 5–2D. Medial displacement and dissection of the posterior attachments of the kidney. Gonadal vessels and ureter divided in preliminary stages of Fig. 5.2C demonstrated.

Fig. 5–2E. Medial dissection completed after specimen resected. Inset depicts lateral closure of the vena cava which may be necessary as discussed in the text.

Extrarenal Wilms'

Tumors with Wilms' histology may rarely arise from tissue with nephrogenic potential over a wide area from the posterior mediastinum down to the inguinal region [29]. A number of such cases have been reported; wide local excision followed by chemotherapy and local irradiation is indicated.

Extensive IVC Tumor Thrombus

Though uncommon, extensive IVC tumor thrombus presents significant hazard not only as a source of hematogenous spread but also as a cause of massive, potentially life-threatening pulmonary embolus during operative manipulation [15,16]. Thus, preoperative evaluation of the cava is critical. If extensive tumor is documented on preliminary studies, right heart catheterization with angiography will document extent of involvement [13]. If documented, a midline incision from sternal notch to pubic provides the best exposure for nephrectomy and embolectomy. Using cardiopulmonary bypass support, the right atrium can be opened and tumor extracted from the atrium and IVC [13,14]. Concurrently, tumor can be extracted from the intraabdominal IVC.

Pulmonary Metastasis at Diagnosis

Children with pulmonary metastases at the time of diagnoses need not be abandoned surgically. Following the workup and documentation of location and number of pulmonary metastases by CT scan, nephrectomy is performed. Gross metastatic disease on chest radiograph probably does not require histologic diagnosis; however, a positive CT scan with a negative chest film may warrant biopsy at operation especially if the lesions are pleurally based [6]. If the ipsilateral lung is involved with a low-lying lesion, transdiaphragmatic biopsy may be feasbile. Alternatively, a separate thoracotomy incision can be employed.

Resection of Pulmonary Metastases

Present treatment of children with pulmonary metastases achieves roughly 50% survival. Persistent pulmonary metastases unresponsive to irradiation and chemotherapy and amenable to resection should be excised by lobectomy or more commonly by wedge resection [30,31].

POSTOPERATIVE CONSIDERATIONS

Convalescence following nephrectomy for Wilms' tumor is usually uncomplicated and short. Though chemotherapeutic drugs, especially adriamycin, can impair wound healing [32], wound complications are rare. Since these tumors are bulky, removal is followed by a tension-free abdominal closure.

COMPLICATIONS OF SURGICAL TREATMENT

While nephrectomy for Wilms' tumor is frequently uneventful and usually followed by an uncomplicated convalescence, the surgeon must be wary of intra- and postoperative problems and complications. Attention can then be directed to their avoidance, minimization, prompt recognition, and treatment. It is incumbent upon the operating surgeon to accurately assess tumor spread and gently remove it. Errors leading to upstaging, burden the patient with more intensive chemo- and radiation therapy and attendant risks.

Virtually all authors emphasize the following operative maneuvers to avoid catastrophic intraoperative complications: 1) secure large bore i.v. access above the diaphragm, 2) wide transperitoneal incision; and 3) relentless dissection with identification of all major intraabdominal vascular structures prior to any irreversible ligations.

Intraoperative Complications

The preoperative diagnosis will be erroneous 5% of the time [6]. This fact should be borne in mind when the operative findings are atypical. Specifically, neuroblastoma may be confused with Wilms' tumor pre-operatively and lead the unwary into exsanguinating hemorrhage. Biopsy of lymph nodes or satellite nodules with frozen section confirmation may make "second-look" laparotomy following chemotherapy less hazardous.

Intraoperative complications can be divided into three groups: hemorrhage, erroneous division of major vascular structures, and injury to adjacent viscera.

Since blood loss can be massive, provision for adequate replacement must be made prior to the fact. Preoperative involvement on the anesthesiologist, ample availability of blood and blood products, central venous access, arterial pressure monitoring, and the occasional use of the auto-transfusion apparatus are all prudent. Technical ability with vascular instruments and techniques is mandatory to safely handle caval bleeding, which can be further complicated by air embolism. For these reasons, frequent intraoperative discussions with the anesthesiologist are important. Caval bleeding from torn branches of the right adrenal gland can be avoided by ligation of all tissue during medial dissection of the upper pole in right-sided lesions.

While there is theoretic advantage in early ligation of the renal vessels, this is frequently difficult. Large tumors distort local anatomy thus making early ligation hazardous. Since virtually all major abdominal blood vessels have been erroneously ligated including the aorta and vena cava, there is no substitute for their methodic identification. As with biliary surgery, no structure should be transected prior to exhaustive delineation of the pertinent anatomy.

During exposure and manipulation of bulky Wilms' tumors, adjacent organs can be injured. The newer self-retaining retractors provide gentle, consistent, and tireless exposure, thus reducing this risk.

Urinary leak following partial nephrectomy is a well-recognized complication. Adequate drainage and bladder decompression are generally sufficient.

Chylous ascites may occur as a consequence of the dissection or lymph node dissection. To reduce the risk, ligatures rather than electrocautery are employed and ultimately prove faster. Drainage is not usually necessary; if chylous ascites accumulate, low fat feedings restricted to medium chain triglycerides [33] or bowel rest and hyperalimentation are generally therapeutic. Should proximal lymphatic obstruction due to tumor cause persistent leak, peritoneovenous shunts may be contemplated [34], though prolonged patency in small children is problematic. Reexploration should be considered as a last resort.

Postoperative Complications

Following any laparotomy, adhesive small bowel obstruction will develop in 2% of children [35]. Early postoperative bowel obstruction may be due to small bowel intussusception [36,37]; awareness of this entity is critical to prompt diagnosis. Treatment is operative reduction.

REFERENCES

1. Jessop, J: Annotations: Extirpation of the kidney. Lancet 1:889, 1877.
2. Kocher T, Longhaus T: Eine nephrotomie wegen nierensarcom, zugleich ein beitrag zur histologie desneiren krebses. Deutsche Ztschr Chir 9:312, 1878.
3. Wilms M: Die mischgeschwülste der nieren. Leipzig: Arthur Georgi, pp 1–90, 1899.
4. Gross RE, Neuhauser EBD: Treatment of mixed tumors of the kidney in childhood. Pediatrics 6:843, 1950.
5. Farber S, Toch R, Sears EM, et al.: Advances in chemotherapy of cancer in man. In Greenstein JP, Hadow A (eds): Advances in Cancer Research, vol. 4. New York: Academic Press, 1954, pp 1–71.
6. Green DM: The diagnosis and management of Wilms' tumor. Pediatr Clin North Am 32:735–754, 1985.
7. Rosenfeld M, Rodgers BM, Talbert JL: Wilms' tumor with acute abdominal pain. Arch Surg 112:1080–1082, 1977.
8. Ramsay NKC, Dehner LP, Coccia PF, et al.: Acute hemorrhage into Wilms' tumor. J Pediatr 91:763–765, 1977.

9. Slovis TL, Phillippart AI, Cushing B, et al.: Evaluation of the inferior vena cava by sonography and venography in children with renal and hepatic tumors. Radiology 140:767–772, 1981.
10. Mahboubi S, Rosenberg HK, D'Angio GJ: Should inferior venacavography be performed in the management of children with Wilms' tumor? Clin Pediatr 21:690–692, 1982.
11. Raffensperger J, Morgan ER. Renal masses. In Swenson O (ed): Swenson's Pediatric Surgery, 4th ed. New York: Appleton-Century Crofts, 1983, pp 315–332.
12. Harrison MR, deLorimer AA, Boswell WO: Postoperative angiographic embolization for large hemorrhagic Wilms' tumor. J Pediatr Surg 13:757–758, 1978.
13. Schullinger JN, Santulli TV, Casarella WJ, et al.: Wilms' tumor: The role of right heart angiography in the management of selected cases. Ann Surg 185:451–455.
14. Luck SR, DeLeon S, Shkolnik A, et al.: Intracardiac Wilms' tumor: Diagnosis and management. J Pediatr Surg 17:551–554, 1982.
15. Akyon MG, Arslan G: Pulmonary embolism during surgery for a Wilms' tumour (nephroblastoma). Br J Anaesthesiol 53:903, 1981.
16. Shurin SB, Gauderer MWL, Dahms BB, et al.: Fatal intraoperative embolization of Wilms' tumor. J Pediatr 101:559–562, 1982.
17. Ladd WE: Embryoma of the kidney (Wilms' tumor). Ann Surg 108:885, 1938.
18. Lemerle J, Vovle PA, Tournade MF, et al.: Preoperative versus postoperative radiotherapy, single versus multiple causes of actinomycin D in the treatment of Wilms' tumor. Cancer 38:647–654, 1976.
19. Donohue, JP, Einhorn LH, Williams SD: Cytoreductive surgery for metastatic testis cancer: Considerations of timing and extent. J Urol 123:818, 1980.
20. Bishop HC, Tefft M, Evans AE, et al.: Survival in bilateral Wilms' tumor—Review of 30 National Wilms' Tumor Study cases. J Pediatr Surg 12:631–638, 1977.
21. Johnson DG: Treatment of Wilms' tumor in children. World J Surg 5:5–13, 1980.
22. White JJ, Golladay ES, Kaizer H, et al.: Conservatively aggressive management with bilateral Wilms' tumors. J Pediatr Surg 11:859–865, 1976.
23. Richards MJ, Miller RC: Radical partial renal irradiation: An alternative to partial nephrectomy in bilateral Wilms' tumor. Cancer 38:2093–2098, 1976.
24. Wiener ES: Bilateral partial nephrectomies for large bilateral Wilms' tumors. J Pediatr Surg 11:867–869, 1976.
25. deLorimier AA, Belzer FO, Kountz SL, et al.: Treatment of bilateral Wilms' tumor. Am J Surg 122:275–281, 1971.
26. Ehrlich RM, Goldman R, Kauffman JJ: Surgery of bilateral Wilms' tumors: The role of renal transplantation. J Urol 111:277–281, 1974.
27. Gay BB, Dawes RK, Atkinson GO, et al.: Wilms' tumor in horseshoe kidneys: Radiologic diagnosis. Radiology 146:693, 1983.
28. Shashikumar VL, Somers LA, Pilling GP IV, et al.: Wilms' tumor in the horseshoe kidney. J Pediatr Surg 9:185–189, 1974.
29. Thompson MR, Emmanuel IG, Campbell MS, et al.: Extrarenal Wilms' tumors. J Pediatr Surg 8:37–41, 1973.
30. Lent MH, Staubitz WJ, Magoss FV, et al.: Surgical therapy of pulmonary metastases for malignancy of genitourinary organs. J Urol 84:746–752, 1960.
31. Haas L, Jackson AD: Lobectomy for pulmonary metastases. Br J Surg 48:516–518, 1961.
32. Devereaux DF, Thibault L, Boretos J, et al.: The quantitative and qualitative impairment of wound healing by adriamycin. Cancer 43:932–938, 1979.
33. Kessel I: Chylous ascites in infancy. Arch Dis Child 27:79, 1952.

34. Vasko JS, Tapper RI: The surgical significance of chylous ascites. Arch Surg 95:355, 1967.
35. Festen C: Postoperative small bowel obstruction in infants and children. Ann Surg 196:580–583, 1982.
36. Ravitch MM: Intussusception in Infants and Children. Springfield, Ill.: Charles C. Thomas, 1959.
37. Mollett DL, Balantine TVN, Grosfeld JL: Postoperative intussusception in infancy and childhood: Analysis of 119 cases. Surgery 86:402, 1979.

Chapter 6
Other Pediatric Renal Tumors

Bruce H. Broecker

Renal tumors other than Wilms' tumor occur very infrequently in children. Those that do may be either primary renal neoplasms or secondary metastatic deposits (Table 6-1).

PRIMARY RENAL TUMORS

Virtually any primary renal tumor may occur during childhood. Excluding Wilms' tumor, the most common neoplasms are mesoblastic nephroma, renal cell carcinoma, sarcoma, and angiomyolipoma.

Mesoblastic Nephroma

Mesoblastic nephroma is the most common renal tumor of the neonatal period. This tumor is discussed separately, along with nephroblastomatosis, in Chapter 3.

Renal Cell Carcinoma

Approximately 1–2% of renal carcinoma occurs in the pediatric age group [1,2]. Renal cell carcinoma is the second most common renal tumor in childhood, following Wilms' tumor. However most Wilms' tumors occur under the age of 10, and during the second decade of life these two tumors occur with equal frequency [1]. The child presents most commonly with the finding of an abdominal mass, but may have the additional findings of hematuria, flank pain, hypertension, or calcification of the mass [1–12].

Pediatric Tumors of the Genitourinary Tract, pages 87–94
© 1988 Alan R. Liss, Inc.

TABLE 6-1. Pediatric Renal Tumors

Primary	Secondary
Malignant	Malignant
Carcinoma	Leukemia
Adenocarcinoma	Lymphoma
Transitional cell carcinoma	Osteogenic sarcoma
Sarcoma	Melanoma
Nephroblastoma	
Rhabdomyosarcoma	
Leiomyosarcoma	
Liposarcoma	
Malignant fibrous histiocytoma	
Hemangioendotheliosarcoma	
Benign	
Angiomyolipoma	
Teratoma	
Oncocytoma	
Adenoma	
Hemangioma	
Hemangiopericytoma	
Lymphangioma	
Leiomyoma	
Ossifying renal tumors of infancy	
Multilocular cyst	
Juxtaglomerular cell tumor	
Malakoplakia	
Cholesteatoma	
Hygroma	

Flank pain and hematuria following minor or major blunt abdominal trauma is a common presentation. Though the age of presentation tends to be older than for children with Wilms' tumor, there is no way to distinguish renal cell carcinoma from Wilms' tumor clinically. This fact at present has little clinical relevance since both tumors are appropriately treated by nephrectomy. Most reviews of renal cell carcinoma have found little difference in their biologic behavior compared to their adult counterpart, and the most significant prognostic variable in both age groups is the stage at presentation. Management is by complete surgical removal when possible. Chemotherapy and radiotherapy unfortunately have minimal effect on this tumor in children as well as adults. The cure rate for localized disease that is completely resected is 80–100%, while for metastatic disease it is 0–20% [1,2,4,7,10]. Most recurrent disease will occur within 2 years of presentation.

Rhabdomyosarcoma

Rhabdomyosarcoma of the kidney has been reported to occur as a distinct entity in children [13,14]. However its distinction from rhabdoid and clear cell sarcoma forms of Wilms' tumor (both unfavorable histologic features) as well as the fetal rhabdomyomatous nephroblastoma (a favorable variant of Wilms' tumor) is often confusing in the literature [13–17]. The tendency of some to segregate these neoplasms from Wilms' tumor categorization is partly based on and strengthened by their distinct natural history [15,16,17]. The clear and rhabdoid sarcomas occur at younger ages and most commonly metastasize to the bone and brain, respectively, rather than lung. They respond poorly to chemotherapy and radiotherapy and carry a poor prognosis. Fetal rhabdomyomatous nephroblastoma, characterized by the presence of fetal striated muscle, also occurs in the younger age group, but has a low incidence of metastatic spread and a favorable prognosis.

Other Sarcomas

All of the forms of sarcoma have been reported to occur in the kidney although they represent less than 3% of renal malignancies and occur almost exclusively in adults. Rare cases have been reported in children, however, including leiomyosarcoma [18,19], liposarcoma [20], malignant fibrous histiocytoma [21,22], and hemangioendotheliosarcoma [23]. These represent isolated case reports, and no conclusions regarding management or prognosis can be drawn beyond those applicable in general to other soft tissue sarcomas in children.

Angiomyolipoma

Angiomyolipoma, also known as renal hamartoma, is a well-recognized renal tumor [24]. It may occur as part of the disease complex of tuberous sclerosis, an entity comprised of mental retardation, epilepsy, glial nodules in the brain, adenoma sebaceum, phakoma of the retina, and hamartomas of the liver, heart, bone or kidney; or it may occur as an isolated finding [25]. Angiomyolipomas in children are usually associated with tuberous sclerosis [26–28]. The tumor is frequently bilateral, multicentric, and large and has a propensity for significant, even life threatening, hemorrhage. Non-surgical management is almost always advocated due to the bilaterality and multicentricity though occasionally surgical resection will be required for refractory hemorrhage. A characteristic appearance on computed tomography as well as the clinical setting of tuberous sclerosis allow one to differentiate angiomyolipoma from renal cell carcinoma or other malignancies with a high degree of confidence [29].

Transitional Cell Carcinoma of the Renal Pelvis

Transitional cell carcinoma (TCCA) of the renal pelvis has been reported by several authors [30–33]. Age in the reported patients has ranged from 3 months to 15 years and as with their counterpart in the bladder (discussed in Chapter 11), they are virtually all low grade and non-invasive. Conservative surgery would seem appropriate when feasible but most will probably require nephroureterectomy for complete excision.

Multilocular Cyst

Multilocular cysts of the kidney occur in both children and adults but with a differing histologic pattern [34–37]. Grossly, the appearance in both age groups is a localized cluster of cysts within an otherwise architecturally normal kidney. It is almost always unilateral. Histologically, however, the multilocular cyst in the pediatric patient is characterized by the presence of blastema in the septae of the cyst rather than the mature fibrous tissue seen in the adult multilocular cyst. It is this blastemal element that may give rise to a Wilms' tumor and is the basis for its categorization by many as a favorable variant of Wilms' tumor. When not associated with a frank nephroblastoma, the multilocular cyst has a benign course, and local excision constitutes adequate treatment.

Miscellaneous Tumors

A wide variety of renal tumors in children have been the subject of isolated case reports in the literature. Among these are teratoma [38,39], oncocytoma [40–43], adenoma [44,45], fibroma [46], leiomyoma [47], hemangioma [48–57], hemangiopericytoma [52], lymphangioma [53,54], ossifying renal tumors of infancy [55], juxtaglomerular cell tumors [56–58], malakoplakia [59], cholesteatoma [60], and hygroma [61]. In most cases these can be distinguished from the more common tumors only after excision and histologic examination.

SECONDARY RENAL TUMORS

Both leukemia and non-Hodgkin's lymphoma may involve the kidneys as metastatic deposits [62–71]. Appropriate therapy for this situation is chemotherapy and/or radiotherapy rather than surgical removal.

Osteogenic sarcoma has also been reported to metastasize to the kidney [72,73] in children, as has malignant melanoma [74].

REFERENCES

Renal Cell Carcinoma
1. Hartman DS, Davis CJ, Madewe JE, et al.: Primary malignant renal tumors in the second decade of life: Wilms tumor versus renal cell carcinoma. J Urol 127:888–891, 1982.

2. Raney RB, Palmer N, Sutow WW, et al.: Renal cell carcinoma in children. Med Pediatr Oncol 11:91–98, 1983.

3. Birken G, King D, Vane D, et al.: Renal cell carcinoma arising in a multicystic dysplastic kidney. J Pediatr Surg 20:619–621, 1985.

4. Lack EE, Cassady JR, Sallan SE: Renal cell carcinoma in childhood and adolescence: A clinical and pathologic study of 17 cases. J Urol 133:882–888, 1985.

5. Rahima M, Barzilay J, Yanai-Inbar I, et al.: Adenocarcinoma of kidney in seven-year-old child. Eight year follow up. Urology 24:182–184, 1984.

6. Chan HS, Daneman A, Gribbin M, et al.: Renal cell carcinoma in the first two decades of life. Pediatr Radiol 13:324–328, 1983.

7. Herschorn S, Hardy BE, Churchill BM: Renal cell carcinoma in children. Can J Surg 22:412–418, 1979.

8. Abrams HJ, Buchbinder ME, Sutton AP: Renal carcinoma in adolescents. J Urol 12:92–94, 1979.

9. Amarjit S, Singh A, Sehgal RK, et al.: Bilateral hypernephroma in a child. J Urol 118:323–234, 1977.

10. Hicks CC, Obrien DP, Majmudar B, et al.: Hypernephroma in children. Urology 6:598–602, 1975.

11. Pochedly L, Suwansirikul S, Penzer P: Renal cell carcinoma with extrarenal manifestations in a 10 month old child. Am J Dis Child 12:528–530, 1971.

12. Kogayashi A, Hoshini H, Onbe Y, et al.: Bilateral renal cell carcinoma. Arch Dis Child 45:141–143, 1970.

Sarcoma

13. Lifschultz BD, Gonzalez-Crussi F, Kidd JM: Renal rhabdomyosarcoma of childhood. J Urol 127:309–310, 1982.

14. Harbaugh JT: Boytryoid sarcoma of the renal pelvis; a case report. J Urol 100:424–426, 1968.

15. Schmidt D, Harms D, Evers KG, et al.: Bone metastasizing renal tumor (clear cell sarcoma) of childhood with epitheliod elements. Cancer 56:609–613, 1985.

16. Suzuki H, Honzumi M, Itoh Y, et al.: Clear cell sarcoma of the kidney seen in a 3 day old newborn. Z Kinderchir 38:422–424, 1983.

17. Wigger HJ: Fetal rhabdomyomatous nephroblastoma—a variant of Wilms tumor. Hum Pathol 7:613, 1976.

18. Blende YM: Plain muscle tumors of the kidney. Indian J Med Sci 6:747–754, 1952.

19. Shen SC, Yunis EJ: Leiomyosarcoma developing in a child during remission of leukemia. J Pediatr 89:780–782, 1976.

20. Itzchak Y, Adar R, Morag B, et al.: Liposarcoma of the renal capsule in a 7 year old girl. Pediatr Radiol 13:182–183, 1975.

21. Burgener FA, Lundman S: Angiographic features of malignant fibrous histiocytoma. Radiology 121:581–583, 1976.

22. Habib W, Gislason GJ: Malignant histiocystic tumor of the kidney. J Urol 94:208, 1965.

23. Dutt AK: Hemangioendotheliosarcoma. Med J Maylaysia, 24:161–163, 1969.

Angiomyolipoma

24. Pode D, Meretik S, Shapiro A, et al.: Diagnosis and management of renal angiomyolipoma. Urology 25:461–467, 1985.

25. Scott MD, Halpern M, Cosgrove MD: Renal angiomyolipoma; Two varieties. Urology 6:768–773, 1975.

26. Bernie JE: Renal angiomyoliphoma in an adolescent: A case report. J Urol 109:492–494, 1973.
27. Mazeman E, Wemeau L, Biserte J, et al.: Renal angiomyolipoma. A report of 11 cases. Eur Urol 6:328–334, 1980.
28. Bret PM, Bretagnolle M, Gaillard D, et al.: Small, asymptomatic angiomyolipomas of the kidney. Radiology 154:7–10, 1985.
29. Sant GR, Heaney JA, Ucci AA, et al.: Computed tomographic findings in renal angiomyolipoma: An histologic correlation. Urology 24:293–296, 1984.

TCCA

30. Karmi S, Averill R, Young JD: Malignant urothelial tumors in childhood. Urology 21:178–180, 1983.
31. Vinocur C, Hitzig G, Marboe C, et al.: Renal pelvic tumors in childhood. Urology 16:393–395, 1980.
32. Koyanagi T, Saski K, Arikado K, et al.: Transitional cell carcinoma of renal pelvis in an infant. J Urol 113:114–117, 1975.
33. Melzer M, Braf Z, Beyar H, et al.: Primary tumors of the renal pelvis and ureter. Int Surg 57:699–702, 1972.

Multilocular Cyst

34. Garrick DJ, Gilbert EF, Beckwith JB, et al.: Congenital cystic mesoblastic nephroma. Hum Pathol 12:1039, 1984.
35. Banner MP, Pollack HM,, Chetten J, et al.: Multilocular renal cysts: Radiologic pathologic correlation. AJR 136:239, 1981.
36. Cho KJ, Thorbury JR, Bernstein J, et al.: Localized cystic disease of the kidney; angiographic pathologic correlation. AJR 132:891, 1979.
37. Coleman M: Multilocular renal cyst. Case report. Ultrastructure and review of the literature. Virchows Arch [A] 387:207, 1980.

Teratoma

38. Ranadive NU, Vaze AM, Deodhar KP, et al.: Primary intrarenal teratoma. A case report. Indian J Cancer 20:295–298, 1984.
39. Dische MR, Johnston R: Teratoma in a horseshoe kidney. Urology 13:435–438, 1979.

Oncocytoma

40. Suherman S, Van-Biervliet JP, Maurus C, et al.: Multiple renal oncocytoma and bilateral cystic kidney. Eur J Pediatr 144:406–409, 1985.
41. Behori R, Green JA, Maharaj R, et al.: Renal oncocytoma. A report of 3 cases. S Afr Med J 67:182–183, 1985.
42. van der Walt JD, Reid HA, Risdon RA, et al.: Renal oncocytoma. A review of the literature and a report of an unusual multicentric case. Virchows Arch 398:291–304, 1983.
43. Pearse HD, Houghton DC: Renal oncocytoma. Urology 13:74–77, 1979.

Adenoma

44. Pfannkuch F, Leistenschnieder W, Nagel R: Problems of assessment in the surgery of renal adenomas. J Urol 125:95–98, 1981.
45. Acharya GV, Chaphekar PM: Benign renal adenoma. A case report of benign adenoma in a child of 2 years. J Postgrad Med 13:125–127, 1967.

Fibroma

46. Hamanaka Y, Okamoto E, Ueda T: Fibroma of the kidney in the newborn. J Pediatr Surg 4:250–255, 1969.

Leiomyoma

47. Fisher KS, van Blerk PJ: Childhood leiomyoma of kidney. Urology 21:74–75, 1983.

Hemangioma

48. Weiner SN, Weiss R, Gauthier B, et al.: Intrarenal hemangioma in the Klippel-Trenaunay syndrome. Urol Radiol 7:48–50, 1985.

49. Mitchell A, Fellows GJ, Smith JC: Partial nephrectomy for renal hemangioma. JR Soc Med 75:766–767, 1982.

50. Samellas W, Morphis LG, Bakopoulos CV: Hemangioma of the kidney. J Urol 116:653, 1976.

51. Summers JL, Keitzer WA: A radiographic clue to the diagnosis of hemangioma of the kidney. J Urol 108:852–853, 1972.

Hemangiopericytoma

52. Lee MR: Renin secreting renal tumors: A rare but remedial cause of serious hypertension. Lancet 2:254, 1971.

Lymphangioma

53. Pickering SP, Fletcher BD, Bryan PJ, et al.: Renal lymphangioma: A cause of neonatal nephromegaly. Pediatr Radiol 14:445–448,1984.

54. Higgins TT, Williams DI, Nash DFE: The urology of childhood. London: Butterworth & Co., 1951.

Ossifying Renal Tumor of Infancy

55. Jerkins GR, Callihan TR: Ossifying renal tumor at infancy. J Urol 135:120–121, 1986.

Juxtaglomerular Cell Tumor

56. Dennis RL, McDougal WS, Glick AD, et al.: Juxtaglomerular cell tumor of the kidney. J Urol 134:334–338, 1985.

57. Squires JP, Ulbright TM, DeSchryver-Kecskemeti K, et al.: Juxtaglomerular cell tumor of the kidney. Cancer 53:516–523, 1984.

58. Conner G, Bennett CM, Lindstrom RR, et al.: Juxtaglomerular cell tumor. Nephron 21:325–333, 1978.

Malakoplakia

59. Trillo A, Lorentz WB, Whilley NO: Malakoplakia of kidney simulating renal neoplasm. Urology 10:472–477, 1977.

Cholesteatoma

60. Ross RR, Lewis HY, Brough AJ: Renal cholesteatoma in a child. J Urol 104:184–188, 1970.

Hygroma

61. Gopal G: A case report of hygroma kidney. Indian Pediatr 113:57–58, 1976.

Metastatic Renal Tumors

62. Patil PS: Renal failure in a Zambian child due to bilateral renal lymphoma. Med J Zambia 18:19–20, 1984.

63. Kumari-Subaiya, S, Lee WJ, Festa R, et al.: Sonographic findings in leukemic renal disease. JCU 12:465–472, 1984.

64. Jafri SZ, Amendola MA, Brady TM, et al.: Angiographic patterns of involvement in renal and perirenal lymphoma. Urol Radiol 6:14–19, 1984.

65. Araki T: Leukemic involvement of the kidney in children: CT features. J Comput Assist Tomogr 6:781–784, 1982.

66. Hartman DS, David CJ, Goldman SM, et al.: Renal lymphoma: Radiologic-pathologic correlation in 21 cases. Radiology 144:759–766, 1982.

67. Falappa P, Trodella L, Maresca G: Lymphomatous involvement of the kidneys: Computed tomography and ultrasound demonstration. Diagn Imaging 49:266–288, 1980.

68. Kushner DC, Weinstein HJ, Kirkpatrick JA: The radiographic diagnosis of leukemia and lymphoma in children. Semin Roentgenol 15:316–334, 1980.

69. Tisnado J, Amendola MA, Beachley MC, et al.: Renal lymphoma, angiographic findings in a child. Rev Interam Radiol 5:55–58, 1980.

70. Goh TS, LeQuesne GW, Wong KY: Severe infiltration of the kidneys with ultrasonic abnormalities in acute lymphoblastic leukemia. Am J Dis Child 132:1204–1205, 1978.

71. Kanfer A, Vandewalle A, Morel-Maroger L, et al.: Acute renal insufficiency due to lymphomatous infiltration of the kidneys: Report of six cases. Cancer 38:2588–2592, 1976.

72. Ayres C, Curry NS, Gordon L, et al.: Renal metastases from osteogenic sarcoma. Urol Radiol 7:39–41, 1985.

73. Gilbert LA, Weiss MA, Gelfand MJ, et al.: Detection of renal metastases of osteosarcoma by bone scan. Clin Nucl Med 8:325–326, 1983.

74. Goldstein HH, Kaninsky S, Wallace S, et al.; Urographic manifestations of metastatic melanoma. Am J Roentgenol Radium Ther Nucl Med 12:801–805, 1974.

Chapter 7
Neuroblastoma

James P. Neifeld

Neuroblastoma is the most common extracranial malignant solid tumor in infancy and childhood. It accounts for as many as 14% of childhood malignancies and as many as 50% of neonatal malignancies. Most patients have metastatic disease at the time of initial diagnosis and, in contrast to the advances made in the management of most childhood cancers, the prognosis for neuroblastoma has remained poor.

Neuroblastoma was first described in the adrenal gland in 1864 by Virchow [1]. During the ensuing 40 years, other case reports described similar tumors. In 1910, Wright demonstrated that neuroblastomas originate from embryonal sympathetic neuroblasts and thus may occur in sympathetic nervous system tissue in any area of the body [2]. The most common site of origin of neuroblastoma, however, remains the adrenal gland (Fig. 7-1) with about 40% of neuroblastomas arising within the adrenal gland, about 25% elsewhere in the abdomen, about one-seventh arising within the chest, and smaller percentages elsewhere in the body [3–5]. Because two-thirds of all children with neuroblastoma have metastatic disease at the time of diagnosis, neuroblastoma remains a significant problem in terms of early diagnosis and treatment.

Neuroblastoma is the most undifferentiated of a spectrum of tumors that includes ganglioneuroblastoma and ganglioneuroma. Ganglioneuroblastoma is a term describing a transitional tumor of sympathetic cell origin that contains both malignant neuroblasts and benign ganglioneuromatous elements [6]. It is thought to represent a maturing tumor which contains ganglion cells, and it has a better prognosis than does neuroblastoma. It is more commonly

Pediatric Tumors of the Genitourinary Tract, pages 95–112

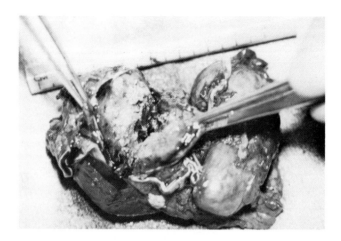

Fig. 7-1. Neuroblastoma arising in the left adrenal gland. Tumor invaded the renal hilum requiring concomitant nephrectomy. Necrotic, hemorrhagic cut interior is visualized.

located in the posterior mediastinum than is neuroblastoma [7], and many patients are asymptomatic, the mass being detected on a chest x-ray performed for other reasons. Clinical presentations may include the presence of an abdominal mass, respiratory symptoms (for mediastinal ganglioneuroblastomas), paraplegia, hypertension, and chronic diarrhea [8,9]. A great majority of these tumors are localized at diagnosis and can be totally resected (Fig. 7-2), following which recurrence is extremely rare. In contrast to neuroblastoma, few patients with ganglioneuroblastoma present with disseminated tumor [7,8]. Those that do will have a clinical course identical to that of neuroblastoma.

Ganglioneuroma represents the differentiated form of neuroblastoma. Ganglioneuromas usually appear much later in life than neuroblastomas and are frequently detected in adolescents or adults [3]. About one-third arise from the thoracic and cervical sympathetic chains, one-third from the adrenals, and one-third from the abdominal and pelvic sympathetic chains (Fig. 7-3). Clinical presentation varies from an asymptomatic mass to neurologic symptoms and even hypertension or diarrhea. Ganglioneuromas are benign tumors that do not metastasize. They are slow-growing and, therefore, may become quite large prior to detection. They are thought to represent the differentiated cell following treatment of neuroblastoma; several infants with a diagnosis of neuroblastoma have later been found to have ganglioneuroma at the site of the previous neuroblastoma, suggesting that maturation is the ultimate fate of

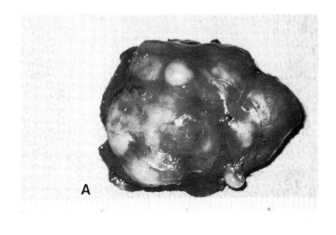

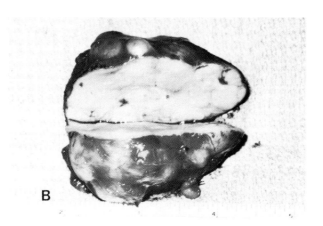

Fig. 7-2. A: Ganglioneuroblastoma of left infrarenal area. **B:** Cut surface is relatively smooth, homogeneous, and does not display the irregularities of neuroblastoma (Fig. 7-1).

some neuroblastomas [3]. Treatment of ganglioneuromas is resection whenever possible, but some tumors may be adherent to vital structures such as the aorta, vena cava, or major nerve trunks, thus precluding safe resection. Nevertheless, partial resection of such tumors will usually result in cure.

EPIDEMIOLOGY

The incidence of neuroblastoma is about one in every 10,000 live births. In newborns dying of other causes, however, the occurrence of small foci of

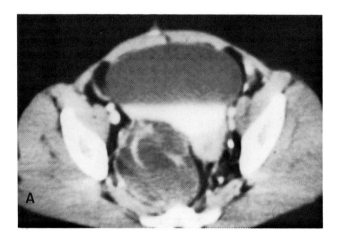

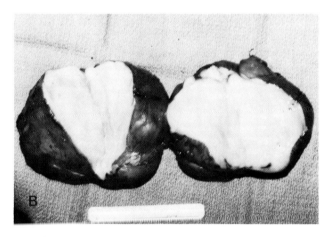

Fig. 7-3. Ganglioneuroma of pelvic sympathetic drain. **A:** Computed tomographic scan shows smooth-walled mass displacing bladder and rectum. **B:** Smooth, regular mass with fatty-like interior architecture.

cells within the adrenal gland that appear identical to neuroblasts is more common, with an average incidence of about one out of 250. Thus, most of these tumors must either disappear, mature, or convert to other forms with increasing age of the child. This may, in part, account for the improved prognosis of neuroblastoma detected in children under the age of 1 year compared to the prognosis of children diagnosed and treated at a later age [10–13].

Although familial neuroblastomas have been reported, it is generally not thought to be hereditary. Other neural crest abnormalities, such as neurofibromatosis [14] and pheochromocytoma, have not been associated with an increased incidence of neuroblastoma development. Therefore, most neuroblastomas probably arise from a mutation of an autosomal dominant gene rather than inherited or environmental factors.

DIAGNOSIS—SIGNS AND SYMPTOMS

The presenting complaints of the patient with neuroblastoma depend on the site of the primary tumor and the extent of dissemination of the tumor. Children with localized disease, which would be unusual for abdominal primary sites, are frequently asymptomatic and have a mass detected either on physical examination (for abdominal primary sites) or on a chest x-ray (for thoracic primary sites). Large tumors may become evident due to symptoms caused by the mass itself; for example, large abdominal tumors may become evident due to early satiety, change in bowel habits, or an increasing abdominal girth. Most abdominal tumors, however, tend to remain asymptomatic until metastatic disease brings the child to the attention of the physician.

Presenting symptoms in children with metastatic neuroblastoma are usually due to the site of metastasis. Proptosis and/or periorbital ecchymosis may be due to metastatic disease to the orbit. Metastases to the long bones may result in disuse of the extremity with subsequent wasting. Cord compression with subsequent weakness of the lower extremities may be due to extradural extension of the tumor or extradural metastasis [15]. Systemic manifestations of neuroblastoma, usually associated with metastatic disease, include weight loss, irritability, and chronic diarrhea. Paraneoplastic syndromes, which are common in other neural crest tumors that produce catecholamines such as pheochromocytoma, are rare in children with neuroblastoma. Accordingly, hypertension is not commonly seen.

STAGING

Proper staging of neuroblastoma depends on evaluation of the extent of the tumor. When neuroblastoma is suspected, documentation of metastatic sites and tumor histology are mandatory prior to treatment.

Laboratory studies should include examination of the peripheral blood, which may document unsuspected anemia or thrombocytopenia due to marrow involvement or platelet trapping. In addition, massive liver replacement may result in the development of coagulopathies. The level of urinary catecholamines or vanillylmandelic acid is elevated in about 80% of patients (although the presence of hypertension is rare) [16]. Bone marrow aspiration and biopsy should be performed in all patients to search for occult metastases.

Diagnostic imaging tests should include a bone scan to determine bony metastases. The most important imaging test is related to imaging of the primary tumor; sonography and computed tomographic (CT) scanning of the primary tumor will show relationships between the tumor, kidney, and adjacent inferior vena cava or aorta in the case of abdominal tumors. In addition, this is useful in imaging the liver and in detecting lymph node metastases. Previously, when intravenous pyelography was the only abdominal imaging test utilized, many patients were explored and found unresectable due to extension across the midline or massive liver disease. The use of CT scanning in these patients may prevent an unnecessary operation and suggest the need for preoperative chemotherapy to reduce tumor bulk, which can facilitate resection of the tumor at a later time.

Several staging systems have been developed for patients with neuroblastoma. They have been formulated by retrospectively reviewing groups of patients with neuroblastoma and correlating their prognosis with the extent of tumor.

The most commonly used staging system is that reported by Evans et al. (Table 7-1) [17]. An interesting group of patients, those in Stage IV-S, represent a special category of Stage IV patients with localized primary tumors and disseminated disease limited to liver, skin, and/or bone marrow. They have an excellent prognosis, with a 3-year survival of about 90% as compared to the usual survival for other Stage IV patients of about 20%.

Other staging systems have also been devised. Although the Pediatric Oncology Group (Table 7-1) and St. Jude Children's Research Hospital (Table 7-1) systems have some similarities to that of Evans et al., they do not consider the IV-S subset separately. The St. Jude system further subdivides patients with disseminated tumor according to bone and/or bone marrow involvement. Thus, it is important to document the staging system utilized as well as the specific sites of metastatic tumor to allow for comparison of results among the various protocols and staging systems.

TREATMENT

Surgery

The guidelines for surgery for neuroblastoma depend on the site of the primary tumor. The basic principle is to totally resect the primary tumor if

TABLE 7-1. Staging Systems for Neuroblastoma

Evans et al. [17]	Pediatric Oncology Group	St. Jude
Stage I: Tumor confined to organ or structure of origin	Stage A: Complete gross resection; intracavitary nodes free of tumor; adherent nodes may be positive	Stage I: Localized tumor, completely resected
Stage II: Tumor extending beyond site of origin, not crossing modline	Stage B: Grossly unresected primary tumor; nodes and liver negative	Stage IIA: Tumor grossly resected; microscopic tumor invasion through capsule
Stage III: Tumor extending beyond midline; nodes may be involved	Stage C: Intracavitary nodes (not adhered to tumor) positive	Stage IIB: Localized, unresectable or partially resectable
Stage IV: Distant metastases to skeleton, bone marrow, soft tissue, etc.	Stage D: Dissemination beyond intracavitary nodes	Stage IIIA: Disseminated tumor but no bone or bone marrow involvement
Stage IV-S: Patients who would be stage I or II but have distant disease confined to liver, skin, or bone marrow		Stage IIIB: Disseminated tumor with one localized bone lesion, but no bone marrow involvement
		Stage IIIC: Disseminated tumor with bone marrow and/or generalized bone involvement

this can be accomplished without removal or permanent damage to any vital structures. If the tumor is resectable, regional lymph nodes should be sampled due to the high incidence of nodal metastases and the important prognostic role these play for the patient. If the tumor is unresectable or there is disseminated disease, a biopsy of the most accessible site from which a diagnosis can be established should be performed and the operation is then terminated.

Thoracic primary tumors are usually located in the posterior mediastinum and may be densely adherent to vertebral bodies [7,8]. If there is any question concerning the mass being in communication with the spinal cord or the dura, a CT scan or myelogram should be performed prior to surgery. This will provide the surgeon with important negative information; if the mass is thought to be a neuroblastoma or ganglioneuroblastoma, the normal spinal cord information will enable one to resect this tumor with confidence that the dural sac and the cord itself will not be injured. Tumors located in the chest will often require sharp dissection to separate the tumor from the spine, but, as long as the bone itself is not involved, this task can be safely performed.

Primary cervical neuroblastomas, although exceedingly rare, may be difficult to totally extirpate with clear margins due to their proximity to important structures [18]. The carotid artery and vagus nerve may be adjacent to or involved by tumor, and thus, removal of all gross tumor with preservation of the neurovascular structures (even leaving tumor cells on these structures), though difficult to advocate for many other tumors, seems reasonable for these patients. Postoperative radiotherapy has been successful in controlling local disease for many patients with this tumor and the long-term, disease-free survival is excellent.

Most neuroblastomas arise within the abdomen, either in an adrenal gland or along a sympathetic chain [19,20]. Abdominal neuroblastomas are often quite advanced when first detected [20] and may be associated with massive lymphadenopathy. Excision of tumors in the adrenal gland will usually require a concomitant nephrectomy in order to remove all gross tumor. Occasional patients may have a segment of bowel adherent to tumor, which should also be resected in order to remove all gross tumor. Accordingly, these patients should be on a bowel prep prior to operation. When the tumor is resectable, lymph nodes in the area of the tumor should be dissected and sent for pathology [21] and, if it is a pelvic primary site, paraaortic lymph nodes at the level of the renal vessels and inferiorly to the aortic bifurcation should also be dissected and sent for pathology. A liver biopsy is generally advocated to assess the liver histologically.

Most patients do not have Stage I or II tumors at initial diagnosis. They may be found to have metastatic disease or locally inoperable disease either prior to surgery or during exploration. After a biopsy has established the diagnosis, the patient should then be closed and receive other therapy [22,23]. This will usually be chemotherapy alone. After induction chemotherapy has been administered, the patient should be restaged with whatever diagnostic modalities were abnormal to begin with and, if the patient was initially locally unresectable, with a CT scan. If the tumor is significantly smaller and no metastases are present, resection of all residual tumor is then a viable option (Fig. 7-4). Even if the patient appears to have had a complete response to chemotherapy, surgery will often document residual microscopic tumor [24]. The same principles of surgery apply as described previously; every attempt should be made to excise all of the residual primary tumor, but en bloc excision of vital organs is generally not advocated. Lymph nodes and liver should be assessed when appropriate.

Complications related to the removal of neuroblastomas are related to the site of the primary tumor and the operation required to remove the tumor

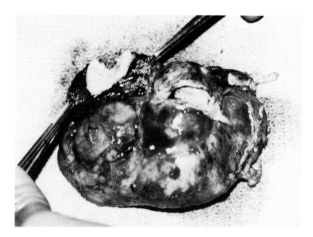

Fig. 7-4. Neuroblastoma following chemotherapy. The cut surface is necrotic.

[25]. Hemorrhage is common if the tumor cannot be totally excised. For those tumors that are totally removed, vascular complications are those that are the most immediately life-threatening to the patient. Tumors that extend across the midline or displace other structures may make identification of the normal anatomy difficult; therefore, protection of vital structures may be challenging. Injuries to the contralateral renal artery, inferior vena cava, celiac artery, or aorta must be repaired using the appropriate vascular techniques. Splenic lacerations may occur during resection of left adrenal neuroblastomas. Whenever possible, the spleen should be salvaged by splenorrhaphy, but there are occasions when splenectomy may be necessary. In that event, pneumovax vaccine must be administered as the patient will be at increased risk of sepsis. The key to prevention of these injuries is careful dissection around the tumor, delineation of proximal and distal areas of normal tissue, then slowly working toward the area where the tumor is most adherent to vital structures. When the aorta or vena cava is involved by tumor, the operation should be terminated and chemotherapy administered. Thus, the principle of "not cutting any bridges" should allow for safe dissection of these tumors.

Radiation Therapy

Radiation therapy was formally an integral modality in the management of neuroblastoma, but more recently it has been used with less frequency. The decreased use of radiation therapy relates to the tolerance of normal tissues in the irradiated area, and severe long-term complications that may become evident after radiotherapy is administered to young children. Marked vertebral body deformities with resultant scoliosis may be caused by radiotherapy given to the paraspinal areas, even with attempted shielding or by rotating the fields. In general, the younger the child, the less the dose of radiation that can be administered. Radiation is used to try to sterilize areas of microscopic residual tumor, as following partial resection of cervical primary tumors. Patients with Stage I or II neuroblastoma generally are not considered candidates for radiotherapy, but children with more advanced disease might be considered candidates if they have localized areas of symptomatic disease. Thus, in these patients, radiotherapy is administered with palliative intent.

Chemotherapy

Although chemotherapy of metastatic neuroblastoma induces a high percentage of complete and partial responses, as yet it has done little to increase the cure rate. Chemotherapy is usually administered in a high dose, intermittent fashion using combinations of drugs. The most effective drugs are cyclophosphamide, dimethyl triazeno imidazole carboxamide (DTIC), vincristine, doxorubicin, daunomycin, VM-26, and cis-platinum.

Various chemotherapy regimens have been attempted with little difference noted in terms of overall survival among patients with disseminated tumor. The Pediatric Oncology Group has used a combination of vincristine, cyclophosphamide, doxorubicin, and cis-platinum [26]. Among 42 previously untreated patients, there were six complete and 18 partial responses (57%). The response durations were very short as only 12% were still responding at 6 months; overall survival was 71% at 6 months but only 45% at 12 months. Even with these poor results, 40 of 42 patients had at least one toxic side effect.

Other investigators have sequentially administered various chemotherapeutic agents to use tumor cell kinetics in an attempt to increase the number of patients experiencing a complete response. One study, reported from the United Kingdom [27], administered vincristine, cyclophosphamide, and sequentially timed cis-platinum and VM-26 (with or without doxorubicin) to 42 patients. Although a response rate of about 75% was reported, the study was marred for several reasons: several Stage II patients, who are known to have a better prognosis, were included; several patients were excluded from survival analysis because they did not adhere to protocol; and exact response criteria were not defined. Nevertheless, the median survival (16 months) suggested the possible value of an approach based on cellular kinetics.

A study reported from the St. Jude Children's Research Hospital described the sequential administration of cyclophosphamide and doxorubicin to 70 patients with disseminated neuroblastoma [23]. Among 68 evaluable patients there were 35 complete and 13 partial responses. The median survivals were 22 months for the complete responders, 14.4 months for the partial responders, and 8.4 months for the non-responders. Thus, the approach of using sequentially administered drugs based on tumor cell kinetics may increase the number of complete responders and improve the length of response durations.

A recent approach to patients with previously treated metastatic neuroblastoma has been the use of supralethal chemotherapy, radiation, and allogeneic or autologous bone marrow reconstitution [28,29]. August et al. used a combination of local irradiation, VM-26, doxorubicin, melphalan, and 1,000 rad total-body irradiation in three fractions. Although three (of ten) patients died in the posttransplant period of fungal infections, four remained in complete clinical remission from 22 to 54 months following marrow transplantation. The morbidity and mortality of this treatment may limit its usefulness [29], and further studies aimed at decreasing the morbidity and increasing the complete response rate, possibly with different combinations of drugs, are necessary before this treatment becomes more widespread.

Although the use of autologous bone marrow is attractive to consider, in many patients the neuroblastoma has already metastasized to the marrow. A possible approach to this problem may be the treatment of a patient's own marrow with monoclonal antibodies directed against the neuroblastoma cell; marrow could be removed, purged of the neuroblastoma cells, and then infused after ablation as described above. This approach has been shown to be feasible in a laboratory setting [30], but clinical trials have not yet been reported.

Another new approach toward the treatment of disseminated neuroblastoma involves the utilization of drugs specifically directed toward inhibition of the catecholamine biosynthetic pathway. The C-1300 murine neuroblastoma, a spontaneously occurring neurogenic tumor in albino A/J mice, exhibits highly reproducible basic growth characteristics and demonstrates biologic behavior similar to that occurring in human neuroblastoma. The C-1300 murine neuroblastoma contains the catecholamine biosynthetic pathway, and dopamine antagonists such as domperidone, pimozide, and spiroperidol have been shown to inhibit macromolecular synthesis in vitro in a dose-response fashion [31]. Furthermore, when the tumor is transplanted into mice, the administration of dopamine antagonists has been demonstrated to prolong disease-free survival when drug administration is begun at the same time as tumor inoculation. Control (untreated) mice had a statistically significant decrease in the time until tumor appearance when compared to treated mice, and treated mice also demonstrated a statistically significant increase in overall survival. These data appear to correlate with the presence of specific membrane-bound dopamine binding activity ("receptor") present on the cell surface of this tumor. Investigations using human neuroblastoma grown in long-term tissue culture also demonstrated a dose-response inhibition of macromolecular precursor incorporation in vitro by the same dopamine antagonists [32]. After inoculation of human neuroblastoma into nude mice, administration of the dopamine antagonist domperidone improved survival when compared to concomitantly inoculated control mice. Dopamine binding activity was present on the cell surface of five of eight human neuroblastoma solid tumors, thereby suggesting the possibility that the presence of this dopamine binding activity might correlate with response to dopamine antagonists.

Additional evidence that human neuroblastoma may be sensitive to drugs that have an effect on the catecholamine biosynthetic pathway has been suggested in other studies. Neurotransmitter-synthesizing enzymes, including tyrosine hydroxylase and choline acetyltransferase, have been demonstrated in some human neuroblastomas [33]. In addition, 6-hydroxydopamine has been shown to be toxic to human neuroblastomas [34] and has also been used to purge bone marrow of neuroblastoma cells [35]. Thus, these data suggest the intriguing possibility that neuroblastomas may be sensitive in vivo to drugs with a direct effect on the catecholamine biosynthetic pathway. Possible future applications might include the in vivo administration of dopamine antagonists to patients with metastatic neuroblastoma, either alone or in combination with cytotoxic chemotherapy. In addition, patients with advanced disease might be candidates for bone marrow harvesting, purging of the marrow with drugs toxic to neuroblastoma cells concomitant with administration of aggressive chemotherapy to the patient, and then autologous marrow reinfusion. Finally, due to the above-mentioned maturation of neuroblastoma to ganglioneuroblastoma and ganglioneuroma that has been suggested in infants and fetal autopsies, it may be possible to administer a maturing agent to patients with neuroblastoma and thus cause the tumor to mature and differentiate to a non-life-threatening form. Investigations are underway, but data are not yet available concerning the possibility of these approaches in children with neuroblastoma.

The failure of surgery alone or with postoperative radiation therapy to cure all patients with apparently localized neuroblastoma has led to the concept that some patients have occult metastases at initial diagnosis and, accordingly, should be treated with systemic therapy. The Children's Cancer Study Group randomized patients with potentially curable neuroblastoma to either cyclophosphamide or observation alone following surgical resection (to which radiation therapy could be added at the discretion of the investigator) [36]. There was no difference in relapse rate for the entire group of patients or according to tumor stage at initial diagnosis. This study, therefore, suggested no benefit of adjuvant cyclophosphamide alone in patients with localized neuroblastoma.

PROGNOSTIC FACTORS

The natural history of neuroblastoma is complex due to the marked variation among individual patients. As alluded to above, patients with neuroblastoma whose tumor is localized (Stages I or II) and totally resected rarely have either local or distant recurrence of tumor. For patients with more advanced disease, the distribution of metastatic disease includes the central nervous system (CNS) (about 50% of patients eventually develop CNS metastases) [37]. Other common sites of metastatic disease include head, neck, liver, pancreas, lymph nodes, bone, lungs, and genitalia. Late recurrence (after 2 years) is uncommon, but patients have been reported to develop metastatic disease more than 15 years after initial treatment [38,39].

Several clinical and laboratory parameters have been demonstrated to be prognostically important for patients with neuroblastoma (Table 7-2). The most important factor is stages. Patients with Stage I or II neuroblastoma have an excellent prognosis; Stage I is not significantly different from Stage II, and patients with such tumors can be expected to be cured in over 90% of cases. The survival with Stage IV neuroblastoma, however, is poor, with only about 20% of patients alive at 3 years. Patients with Stage III neuroblastoma have an intermediate prognosis, with just over half the patients alive 3 years following initial diagnosis. These data suggest, therefore, that patients whose tumors can be removed leaving no macroscopic or microscopic residual will have a much better prognosis than those patients whose tumors are not totally excised.

A second important prognostic factor is patient age. Children who are diagnosed prior to the age of 1 year have a much better prognosis than

TABLE 7-2. Neuroblastoma Prognostic Factors

	Favorable	Unfavorable
Stage	Low (I or II)	High (IV)
Age at diagnosis	< 1	> 1
Primary tumor site	Neck, thorax	Abdomen
Serum ferritin	Low	High

patients with a diagnosis after that age, even when their stages are similar. Many of these younger children have tumors that undergo spontaneous regression, a poorly understood phenomenon which may be related to the high incidence of occult neuroblastoma detected in stillborns or young children dying of unrelated causes. As an example, the 2-year survival in children under the age of 1 year with Stage IV disease is about 50%, compared to less than 10% in older children. Stage IV-S disease is usually found in children less than 1 year of age, which may account for the long-term survival of many of these patients even when not given systemic therapy [13].

The third important prognostic factor is the site of the primary tumor. Tumors arising in the chest or in the neck have a better prognosis than tumors arising within the abdomen. This may, in part, be due to the fact that cervical or thoracic tumors are diagnosed when smaller and at an earlier stage than abdominal tumors, but there may also be a slightly different natural history to these other tumors. The large number of ganglioneuroblastomas and ganglioneuromas found in the thorax compared to the abdomen suggests the possibility that intrathoracic neuroblastomas may be more prone to benign differentiation than are their abdominal counterparts. Nevertheless, for whatever reason, the fact remains that over 80% of thoracic and cervical neuroblastomas can be cured by surgery alone or with postoperative irradiation when the margins are microscopically involved.

Several other symptoms and signs have been associated with poor prognosis. Patients who present with failure to thrive, anemia, lymphadenopathy, and/or marrow involvement also have a poor prognosis.

TUMOR MARKERS

Biochemical products related to catecholamine synthesis and degradation have long been measured in children with neuroblastoma. Catecholamines represent the classic marker used in this tumor; neuroblastomas contain the biochemical pathway that progresses from phenylalanine to tyrosine to dopa with subsequent decarboxylation to dopamine and then conversion to the catecholamines. Approximately 80% of patients with neuroblastoma have elevated levels of vanillylmandelic acid in their urine, despite the fact that they demonstrate no clinical manifestations of elevated serum levels of catecholamines [16]. The more differentiated patterns of catecholamine metabolism, both in the tumor and in the urine, have been associated with age less than 1 year at diagnosis and a less advanced clinical stage. These patients have a favorable prognosis. In addition to absolute values, a ratio of vanillylmandelic acid/homovanillic acid greater than 1.5 indicates a better prognosis. Thus, measurement of urine catecholamines may be useful in defining the patient's prognosis.

Serum ferritin was measured at the time of diagnosis in a large group of patients with neuroblastoma treated by the Children's Cancer Study Group [40]. Ferritin is rarely elevated in patients with Stage I or II disease, but was elevated in 37 and 54% of those patients with Stage III and IV neuroblastoma; respectively. Among those patients with Stage III and IV tumor, analysis of progression-free survival demonstrated that elevated serum ferritin was associated with a significantly worse prognosis than was normal serum ferritin, and that this correlation was independent of stage and age at diagnosis. Among patients with Stage III disease, the 2-year progression-free survival was 76% if their initial serum ferritin was normal but only 23% when their initial serum ferritin was abnormal. Other investigations suggest that Stage IV-S neuroblastoma patients have normal serum ferritin levels and that these can aid in distinguishing Stage IV from Stage IV-S [41]. Serial serum ferritin levels were measured in a group of patients treated at the Memorial Sloan-Kettering Cancer Center. Although serum ferritin did increase with increasing numbers of blood transfusions, the results also suggested that the amount of tumor contributed to increasing serum ferritin levels [42]. Their data suggest that serial measurements of serum ferritin may be useful in detecting early signs of recurrence of neuroblastoma following treatment.

Several other tumor markers have been investigated for their usefulness in patients with neuroblastoma. Serum neuron-specific enolase has been shown to rise steadily with increasing stage of tumor, although the IV-S variant has much lower serum levels than does Stage IV neuroblastoma [43]. Low levels of serum neuron-specific enolase correlate with a good disease-free survival, whereas high levels have a poor survival. Among patients undergoing serial analysis of serum samples, patients with an elevated level of neuron-specific enolase achieved near normal levels during remission, but the recurrences did not appear to be predicted by a rise in the level of the serum neuron-specific enolase. These data suggest that patients with neuroblastoma may benefit from having a serum neuron-specific enolase measured, as normal levels suggest a more benign clinical course of the tumor.

SUMMARY

Neuroblastoma remains a tumor often diagnosed late in its course; surgery is the mainstay of treatment and is curative for most patients with Stage I or II disease. Patients with more advanced tumor, however, have a poor prognosis despite the administration of the most effective chemotherapy, which includes cyclophosphamide, DTIC, vincristine, and doxorubicin. The major prognostic variables include stage of the tumor at diagnosis, age of the patient, and site of the primary tumor.

REFERENCES

1. Virchow R: Hyperplasie der Zirbel und der Nebennieren. In: Die Krankhaften Geschwülste, vol. 2. Berlin: A. Hirschwald, 1964–1965, p 149.
2. Wright JH: Neurocytoma or neuroblastoma, a kind of tumor not generally recognized. J Exp Med 12:556–561, 1910.
3. Pochedly C (ed): Neuroblastoma. Toronto: Publishing Sciences Group, 1976.
4. Rosen EM, Cassady JR, Frantz CN, et al.: Neuroblastoma: The Joint Center for Radiation Therapy/Dana-Farber Cancer Institute/Children's Hospital experience. J Clin Oncol 2:719–732, 1984.
5. Thomas PRM, Lee JY, Fineberg BB, et al.: An analysis of neuroblastoma at a single institution. Cancer 53:2079–2082, 1984.
6. Robertson HE: Das Ganglioneuroblastom ein besonderer Typus im System der Neurome. Virchows Arch [A] 220:147–168, 1915.
7. Carachi R, Campbell PE, Kent M: Thoracic neural crest tumors: A clinical review. Cancer 51:949–954, 1983.
8. Adam A, Hochholzer L: Gangioneuroblastoma of the posterior mediastinum: A clinicopathologic review of 80 cases. Cancer 47:373–381, 1981.
9. Kedar A, Glassman M, Voorhess ML, et al.: Severe hypertension in a child with ganglioneuroblastoma. Cancer 47:2077–2080, 1981.
10. Kretschmar CS, Frantz CN, Rosen EM, et al.: Improved prognosis for infants with Stage IV neuroblastoma. J Clin Oncol 2:799–803, 1984.
11. Stokes SH, Thomas PRM, Perez CA, et al.: Stage IV-S neuroblastoma: Results with definitive therapy. Cancer 53:2083–2086, 1984.
12. Hann H-WL, Evans AE, Cohen IJ, et al.: Biologic differences between neuroblastoma stages IV-S and IV. N Engl J Med 305:425–429, 1981.
13. Evans AE, Baum E, Chard R: Do infants with Stage IV-S neuroblastoma need treatment? Arch Dis Child 56:271–274, 1981.
14. Kushner BH, Hajdu SI, Helson L: Synchronous neuroblastoma and von Recklinghausen's disease: A review of the literature. J Clin Oncol 3:117–120, 1985.
15. Punt J, Pritchard J, Pincott JR, et al.: Neuroblastoma: A review of 21 cases presenting with spinal cord compression. Cancer 45:3095–3101, 1980.
16. Graham-Pole J, Salmi T, Anton AH, et al.: Tumor and urine catecholamines (CATs) in neurogenic tumors: Correlations with other prognostic factors and survival. Cancer 51:834–839, 1983.
17. Evans AE, D'Angio GJ, Randolph J: A proposed staging system for children with neuroblastoma. Cancer 27:374–378, 1971.
18. Cushing BA, Slovis TL, Philippart AI, et al.: A rational approach to cervical neuroblastoma. Cancer 50:785–787, 1982.
19. Koop CE, Schnaufer L: The management of abdominal neuroblastoma. Cancer 35:905–909, 1975.

20. Grosfeld JL, Baehner RL: Neuroblastoma: An analysis of 160 cases. World J Surg 4:29–38, 1980.

21. Hayes FA, Green A, Hustu HO, et al.: Surgicopathologic staging of neuroblastoma: Prognostic significance of regional lymph node metastases. J Pediatr 102:59–62, 1983.

22. Smith EI, Krous HF, Tunell WP, et al.: The impact of chemotherapy and radiation therapy on secondary operations for neuroblastoma. Ann Surg 191:561–569, 1980.

23. Green AA, Hayes FA, Hustu HO: Sequential cyclophosphamide and doxorubicin for induction of complete remission in children with disseminated neuroblastoma. Cancer 48:2310–2317, 1981.

24. Sitarz A, Finklestein J, Grosfeld J, et al.: An evaluation of the role of surgery in disseminated neuroblastoma: A report from the Children's Cancer Study group. J Pediatr Surg 18:147–151, 1983.

25. Azizkhan RG, Shaw A, Chandler JG: Surgical complications of neuroblastoma resection. Surgery 97:514–517, 1985.

26. Shuster JJ, Land VJ, Nitschke R, et al.: Phase II study of four-drug chemotherapy for metastatic neuroblastoma: A Pediatric Oncology Group Study. Cancer Treat Rep 67:187–188, 1983.

27. Shafford EA, Rogers DW, Pritchard J: Advanced neuroblastoma: Improved response rate using a multiagent regimen (OPEC) including sequential cisplatin and VM-26. J Clin Oncol 2:742–747, 1984.

28. August CS, Serota FT, Koch PA, et al.: Treatment of advanced neuroblastoma with supralethal chemotherapy, radiation, and allogeneic or autologous marrow reconstitution. J Clin Oncol 2:609–616, 1984.

29. August CS, Bayever E, Levy Y, et al.: Eight years' experience in neuroblastoma patients transplanted after relapse. Proc AACR 27:203, 1986.

30. Saarinen UM, Coccia PF, Gerson SL, et al.: Eradication of neuroblastoma cells in vitro by monoclonal antibody and human complement: Method for purging autologous bone marrow. Cancer Res 45:5969–5975, 1985.

31. McGrath PC, Neifeld JP: Inhibition of murine neuroblastoma growth by dopamine antagonists. J Surg Res 36:413–419, 1984.

32. McGrath PC, Neifeld JP: Inhibition of human neuroblastoma by dopamine antagonists. Surgery 98:135–141, 1985.

33. Yokomori K, Tsuchida Y, Saito S: Tyrosine hydroxylase and choline acetyltransferase activity in human neuroblastoma. Cancer 52:263–272, 1983.

34. Tiffany-Castiglioni E, Perez-Polo JR: Evaluation of methods for determining 6-hydroxy-dopamine cytotoxicity. In Vitro 16:591–599, 1980.

35. Reynolds CP, Reynolds DA, Frenkel EP, et al.: Selective toxicity of 6-hydroxydopamine and ascorbate for human neuroblastoma in vitro: A model for clearing marrow prior to autologous transplant. Cancer Res 42:1331–1336, 1982.

36. Evans AE, Albo V, D'Angio GJ, et al.: Cyclophosphamide treatment of patients with localized and regional neuroblastoma: A randomized study. Cancer 38:655–660, 1976.

37. de la Monte SM, Moore WG, Hutchins GM: Nonrandom distribution of metastases in neuroblastic tumors. Cancer 52:915–925, 1983.

38. Richards MJS, Joo P, Gilbert EF: The rare problem of late recurrence in neuroblastoma. Cancer 38:1847–1852, 1976.

39. Sutherland CM, Krementz ET, Harkin JC, et al.: Recurrence of neuroblastoma following prolonged remission. Arch Surg 116:474–475, 1981.

40. Hann H-WL, Evans AE, Siegel SE, et al.: Prognostic importance of serum ferritin in patients with Stages III and IV neuroblastoma: The Children's Cancer Study Group experience. Cancer Res 45:2843–2848, 1985.
41. Hann H-WL, Evans AE, Cohen IJ, et al.: Biologic differences between neuroblastoma Stages IV-S and IV: Measurement of serum ferritin and E-rosette inhibition in 30 children. N Engl J Med 305:425–429, 1981.
42. Potaznik D, de Sousa M, Helson L, et al.: Ferritin in neuroblastoma. Impact of tumor load and blood transfusions. Cancer Invest 3:327–338, 1985.
43. Zeltzer PM, Marangos PJ, Evans AE, et al.: Serum neuron-specific enolase in children with neuroblastoma: Relationship to stage and disease course. Cancer 57:1230–1234, 1986.

Chapter 8
Pediatric Adrenal Neoplasms

M. David Gibbons, Gian Antonio M. Manzoni, and Richard H. Byrne

The adrenal gland may give rise to three different types of tumors. Neuroblastomas, discussed in Chapter 7, are by far the most common. Adrenocortical tumors and pheochromocytomas, the remaining two types, will be presented in this chapter. Pediatric pheochromocytomas are exceedingly rare, and the majority of our discussion will be limited to adrenocortical tumors.

ADRENOCORTICAL TUMORS

Adrenocortical tumors in children are rare and comprise approximately 0.0002% of childhood neoplasms. Unlike their adult counterparts, these tumors are usually functional, and their clinical presentation makes the distinction between adrenocortical carcinoma and benign conditions difficult. Clinical signs of virilism, Cushing's syndrome, feminization, and hyperaldosteronism in the child should alert the clinician to the possibility of this potentially devastating and lethal disease.

Approximately 350 cases of adrenocortical carcinoma have been described [1–3]. There is a female:male predominance of approximately 2–3:1. Although the children often present with mixed clinical syndromes, virilism predominates in two-thirds and Cushing's syndrome in the remainder [1]. Feminization occurs infrequently [4–11]. Only rare case reports of aldosterone secretory tumors exist [12,13]. Primary non-functional carcinomas have been infrequently described [14–17], and these usually present as asymptomatic abdominal masses.

Pediatric Tumors of the Genitourinary Tract, pages 113-137

Adrenocortical tumors occur in association with a variety of hereditary conditions including 21-hydroxylase deficiency congenital adrenal hyperplasia [18–20], multiple endocrine adrenomatosis I [21], and Beckwith-Weidemann syndrome [22], suggesting a genetic predisposition in these rare cases. The association of adrenal tumors with other congenital abnormalities such as hemihypertrophy, astrocytoma, cutaneous lesions, abnormalities of the contralateral adrenal, and urinary tract anomalies may suggest oncogenic factors occurring during embryonic development [15,19,23,24]. The family history is important and sibship occurrence has been reported [25,26]. A strong family history of neoplasia has been noted in a few cases [3,27]. The etiology of the tumor in the vast majority of cases is obscure.

Clinical Presentation

Virilizing adrenal tumors are most common (Table 8-1). These tumors usually occur after 2 years of age, but may rarely be seen in infants [1,28–30]. They characteristically secrete large amounts of dehydroepiandrosterone (DHA), a 17-ketosteroid, which, although a weak androgen, may be partly responsible for the clinical features. DHA can also be converted to delta-4-androstenedione and testosterone, two more potent androgens, and these may play a masculinizing role.

The common manifestations of excessive androgen production, including increased muscle mass and rapid growth with accelerated epiphyseal development in the preadolescent child, are usually seen [1,30,31]. The male child exhibits the classic signs of precocious puberty (i.e., enlargement of the penis; pubic, axillary, and facial hair; scrotal wrinkling and stippling; and acne). The testes usually remain bilaterally small. This is an important point in differentiating between adrenal tumors, Leydig cell tumors, or sexual precocity. A unilateral Leydig cell tumor produces an enlarged testis, whereas

TABLE 8–1. Adrenal Causes for Virilization

Premature adrenarche
CAH
    21-hydroxylase
    11 β-hydroxylase
    3β-hydroxysteroid dehydrogenase deficiency
ACTH excess
    Cushing's disease (pituitary)
    Ectopic secretion
Adrenal tumors
    Adenoma
    Adenocarcinoma

the testes in sexual precocity are symmetrical and enlarged. Bilateral testicular enlargement with adrenocortical carcinoma, however, has been noted in rare cases [3,32]. In girls, enlargment of the clitoris and labia majora, the appearance of pubic and axillary hair, seborrhea, and acne are common presenting signs.

In males, the differential diagnosis consists of sexual precocity, interstitial cell tumors of the testes, or the delayed appearance of congenital adrenal hyperplasia (CAH). The testicular exam will help differentiate adrenal tumors from precocious puberty and Leydig cell tumors. Precise laboratory studies are necessary to differentiate between CAH and adrenal neoplasms. In females, virilization can be caused by ovarian arrhenoblastoma, CAH, or rarely, acquired adrenal hyperplasia, as well as tumors of the adrenal cortex. The normal appearance of premature pubarche (the early appearance of axillary and pubic hair) [33] may mimic the signs of adrenal tumor. As a general rule, posterior labial fusion, commonly seen in virilizing congenital adrenal hyperplasia, is not noted in adrenal tumors [3].

The clinical features of Cushing's syndrome predominate in approximately one-third of cases (Table 8-2). Cancer of the adrenal cortex is probably the most common non-iatrogenic cause of Cushing's syndrome in infancy and early childhood [34–37], although other causes are adrenal adenoma and hyperplasia. The manifestations of Cushing's syndrome are the result of excessive cortisol production. Protein catabolism and diversion of amino acids to gluconeogenesis and ultimately increased fat deposition leads to the typical symptoms. Cushing's syndrome caused by adrenocortical tumors is rare in its pure form, and some effects of the hypercortisolism may be masked by excessive androgens.

The most common clinical sign is progressive obesity, which may become massive. Fatty deposits tend to occur centrally, in the cheeks, trunk, and pectoral girdle, resulting in the well-known "buffalo hump" and "moon facies." In infants, the obesity tends to be generalized. In older children, thinning of the extremities, secondary to muscle wasting, may be seen. Muscle weakness may be a predominant feature. Other features of the complete syndrome include growth arrest, osteoporosis, facial plethora with downy facial hair, acne, and seborrhea. Pink to violaceous striae of the abdomen and legs may be seen in older children, but are commonly absent in infants and young chldren. It should be noted that growth arrest may be masked by excessive androgen stimulation of the epiphyses. Hypertension and cardiomegaly have been noted and are probably secondary to the mineralocorticoid effects of excessive corticosterods.

Feminizing adrenal tumors are extremely rare. Unlike the other types, there is male predominance, but cases have been reported in females [4,9–11].

TABLE 8–2. Principal Features in 13 Cases of Cushing's Disease in Children[1]

	No.
Truncal obesity, moonface, buffalo hump	13
Short stature, 10th percentile or less	11
Hirsutism	11
Acne	11
Flushed cheeks	10
Hypertension[2]	10
Osteoporosis	7
Cutaneous striae	7
Headache	6
Emotional lability	6
Weakness	6
Ecchymosis	5
Premature appearance of pubic and axillary hair	5
Pigmentation (preoperatively)	4
Amenorrhea	3[3]
Renal stones	2
Symptomatic diabetes mellitus	1
Diabetic glucose tolerance test	5[4]

[1]From Reference 37.
[2]Diastolic pressure of 90 mmHg or greater.
[3]A total of four at risk.
[4]A total of five tested.
(From McArthur RG, Cloutier MD, Hayles AB, et al: Cushing's disease in children: findings in 13 cases. Mayo Clin Proc 47:318, 1972.)

TABLE 8–3. Major Metastatic Sites for Adrenocortical Carcinoma

	Percentage
Pulmonary	60
Liver	54
Nodes (regional mediastinal, etc.)	47
Abdominal (local, peritoneal, pancrease, retroperitoneal, opposite adrenal)	43
Bones (pelvis, spine, extremities, ribs, skull)	33
Kidneys	20
Brain	10

TABLE 8–4. Adrenocortical Carcinoma

Staging Criteria	
T1	Tumor $\leqslant$ 5 cm, no invasion
T2	Tumor < 5 cm, no invasion
T3	Tumor, any size, locally invading to but not involving adjacent organs
T4	Tumor, any size, locally invading adjacent organs
N0	No regional nodes
N1	Positive regional nodes
M0	No distant metastatic disease
M1	Distant metastatic disease
Stage	
I	T1 N0 N0
II	T2 N0 M0
III	T1 or T2 N1 M0, T3 N0 M0
IV	Any T, any N M1, T3 N1, T4

Gynecomastia is one of the most prominent findings, although signs of virilism, such as acne and facial hair, are also common.

Diagnostic Evaluation

Biochemical. The diagnosis of adrenal hyperfunction is biochemical, based on measurement of urinary 17-keto steroids, 17-hydroxycorticosteroids, DHA, and free cortisol [38,39]. More recently radioimmunoassays for serum dehydroepiandrosterone sulfate, testosterone, and cortisol have been utilized, eliminating the need for timed urine collections [3,40–43]. In those rare patients with feminization, estrogen levels will be elevated [44,45].

Radiographic. Radiologic evaluation is necessary to localize the lesion prior to treatment. The primacy of intravenous urography [46], capable of detecting masses greater than 2–3 cm in diameter, has recently been replaced by arteriography, computerized tomography [47], or ultrasound [48] for localization and evaluation. The use of radiocholesterol scanning has not been reported in children, but has shown limited usefulness in adults [49].

Treatment

Definitive therapy of adrenocortical carcinoma is surgical resection. The approach of choice is an anterior transverse incision, enabling the surgeon to thoroughly explore the abdomen and the contralateral adrenal gland. Pre- and perioperative cortisol replacement is essential as the function of the contralateral gland is often suppressed.

Complementary treatment may consist of chemotherapy or radiotherapy. The choice of therapy after resection is based on pathological and clinical assessment of the individual patient. Tumor size greater than 5 cm in diameter seems to be the single best determinant of potential malignancy [50]. Staging of this tumor is based on this finding. Other factors felt to be important in the determination of malignancy are mitotic activity, capsular invasion, and permeation of vascular spaces [51].

There is no convincing data on the efficacy of radiotherapy in the adjunctive treatment of this disease [52–56]. It is advocated by some and condemned by others.

Chemotherapy has been found helpful in the management of patients whose tumors are not completely resected and in whom there is evidence of metastatic disease. Persistently elevated hormonal levels or hormone-related symptoms or radiographic evidence of metastases are other indications for an attempt at chemotherapeutic control or aggressive surgical management of approachable metastases.

Mitotane (op'DDD) has been used extensively in the treatment of adrenocortical carcinoma in adults and has been used with some success in children. Its mode of action is the selective necrosis of the adrenal, and its efficacy in treatment of metastatic disease was first demonstrated by Bergenstal in 1960 [57]. The toxicity of mitotane can limit its usefulness, with 83% of patients suffering gastrointestinal side effects, and 41% neurotoxicity in one review [58]. Administration of op'DDD may mask biochemical evidence of metastatic disease [3]. Chemotherapeutic agents other than mitotane have been utilized in individual cases. These include vinblastine, L-arcolysine, methotrexate, 5-fluorouracil, medroxyprogesterone, hydroxyurea, daunomycin, cyclophosphamide, MCNU, adriamycin, and cisplatinum. These reports are purely anecdotal and have only rarely changed the prognosis of the disease.

Metastatic disease can be widespread. Common sites are liver, lung, abdomen, bone, kidney, lymph nodes, and brain [53–59].

CONCLUSIONS

Adrenocortical carcinoma, although rare, must be suspected in patients exhibiting signs and symptoms of adrenal hyperfunction. Accurate endocrinologic laboratory assessment and radiologic localization is mandatory prior to treatment. Curative surgical resection must be aggressive following adequate staging. The precise role of postoperative therapy is unclear following palliative or curative resection.

PHEOCHROMOCYTOMA

Pheochromocytoma is a tumor developing from the chromaffin tissue of the adrenal medulla and less frequently in the cells of the extraadrenal paraganglion system. It was first described in 1886 by Frankel [60] and given its name pheochromocytoma or "black celled tumor" in 1912 by Pick [61], but it was not until 1922 that Labbe et al. clearly demonstrate its association with hypertension of a paroxysmal nature [62]. From the work of von Euler in 1946 [63], Holton in 1949 [64], and Goldenberg et al. in 1950 [65] it has become clear that the clinical manifestations are related to the secretory output of catecholamines by the tumor. During the 1920s Charles Mayo in the United States [66] and Roux in France [67] obtained the first successful surgical removal of pheochromocytomas.

The first case of pheochromocytoma in a child was reported by Marchetti in 1904 [68]. This was found in the post-mortem examination in a 15-year-old boy who died of typhoid fever. Since then many other cases of unilateral, bilateral, and extraadrenal pheochromocytomas have been reported, giving this rare tumor its own characteristics in the pediatric population.

Pheochromocytoma is a rare disorder with incidences varying between 0.1 and 0.01% of the hypertensive population and approximately 2 in 100,000 of the adult population [69]. Occurring in all age groups, about 10% are diagnosed in children, occasionally presenting with unique chracteristics. Three distinct groups are recognized: primary sporadic, malignant metastatic, and familial pheochromocytoma (Table 8-5).

Primary sporadic (benign) pheochromocytoma is the most frequent form (90%) and generally occurs as a single lesion of the adrenal medulla. Boys

TABLE 8–5. Pheochromocytoma Classification

Primary sporadic (benign) (90%)
Metastatic (malignant) (10%)
   Sporadic
   Familial
Familial
   With no associated syndrome
   Neuroectodermal disorders
      von Hippel-Lindau
      von Recklinghausen's neurofibromatosis
      Tuberous sclerosis
      Sturge-Weber's
   Multiple endocrine neoplasia (MEN)
      Type 2a (Sipple)
      Type 3 (2b)[1]
   Multiple tumors (non-MEN)[1]
      Gastric epithelioid
      leiomyosarcoma, pulmonary
      chondroma

[1]Usually sporadic, non-familial.

are affected twice as often as girls. Käser has noticed a considerably higher female to male ratio in children than in adults and has suggested an autosomal recessive inheritance [69]. Metastatic malignant pheochromocytoma has an incidence exceeding 10% in adults [70], while in children it usually is less than 6% although some have reported a higher incidence [71]. It can present either in the sporadic or familial form. The diagnosis of malignant pheochromocytoma depends on pathologic demonstration of tumor in an area where chromaffin tissue does not normally exist (lymph nodes, lung, liver, bone) or clinical course characterized by recurrence or metastasis of an initially benign form [72].

About 10% of children with pheochromocytoma have an associated familial condition. The mode of inheritance seems to be autosomal dominant with a high degree of penetrance [73]. It can present as an isolated familial disease or in association with other syndromes. Neuroectodermal disorders (von Recklinghausen's neurofibromatosis, von Hippel-Lindau disease, Sturge-Weber syndrome, and tuberous sclerosis) were some of the earliest familial conditions recognized to be associated with pheochromocytoma [74-78]. Sipple has described association of pheochromocytoma, usually bilateral, with medullary carcinoma of the thyroid gland and parathyroid gland hyperplasia or tumors [multiple endocrine neoplasia (MEN) type 2a] [93]. Patients with MEN type 3 or 2b have submucosal neuromas (lips, tongue, eyelids, and gastrointestinal tract), and frequently marfanoid habitus with either medullary thyroid cancer alone or associated with adrenal medullary disease. The type 2b seems to be more frequently sporadic than familial. It has been clearly demonstrated that adrenal medullary hyperplasia is a precursor of pheochromocytoma in MEN-2 syndromes [80,81] and a policy of bilateral adrenalectomy in this group has been suggested [68].

A syndrome of gastric leiomyosarcoma, pulmonary chondroma, and functioning extraadrenal paraganglioma (pheochromocytoma) [81] has been described in the non-MEN group, with associated multiple rare neoplasms. All the described cases were sporadic, with female prevalence and tendency to tumor multicentricity.

The chromaffin paraganglia develop from the primary sympathetic chains, which themselves derive from the neural crest of the brain stem. They undergo somite metamerisation and, hence, are precursors of the intra- and extraadrenal medullary paraganglia. The most frequent paraganglion formation in adults is the adrenal medulla. The presumptive paraganglion cells migrate along the aorta, its collaterals explaining the occurrence of the various thoracoabdominal locations of the tumor. Four main groups can therefore be identified: adrenal, extraadrenal, simultaneous adrenal and extraadrenal, and extraadrenal metastatic (malignant) (Table 8-6).

TABLE 8-6. Pheochromocytoma Location

Adrenal
  Unilateral
  Bilateral
Extraadrenal
  Single
    Bladder
    Zückerkandl's organ
  Multiple
    Paraganglion region
      Neck
      Thorax, mediastinum
      Abdomen
Adrenal and extraadrenal
Extraadrenal metastatic (malignant)

The adrenal medulla is the most common site (70%) and usually is unilateral with no difference in side prevalence. In children, about 30% are extraadrenal, either single or multiple. The most common extraadrenal site is the bladder, and girls are more affected than boys. [82,83]. Hematuria may be present in addition to the usual symptoms. Hypertensive crises may accompany micturition. Most of these tumors are benign, but malignant forms with metastases have been reported [84,85].

Other extraadrenal sites include the abdominal, thoracic, and cervical paraganglia including Zuckerkandl's organ. The midline, especially at the bifurcation of the aorta, and the left side are usually predominantly involved, either with single or multiple tumors [86]. The simultaneous occurrence of adrenal and extraadrenal pheochromocytoma is a rare phenomenon with only a few reported pediatric cases [87,88].

In the metastatic (malignant) pheochromocytoma there is extraadrenal identification of chromaffin cells at sites that do not usually contain such tissue. The most commonly reported sites are lymph nodes, lungs, liver, and bones.

Clinical Presentation

Most (80%) children with pheochromocytomas are hypertensive. Approximately 7% of hypertensive children will have a pheochromocytoma. In up to 50% of adult patients hypertension is paroxysmal with normotensive symptom-free intervals between attacks, while hypertension in the pediatric population tends to be sustained (92%). Paroxysmal hypertensive crises may also be superimposed on an already elevated blood pressure. Other common symptoms include tachycardia, flushing, sweating, apprehension, headaches, blurred vision, seizures, tremor, and fainting. Polydipsia, polyuria, weight loss, and constipation have been reported with variable incidence (Table 8-7) [71,74,86]. The earliest onset of symptoms was in a 1-month-old boy, but generally they begin later (9–10 years of age). The longest duration of specific symptoms apparently was 3.5 years [86].

The signs and symptoms of pheochromocytoma reflect the hypermetabolism secondary to the secretion of epinephrine and norepinephrine by the tumor. In general the majority of extraadrenal tumors are pure norepinephrine producers, while the tumors that arise in the adrenal medulla produce both catecholamines. Very rarely pure epinephrine-producing tumors, either adrenomedullary or extramedullary, are encountered. In children it has been

TABLE 8-7. Symptoms and Signs of Pheochromocytoma*

	Approximate percent	
	Adult	Child
Symptoms		
Persistent hypertension	65	92
Paroxysmal hypertension	30	8
Headache	80	81
Sweating	70	68
Palpitation, nervousness	60	34
Pallor of face	40	27
Tremor	40	
Nausea	30	56
Weakness, fatigue	25	27
Weight loss	15	44
Abdominal or chest pain	15	35
Dyspnea	15	16
Visual changes	10	44
Constipation	5	8
Raynaud's phenomenon	5	
Convulsions	3	23
Polydipsia, polyuria		25
Puffy, red, cyanotic hands		11
Signs		
BMR over +20 percent	50	83
Fasting blood sugar over 120 mg/100 ml	40	40
Glycosuria	10	3
Eye ground changes	30	70

*From Hume DM in Astwood EB, and Cassidy CE (eds): Clinical Endocrinology. Volume II. New York: Grune and Stratton, 1968. In Scott HW and Sabiston DC: The Pituitary and the Adrenal. 11th ed. p. 779.

observed that the product of most pheochromocytomas is predominantly norepinephrine [89].

Diagnostic Evaluation

The most widely used modality for detection of pheochromocytoma is measurement of urinary catecholamines or their metabolites, vanillylmandelic acid (VMA) and metanephrines [90]. These tests are relatively easy to perform, readily available, and have a combined accuracy of approximately 100% [91,92]. Urinary metanephrines alone are elevated in 95% of cases and provide a more reliable clue to the presence of pheochromocytoma than either urinary VMA or free catecholamines.

There are different opinions on the reliability of plasma catecholamine levels in predicting the presence of tumor [93,94]. The metabolism of catecholamines in patients with pheochromocytoma may be modified by either a lack or an excess of metabolizing enzymes. Therefore in equivocal cases the most logical approach would include both determinations with the addition of the fractionated free catecholamines [91,95].

Provocative or suppressive tests, although still used in equivocal cases in adults [91,95], have not been reported in the pediatric population. Selective and multiple vena cava sampling, as well, do not provide more discriminating data for tumor localization than other invasive or non-invasive techniques [96,97].

Localization techniques have undergone considerable change during the last 30 years. Computed tomography (CT) is the initial localizing procedure [91,98-101]. It is non-invasive and demonstrates 95% of intraadrenal tumors. Adrenal lesions less than 2 cm in diameter and some extraadrenal tumors larger than 2 cm in diameter may not be visualized, however. Previously excretory urography (bolus nephrotomography) was used to identify the site of the lesion, with an accuracy in only 55% [102]. Arteriography [103,104], although potentially hazardous and invasive, and high resolution ultrasound [105] have also been used for localization but are (now) of limited usefulness in the pediatric age group (Figs. 8-1-8-4).

The major persisting problems in tumor location are detection of adrenal hyperplasia and small adrenal pheochromocytomas in patients with MEN type 2, location of extraadrenal sites, location of residual and/or recurrent tumor, and detection and delineation of metastatic malignant pheochromocytoma.

Radioisotope imaging with ^{131}I-meta-iodobenzylguanidine (MIBG) [106] has provided a new approach to the localization of pheochromocytoma [107-109]. A guanethidine analog with affinity for the chromaffin tissue, MIBG is

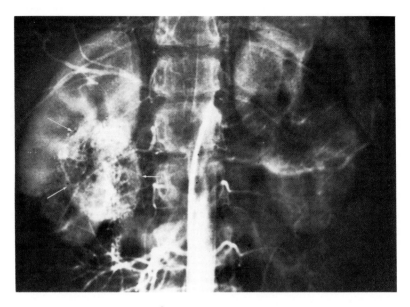

Fig. 8-1. A 6-year-old girl with right, parahilar pheochromocytoma. Note neovascularity.

an adrenergic neuron-blocker and an inhibitor of catecholamine uptake. A typical intraadrenal tumor concentrates 2–4% of the administered radiopharmaceutical. Images are recorded 24, 48, and 72 hours after an intravenous injection of MIBG (20–40 MBq or 0.5–1 MCi) and 90% of tumors are demonstrated at 24 hours. Recent experience in more than 500 patients with pheochromocytoma examined by MIBG imaging indicates a very high diagnostic sensitivity (about 85%), specificity (about 98%), and clinical accuracy (about 92%) [110] (Table 8-8).

Labeled MIBG has also been used to treat patients with functioning malignant metastases from pheochromocytoma [111,112] with encouraging results. It has also been successful in the imaging of other chromaffin tumors (neuroblastoma and carcinoid) [113,114].

Perioperative Management

Surgical management includes prevention of the complications of acute hypertensive crisis, cardiac arrhythmias, and shock, all potentially fatal for the child. It is mandatory to delay tumor removal until adequate preoperative preparation of the patient has been achieved. This should include an initial alpha-sympathetic blockade (phenoxybenzamine) usually started 1 week before surgery [71]. In the pediatric population, hypertension tends to be more severe and sustained than in adults and may lead to blood volume contraction. Blood transfusion is usually required during preoperative adrenergic blockage as indicated by a fall in hematocrit.

Opinions are divided about the additional benefits of beta-sympathetic blockade [71,115–117]. In the pediatric patient, these tumors tend to be norepinephrine-secreting, causing rare ventricular extrasystoles and tachycardia, which are more readily tolerated than in adults [115]. In the Mayo Clinic protocol, however, propanolol is added to the alpha-blockade 3 days before surgery, the final dose being given on the morning of surgery [116].

The induction of general anesthesia is particularly critical. Adequate sedation is mandatory to avoid apprehension with secondary severe hypertension [118]. Usually sodium thiopentone (thiopental) is given for induction with a non-depolarizing agent (pancuronium) for intubation and muscular relaxation. General anesthesia is maintained with isoflurane or enflurane while halohane is not employed because of its adverse property of sensitizing the myocardium to the arrhythmic activity of catecholamines.

During the removal of a pheochromocytoma, two anesthetic stages are critical [118]. During the first, isolation of the tumor and the ligation of its blood supply, the goal is the control of systemic blood pressure. During the second stage, following tumor removal, efforts are made to sustain blood pressure. During manipulation of the tumor, acute increases in systemic blood pressure may occur and these may be controlled either with phentolamine or nitroprusside. Cardiac arrhythmias are rare but xylocaine or propranolol may be used if they occur. Once the tumor is removed, a precipitous fall in blood pressure may occur. If this is not observed, it is most advisable to search for a second tumor [115]. Blood or fluids should be administered until the patient is hemodynamically stable.

The principal goals of the operative procedure include a wide exposure that permits examination of both adrenal glands and of the paraspinal axis and non-manipulative dissection in the removal of the pheochromocytoma [74,115,119,120]. An anterior transperitoneal approach either with a transverse supraumbilical or a thoracoabdominal incision will accomplish these goals. Careful, gentle dissection and minimal manipulation with early control of the venous drainage is necessary to reduce the release of catecholamines [119]. Exploration of both adrenals, the paraaortic area, and the retroperitoneal space is mandatory because of the possible presence of bilateral adrenal involvement and/or coexisting tumor in an extraadrenal location [120,121]. Total adrenalectomy is required and in the presence of suspected bilateral tumor, biopsy of the opposite adrenal is necessary.

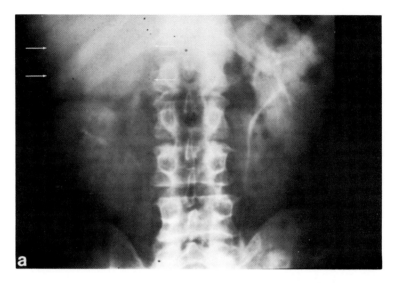

Fig. 8-2. A 7-year-old girl with right adrenal pheochromocytoma. **a:** IVP, suprarenal mass. **b:** Angioneovascularity, splayed adrenal vasculature. **c:** Angioneovascularity.

In patients with MEN-2a syndrome there is a high incidence of bilaterality. Because of the risk of local recurrence and the development of additional pheochromocytomas, bilateral adrenalectomy is strongly suggested [122].

In all recent reports in pediatric series [84,115,119–121] the surgical mortality has been reduced to zero, undoubtedly due to adequate preoperative management, safe anesthesia, and careful surgical technique now practiced.

Conclusions

Pheochromocytoma in the pediatric age group remains a challenging lesion to diagnose, localize, and succesfully remove. The recent advances are related to improvement in the localization of the tumor. Adequate preoperative preparation with careful anesthetic and surgical technique has led to safe surgical treatment. The prognosis in children with successfully resected pheochromocytoma will ultimately depend on tumor characteristics, the presence of associated conditions, and the occurrence of undiagnosed or missed pheochromocytoma. Long-term followup should be recommended.

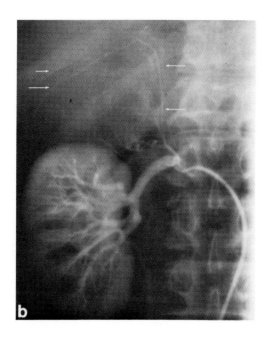

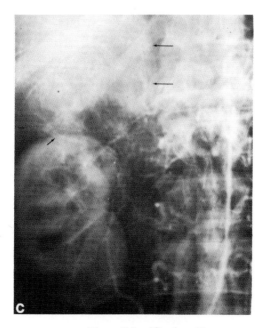

Figure 8-2. (Continued.)

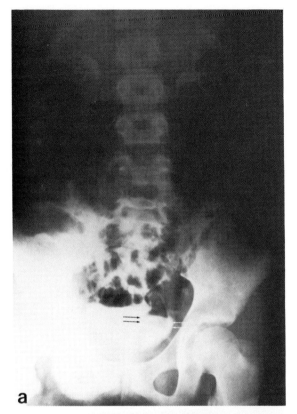

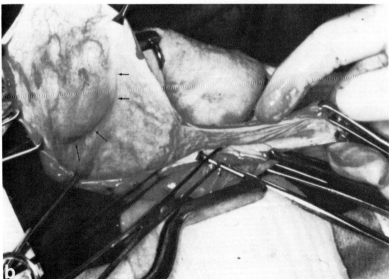

Fig. 8-3. A 13-year-old girl with blurring of vision, headaches, and hypertension with voiding. **a**: IVP suggests mass, left bladder dome. **b**: At exploration, vesical pheochromocytoma on left posterolateral bladder wall. Note tumor is submucosal. **c**: Segmental cystectomy specimen with submucosal mass. **d**: Note intramural location of bladder pheochromocytoma.

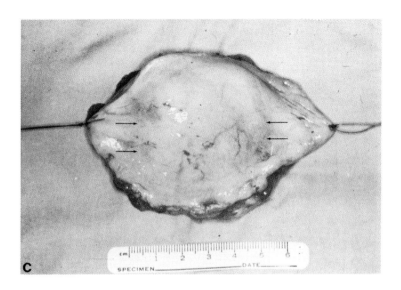

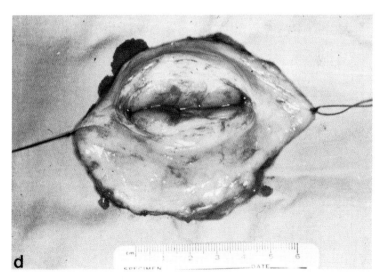

Figure 8-3. (Continued.)

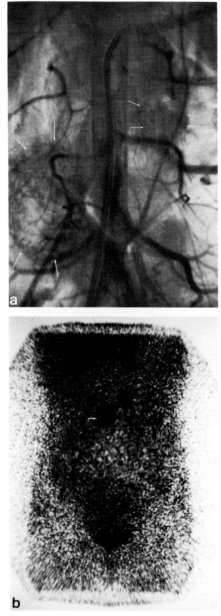

Fig. 8–4. A 10-year-old girl with two paraaortic pheochromocytomas, arising from organ of Zückerkandl. **a**: Flush aortogram, large right paracaval and smaller left paraaortic pheochromocytoma. **b**: MIBG scan demonstrates two areas of increased uptake in tumor masses.

TABLE 8–8. Summary of Overall Results at the University of Michigan and
Comparison With Other Series Using MIBG to Localize Pheochromocytoma[1]

	Sens[2]	Spec[3]	Neg PDA[4]	Post PDA[5]	Prevalence
Michigan (overall)[6]	87.4	98.9	94.8	97.4	30.2
Southamptom	88	95	88	95	52
Mayo Clinic	79	96	85	94	45
Tours	89	94	94	89	33
(Combined German Experience)	88	99	94	98	34

[1]From Reference 110.
[2]Sens = sensitivity.
[3]Spec = specificity.
[4]Neg PDA = negative predictive accuracy.
[5]Post PDA = positive predictive accuracy.
[6]Based on number of cases studied.

From: Shapiro B. J Nucl Med 26:576–585, 1985.

TABLE 8–9. Principal Differences Between Adult and Pediatric Pheochromocytoma

	Pediatric (%)	Adult (%)
Familial plus MEN-2 incidence	10	2.5
Bilaterality	24	7
Bilateral, multiple, extraadrenal	50	5
Malignancy	6	5–10
Hypertension sustained	92	40
Paroxysmal	8	50

REFERENCES

1. Hayles AB, Hahn HB, Sprague RG, et al.: Hormone secreting tumors of the adrenal cortex in children. Pediatrics 37:19, 1966.
2. Bulger AR, Correa RJ: Experience with adrenal cortical carcinoma. Urology 10:12, 1977.
3. Lee PDK, Winter RJ, Green OC: Virilizing adrenocortical tumors in childhood: Eight cases and a review of the literature. Pediatrics 76:437, 1985.
4. Bacon GE, Lowrey GH: Feminizing adrenal tumor in a 6-year-old boy. J Clin Endocrinol 25:1403, 1965.
5. Bhettay E, Bonnici F: Pure oestrogen-secreting feminizing adrenocortical adenoma. Arch Dis Child 52:241, 1977.
6. Howard CP, Takashashi H, Hayles AB: Feminizing adrenal adenoma in a boy. Proc Mayo Clin 52:354, 1977.
7. Kepler EJ, Walters W, Dixon RK: Menstruation in a child aged nineteen months as a result of tumor of the left adrenal cortex: Successful surgical treatment. Proc Mayo Clin 13:362, 1938.

8. Mosier HD, Goodwin WE: Feminizing adrenal adenoma in a 7-year-old boy. Pediatrics 27:1016, 1961.
9. Smith AH: A case of feminizing adrenal tumor in a girl. J Clin Endocrinol 18:318, 1958.
10. Comite F, Schiebinger RJ, Albertson BD, et al.: Isoxesual precocious pseudopuberty secondary to a feminizing adrenal tumor. J Clin Endocrinol Metab 58:435, 1984.
11. Halmi KA, Lascari AD: Conversion of virilization to feminization in a young girl with adrenal cortical carcinoma. Cancer 27:931, 1971.
12. Grane MG, Holloway JE, Winsor WG: Aldosterone-secreting adenoma: Report of a case in a juvenile. Ann Intern Med 54:280, 1961.
13. Ganguly A, Bergstein J, Grim CE, et al.: Childhood primary aldosteronism due to an adrenal adenoma: Preoperative localization by adrenal vein catheterization. Pediatrics 65:605, 1980.
14. Zaitoon MM, Mackie GG: Adrenal cortical tumors in children. Urology 12:645, 1978.
15. Graff DB, Buchino JJ: A child with hemihypertrophy and a right flank mass. J Pediatr 100:500, 1982.
16. Fukushima DK, Gallagher TF: Steroid production in "non-functioning" adrenal cortical tumor. J Clin Endocrinol 23:923, 1963.
17. Heinbacker P, O'Neal LW, Ackerman LV: Functioning and non-functioning adrenocortical tumors. Surg Gynecol Obstet 105:21, 1957.
18. Bangioranim AM: Neoplasms associated with congenital adrenal hyperplasia. J Pediatr 100:507, 1982.
19. Fraumeni JM, Miller RW: Adrenocortical neoplasms with hemihypertrophy, brain tumors and other disorders. J Pediatr 70:129, 1967.
20. Duck SC: Malignancy associated with congenital adrenal hyperplasia. J Pediatr 99:423, 1981.
21. Schimke RN: Endocrine gland neoplasia. In Emery AEH (ed): Genetics and Cancer in Man. New York: Churchill Livingstone, 1978, pp 47–62.
22. Kosseff AL, Herrman J, Gilbert EF, et al.: Studies of malformation syndromes of man. XXIX: The Wiedemann and Beckwith Syndrome. Clinical, genetic and pathogenetic studies of 12 cases. Eur J Pediatr 123:139, 1976.
23. Haicken BN, Schulman NH, Schneider KM: Adrenocortical carcinoma and congenital hemihypertrophy. J Pediatr 83:284, 1973.
24. Miller RW: Peculiarities in the occurrence of adrenal cortical carcinoma. Am J Dis Child 132:235, 1978.
25. Steiner MM: Modern concepts of urologic endocrinology. J Urol 81:1, 1959.
26. Mahlondji M, Ronaghy H, Dutz W: Virilizing adrenal carcinoma in two sibs. J Med Genet 8:160, 1971.
27. Kenny FM, Hashida Y, Askari HA, et al.: Virilizing tumors of the adrenal cortex. Am J Dis Child 115:445, 1968.
28. Cubill GF, Melicon MM, Darby HH: Adrenocortical tumors: The types of nonhormonal and hormonal tumors. Surg Gynecol Obstet 74:281, 1942.
29. Garrett RA: Adrenocortical carcinoma in children. J Urol 66:477, 1951.
30. Cooper JD, Maldonado L, Earl JM: Adrenocortical carcinoma with virilism in an infant under one year of age. Am J Dis Child 113:730, 1967.
31. Sobel EH, Lee CM, Esselboru VM, et al.: Functioning adrenal tumors in childhood. Am J Dis Child 86:733, 1953.
32. Drago JR, Olstein JS, Tesluk H, et al.: Virilizing adrenal cortical carcinoma with hypertrophy of spermatic tubule in childhood. Urology 14:70, 1979.

33. Wilkens L: The Diagnosis and Treatment of Endocrine Disorders in Childhood and Adolescence, 3rd ed. Springfield, Ill.: Charles C Thomas, 1965.

34. Gilbert MG, Cleveland WW: Cushing's syndrome in infancy. Pediatrics 46:217, 1970.

35. Grim GH, Gilbert EF: Cushing's syndrome in children associated with adrenocortical carcinoma: A case report with a review of the literature. Am J Dis Child 92:297, 1956.

36. Loridan L, Senior B: Cushing's syndrome in infancy. J Pediatr 75:349, 1969.

37. McArthur RG, Cloutier MD, Hayles AB, et al.: Cushing's disease in children: Findings in thirteen cases. Proc Mayo Clinic 47:318, 1972.

38. Chambers WL: Adrenal Cortical carcinoma in a male with excess gonadotrophin in the urine. J Clin Endocrinol 9:451, 1949.

39. Lipsett MB, Weson H: Adrenocortical cancer: Steroid biosynthesis and metabolism evaluabted by urinary metabolites. J Clin Endocrinol 22:906, 1962.

40. Cahen LA, Villee DB, Powers ML, et al.: A virilizing adrenocortical tumor in a female infant: In vivo and in vitro biochemical characteristics. J Clin Endocrinol Metab 47:300, 1978.

41. Suez JM, Lorans B, Morera AM, et al.: Studies of androgens and their precursors in adrenocortical virilizing carcinomas. J Clin Endocrinol Metab 32:462, 1971.

42. Suez JM, Rivarola MA, Migeon CJ: Studies of androgens in patients with adrenocortical tumors. J Clin Endocrinol Metab 27:615, 1967.

43. Villee EB, Rotner H, Kliman B, et al.: Androgen synthesis in a patient with virilizing adrenocortical carcinoma. J Clin Endocrinol Metab 27:1112, 1967.

44. Axelrod LR, Goldzieher JW, Woodhead DM: Steroid biosynthesis in feminizing adrenal carcinomas. J Clin Endocrinol Metab 29:1481, 1968.

45. Wotiz HH, Chattoray SC, Gabrilone JL: Urinary estrogen titers in a patient with feminizing adrenocortical carcinoma. J Clin Endocrinol 28:192, 1968.

46. Pickering RS, Hartman GW, Weeks RE, et al.: Excretory urographic localization of adrenal cortical tumors and pheochromocytomas. Radiology 114:345, 1975.

47. Solomon A, Kreel L: Computed tomographic assessment of adrenal masses. Clin Radiol 31:137, 1980.

48. Sample WF, Sarti DA: Computed tomography and grey scale ultrasonography of the adrenal gland: A comparative study. Radiology 128:377, 1978.

49. Schteingart DE, Seabold JE, Gross MD, et al.: Iodocholesterol adrenal tissue uptake and imaging in adrenal neoplasms. J Clin Endocrinol Metab 52:1156, 1981.

50. Scott HW, Abumrad NN, Onth DN: Tumors of the adrenal cortex and Cushing's syndrome. Ann Surg 201:586, 1984.

51. King DR, Lack EE: Adrenal cortical carcinoma: A clinical and pathologic study of 49 cases. Cancer 44:239, 1979.

52. Stewart DR, Monis-Jones PH, Jolley A: Carcinoma of the adrenal gland in children. J Pediatr Surg 9:59, 1974.

53. Sullwin M, Boilseu M, Hodges CV: Adrenocortical carcinoma. J Urol 120:660, 1978.

54. Lubitz JA, Freeman L, Okin R: Mitotane use in inoperable adrenal cortical carcinoma. JAMA 223:1109, 1973.

55. Ritchie JP, Gittes RF: Carcinoma of the ardrenal cortex. Cancer 45:1957, 1980.

56. Sprague RG, Kosle WF, Priestly JT: Management of certain hyperfunctioning lesions of the adrenal cortex and medulla. JAMA 151:629, 1953.

57. Bergenstal DM, Hertz R, Lipsett MB, et al.: Chemotherapy of adrenocortical cancer with op'DDD. Ann Int Med 53:672, 1960.

58. Hutler AM, Kayhor DE: Adrenal cortical carcinoma: Results of treatment with op'DDD in 138 patients. Am J Med 41:581, 1966.

59. Huyjan RA, Hickey RC, Samason NA: Adrenocortical carcinoma: A study of thirty-two patients. Cancer 35:549, 1975.

60. Frankel F: Ein fall von doppelseitigen, vollig latent verlaufenen nebbenierentumor und gleichzeitiger nephritis mit veranderungen am circulations-apparat und retinitis. Arch Pathol Anat 103:244, 1886.

61. Pick L: Das ganglioma embryonale sympathicium. Klin Wochenschr 19:16, 1912.

62. Labbe M, Tinel J, Doumer A: Crises solaires et hypertension paroxystique en rapport avec une tumeur surrenale. Bull Soc Med Hop Paris 46:982, 1922.

63. von Euler US: Specific sympathomimetic ergone in adrenergic nerve fibres (sympathin) and its relations to adrenaline and nor-adrenaline. Acta Physiol Scand 12:73, 1946.

64. Holton P: Noradrenaline in adrenal medullary tumors. Nature 163:217, 1949.

65. Goldenberg M, Aranow H, Jr, Smith AA, Faber M: Pheochromocytoma and essential hypertensive vascular disease. Arch Intern Med 86:823, 1950.

66. Mayo CH: Paroxysmal hypertension with tumor of retroperitoneal nerve. JAMA 89:1047, 1927.

67. Roux C: Cited by Barbeau A, et al.: Le pheochromocytome bilateral presentation d'un cas et revue de la literature. Un Med Can 87:165, 1958.

68. Marchetti G: Cited by Hume DM: Pheochromocytoma in the adult and in the child. Am J Surg 99:458, 1960.

69. Käser HE, Wagner H: Chromaffin tumors in childhood: Experience with 29 cases. In Raybaud C, Clement R, Lebruil G, et al. (eds): Pediatric Oncology. Amsterdam: Excerpta Medica, 1982, pp 240–244.

70. ReMine WH, Chong GC, van Heerden JA, et al.: Current management of pheochromocytoma. Ann Surg 179:740, 1974.

71. Gilchrist GS, Telander RL: Adrenal medulla and sympathetic chain. In Kelalis PP, King LR, Belman AB (eds): Clinical Pediatric Urology, 2nd ed; vol. 2. Philadelphia: WB Saunders, 1985, pp 1265–1271.

72. Mahoney EM, Harrison JH: Malignant pheochromocytoma: Clinical course and treatment. J Urol 118:225, 1977.

73. Van Way CW, III, Scott HW, Jr., Page DL, et al.: Pheochromocytoma. In Ravitch MM (ed): Current Problems in Surgery. Chicago: Year Book Medical Publishers, 1974, pp 35–36.

74. Scott HW, Jr.: The pituitary and the adrenals. In Sabiston DC, Jr. (ed): Textbook of Surgery: The Biological Basis of Modern Surgical Practice, 11th ed. Philadelphia: WB Saunders, 1977, pp 776–783.

75. Tisherman SE, Gregg FJ, Danowski TS: Familial pheochromocytoma. JAMA 182:150, 1962.

76. Sizemore GW, Heath H, Carney JA: Multiple endocrine neoplasia type 2. Clin Endocrinol Metab 9:29, 1980.

77. Glowniak JV, et al.: Familial extra-adrenal pheochromocytoma: A new syndrome. Arch Int Med 145:257, 1985.

78. Ansari AN: Familial extra-adrenal pheochromocytoma. Arch Int Med 145:228, 1985.

79. Sipple JH: The association of pheochromocytoma with carcinomas of the thyroid gland. Am J Med 31:163, 1961.

80. Carney JA, Sizemore GW, Tyce GM: Bilateral adrenal medullary hyperplasia in multiple endocrine neoplasia, type 2: The precursor of bilateral pheochromocytoma. Mayo Clin Proc 50:3, 1975.

81. Carney JA: The triad of gastric epithelioid leiomyosarcoma, functioning extra-adrenal paraganglioma, and pulmonary chondroma. Cancer 43:374, 1979.

82. Albores-Saavedra J, Maldonado ME, Ibarra J, et al.: Pheochromocytoma of the urinary bladder. Cancer 23:1110, 1969.
83. Schutz W, Vogel E: Pheochromocytoma of the urinary bladder: A case report and review of the literature. Urol Int 39·250, 1984.
84. Higgins PM, Tressider GC: Pheochromocytoma of the urinary bladder. Br Med J 2.274, 1966.
85. Meyer JJ, Sane SM, Drake RM: Malignant paraganglioma (pheochromocytoma) of the urinary bladder: Report of a case and review of the literature. Pediatrics 63:879, 1979.
86. Stackpole RH, Melicow MM, Uson AC: Pheochromocytoma in children: Report of 9 cases and review of the first 100 cases published with follow-up studies. J Pediatr 63:315, 1963.
87. Gibbs MK, Carney JA, Hayles AB, et al.: Simultaneous adrenal and cervical pheochromocytoma in childhood. Ann Surg 185:273, 1977.
88. Cone TE, Jr.: Recurrent pheochromocytoma: Report of a case in a previously treated child. Pediatrics 21:994, 1958.
89. Freier DT, Tank ES, Harrison TS: Pediatric and adult pheochromocytoma: A biochemical and clinical comparison. Arch Surg 107:252, 1973.
90. Bravo EL, Tarazi RC, Gifford RW, et al.: Circulating and urinary catecholamines in pheochromocytoma: Diagnostic and pathophysiologic implications. N Engl J Med 301:682, 1979.
91. Kaufman BH, Telander RL, van Heerden JA, et al.: Pheochromocytoma in the pediatric age group: Current status. J Pediatr Surg 18:879, 1983.
92. van Heerden JA, Sheps SG, Hamberger B, et al.: Pheochromocytoma: Current status and changing trends. Surgery 91:367, 1982.
93. Plouin PF, Duclos JM, Menard J, et al.: Biochemical tests for diagnosis of pheochromocytoma: Urinary versus plasma determinations. Br Med J 282:853, 1981.
94. Kopin IJ, Lake RC, Ziegler M: Plasma levels of norepinephrine. Ann Intern Med 88:671, 1978.
95. Bravo EL, Gifford RW: Pheochromocytoma: Diagnosis, localization and management. N Engl J Med 311:1298, 1984.
96. Lenoir GR, Comoy E, Guillot M, et al.: Is "vena cava sampling" useful for tumor localization in children with pheochromocytoma. In Raybaud C, Clement R, Lebreuil G, et al. (eds): Pediatric Oncology. Amsterdam: Excerpta Medica, 1982, pp 231–35.
97. Allison DJ, Brown MJ, Jones DH, et al.: Role of venous sampling in locating a pheochromocytoma. Br Med J 286:1122, 1983.
98. Abrams HL, Siegelman SS, Adams DF, et al.: Computed tomography versus ultrasound of the adrenal gland: A prospective study. Radiology 143:121, 1982.
99. Stewart BH, Bravo EL, Haaga J, et al.: Localization of pheochromocytoma by computed tomography. N Engl J Med 299:460, 1978.
100. Laursen K, Damgaard-Pedersen K: CT for pheochromocytoma diagnosis. AJR 134:277, 1980.
101. Thomas JL, Bernardino ME, Samaan NA, et al.: CT of pheochromocytoma. AJR 135:477, 1980.
102. Pickering RS, Hartman GW, Weeks RE, et al.: Excretory urographic localization of adrenal cortical tumors and pheochromocytoma. Radiology 114:345, 1975.
103. Rossi P, Young IS, Panke WF: Techniques, usefulness and hazards of arteriography of pheochromocytoma: Review of 99 cases. JAMA 205:547, 1968.
104. Kinkhabwala MN, Conradi H: Angiography of extra-adrenal pheochromocytoma. J Urol 108:666, 1972.

105. Bowerman RA, Silver TH, Jaffe MJ, et al.: Sonography of adrenal pheochromocytoma. AJR 137:1227, 1981.
106. Wieland DM, Wu JL, Brown LE, et al.: Radiolabelled andrenergic neuron blocking agents: Adrenomedullary imaging with ^{131}I iodobenzylguanidine. J Nucl Med 21:349, 1980.
107. Sisson JC, Frager MS, Valk TW, et al.: Scintigraphic localization of pheochromocytoma. N Engl J Med 305:12, 1981.
108. Ackery DM, Tippett PA, Condon BR, et al.: New approach to the localization of pheochromocytoma: Imaging with iodine-131-metaiodobenzylguanidine. Br Med J 288:1587, 1984.
109. Fischer M, Vetter W, Winterberg B, et al.: Scintigraphic localization of pheochromocytoma. Clin Endocrinol 20:1, 1984.
110. Shapiro B, Copp JE, Sisson JC, et al.: Iodine-131 metaiodobenzylguanidine for the locating of suspected pheochromocytoma: Experience in 400 cases. J Nucl Med 26:576, 1985.
111. Shapiro B, Sisson JC, Lloyd R, et al.: Malignant pheochromocytoma: Clinical, biochemical and scintigraphic characterization. Clin Endocrinol 20:189, 1984.
112. Sisson JC, Shapiro B, Beierwalters WH, et al.: Radiopharmaceutical treatment of malignant pheochromocytoma. J Nucl Med 24:197, 1984.
113. Kimming B, Brandeis WE, Eisenhut M: Scintigraphy of a neuroblastoma with 131-I metaiodobenzylguanidine. J Nucl Med 1:773, 1984.
114. Fischer M, Kamanbroo D, Sonderkamp H, et al.: Scintigraphic imaging of carcinoid tumors with 131 I-metaiodobenzylguanidine. Lancet 2:165, 1984.
115. Stringel G, Ein SH, Creighton R, et al.: Pheochromocytoma in children—an update. J Pediatr Surg 15:496, 1980.
116. Ellis D, Gartner JC: The intraoperative management of childhood pheochromocytoma. J Pediatr Surg 15:655, 1980.
117. Kaufman BH, Telander RL, van Heerden JA, et al.: Pheochromocytoma in the pediatric age group: Current status. J Pediatr Surg 18:879, 1983.
118. Wotherspoon GP, Overton JH, Lomaz JG: Pheochromocytoma in a child. Anaesthesiol Intens Care 2:83, 1974.
119. Bloom DA, Fonkalsrud EW: Surgical management of pheochromocytoma in children. J Pediatr Surg 12:157, 1977.
120. Heikkinen ES, Akerbom HK; Diagnostic and operative problems in multiple pheochromocytoma. J Pediatr Surg 12:157, 1977.
121. Ellis D, Gartner JC: The intraoperative management of childhood pheochromocytoma. J Pediatr Surg 15:655, 1980.
122. Prevot J, Olive D, Schmitt M, et al.: Surgical considerations and multiple localization of pheochromocytoma in childhood. In Paybaud C, Clement R, Lebreuil G, et al. (eds): Pediatric Oncology. Amsterdam: Excerpta Medica, 1982, pp 236–239.
123. Young TL, Miller RW: Incidence of indigent tumors in U.S. children. J Pediatr 86:254, 1975.
124. Barrington JD, Stephens CA: Virilizing tumors of the adrenal gland in childhood: Report of eight cases. J Pediatr Surg 4:291, 1969.
125. DeCourt J, Anoussakis C: Les tumeurs virilisantes de la corticosurr nale chez l'enfant avant l'age de la pubertie. Sem Hop Paris 45:817, 1969.
126. Gross RE: Neoplasia producing endocrine distrubance in childhood. Am J Dis Child 59:579, 1940.

127. Lerinia Hernandez A, Reynoso Garcia M: Adrenal cortical suprarenal carcinoma in children. Bol Med Hosp Infant Mex 37:399, 1980.
128. Scarpa-Smith C, Thornton N, Coffey EL, et al.: Virilizing adrenal tumors in children. Am J Dis Child 97:78, 1959.
129. Stewart DR, Morris Jones PH, Jobeys A: Carcinoma of the adrenal gland in children. J Pediatr Surg 9:59, 1974.
130. Kay R, Schumacher P, Turk ES: Adrenocortical carcinoma in children. J Urol 130:1130, 1983.
131. Benailly M, Schweisguth O, Job JC: Les tumeurs cortico-surr nales de l'enfant. Etude ritrospective de 34 cas observes de 1954 à 1973. Arch Franc Pediat 32:441, 1975.
132. Bürich JR: Nebennierenriden tumoren mit wirkung auf die Sexualsphare. Minerva Pediatr 17:725, 1965.
133. Levine LS, New MI: Neoplasms associated with congenital adrenal hyperplasia. J Pediatr 100:506, 1982.
134. Fukushima DK, Bradlow HC, Hellman L, et al.: Origin of pregnanetriol in adrenal carcinoma. J Clin Endocrinol 23:267, 1963.
135. Martin FI: Evidence of a hormonal influence on the steroid output of adrenal carcinoma. Am J Med 32:795, 1962.
136. Matsukura S, Kakita T, Sueoka S, et al.: Multiple hormone receptors in the adenylate cyclase of human adrenocortical tumors. Cancer Res 40:3768, 1980.
137. Hoevels J, Ekelind L: Angiographic findings in adrenal masses. Acta Radiol Diagr 20:337, 1979.
138. Bravo EL, Tarazi RC, Fuad FM, et al.: Clonidine-suppression test: A useful aid in the diagnosis of pheochromocytoma. N Engl J Med 305:623, 1981.
139. Carney JA, Sizemore GW, Tyce GM: Bilateral adrenal medullary hyperplasia in multiple endocrine neoplasia, type 2: The precursor of bilateral pheochromocytoma. Mayo Clin Proc 55:271, 1980.

Chapter 9
Rhabdomyosarcoma—Medical Aspects

Harold M. Maurer

Rhabdomyosarcoma (RMS) is a malignant tumor of the same mesodermal tissues that give rise to striated skeletal muscle. It is the most common soft tissue sarcoma of childhood, and it accounts for 5–15% of all malignant solid tumors and 4–8% of all malignant disease in patients under 15 years of age. It ranks seventh among the malignant tumors of childhood, preceded by leukemia, tumors of the central nervous system, lymphoma, neuroblastoma, Wilms' tumor, and bone cancer. The annual incidence in the United States is estimated to be 4.4 per million white children and 1.3 per million black children under age 15; the ratio of males to females is 1.4:1 [1–3].

Rhabdomyosarcoma can arise virtually anywhere in the body and tends to disseminate early in the course of disease. Each site of origin has its own peculiarities of disease evolution and set of therapeutic problems. The primary site of tumor origin in order of frequency are: the head and neck region (38%, of which 10% are located in the orbit); genitourinary region (21%); the extremity (18%); the trunk (7%); the retroperitoneum (7 %); the intrathoracic region (3%); the gastrointestinal tract, including liver and biliary tract (3%); the perineum-anus (2%); and other sites (1%).

EPIDEMIOLOGIC CHARACTERISTICS

There is a high occurrence of soft tissue sarcomas in families of children with RMS [4]. There also is a high frequency of carcinoma of the breast and other sites, and of brain tumors. RMS may be seen as a malignant complication of neurofibromatosis. Osteosarcoma, acute myelocytic leukemia, brain

Pediatric Tumors of the Genitourinary Tract, pages 139–151
© 1988 Alan R. Liss, Inc.

tumors, and sarcoma of the trachea have developed as a second malignant neoplasm in patients with RMS, indicating the effects of genetic predisposition and/or therapy.

Gufferman et al. have reported possible etiologic factors in RMS. In a case-control study of RMS carried out in North Carolina, they found an association between fathers' (but not mothers') cigarette smoking and an increased risk of RMS in the child [5]. There was an inverse relationship between a child's immunization status and RMS risk and a positive association between RMS and preventable infectious diseases, environmental exposures to chemicals, mother's age at subject's birth, and family history of asthma; there was an inverse association between RMS and socioeconomic status. A larger case-control study in conjunction with the Intergroup Rhabdomyosarcoma Study (IRS) is being done to confirm these and investigate other potential etiologic environmental factors.

CONGENITAL ANOMALIES

Congenital anomalies have been identified in approximately one-third of children and adolescents autopsied with RMS [6]. Anomalies involve the central nervous, genitourinary, gastrointestinal, and cardiovascular systems. Included among these anomalies are the Rubinstein-Taybi syndrome, neurofibromatosis, single horseshoe kidney, hemi-hypertrophy, and Arnold-Chiari malformation. The similarity in some congenital anomalies in RMS and Wilms' tumor suggests that similar molecular genetic events may be occurring in both childhood malignancies. Recent molecular investigations have demonstrated homozygosity for a mutant allele locus on chromosome 11 [7].

HISTOLOGIC CLASSIFICATION

With the exception of sarcoma botryoids, which appear as grape-like clusters, there is little variation among RMS subtypes grossly and no gross characteristics that distinguish it from other malignant soft tissue tumors. Typically, the tumors are firm, vary in size, are well circumscribed but not encapsulated, and infiltrate extensively into the surrounding tissue.

There are four classic histologic forms of RMS and two other histologic types that are sometimes lumped with RMS. The embryonal form is the most common cell type and accounts for 57% of these six cell types. It is seen in approximately 75% of head and neck and genitourinary tumors. The alveolar cell type is the next most common form and accounts for 19% of the cases. It is found often in tumors of the trunk, extremity, and perianal region and has the poorest prognosis. Accounting for 6% of the cases is the botryoid cell type, which is actually a variant of the embryonal form, and is seen most often in the genitourinary region. It usually is seen in patients under age 6. The pleomorphic type is usually considered the adult form and occurs in 1% of cases. It is located mostly in the extremity and trunk. Extraosseous Ewing's sarcoma and undifferentiated sarcoma, type indeterminate, are sometimes submitted as RMS variants and lumped with the four classic types. They account for 7 and 10%, respectively. The former type is more common in children over age 6 and found frequently in the extremity and trunk. The latter accounts for approximately 35% of cases under the age of 1 year. Both types are indistinguishable from the embryonal form in terms of response to radiation and chemotherapy and prognosis.

Electron microscopy may be helpful when the diagnosis is questionable. It makes possible the identification of structural components of skeletal muscle differentiation, including actin-myosin-Z-band arrangements of various combinations of these elements.

Immunohistochemistry may be valuable in establishing or confirming a diagnosis of RMS. Antigenic markers that have been studied include myoglobin, skeletal muscle myosin, creatinine kinase (CK), MM, CKBB, desmin, vimentin, calcium-magnesium-dependent ATPase, and calsequestrin; the detection of myoglobin, myosin, CKMM, and desmin has been most commonly reported.

The IRS has identified a cytologic classification that may have prognostic significance [8]. The three forms in this scheme are anaplastic, monomorphous, and mixed. Preliminary findings suggest that anaplastic and monomorphous forms have a poor prognosis when compared to the mixed type. Further studies are being done to verify and extend these observations.

CLINICAL STAGING CLASSIFICATION

The IRS Clinical Grouping classification is the most widely used scheme for "staging" RMS. This system depends largely on the resectability of the primary tumor plus the status of the regional lymph nodes, rather than on any anatomic or histologic criteria. This system, shown in Table 9-1, does have prognostic validity despite the shortcoming that group assignment is based on the type of surgery performed. The International Union Against Cancer (UICC) TNM pretreatment staging classification is widely used in Europe, but does not have a firm basis if one uses the survival data from the large IRS series [9,10]. Donaldson and Belli have proved a pretreatment staging system that emphasizes invasiveness, nodal status, and the presence

TABLE 9-1. IRS Clinical Group Classification

Group I:
Localized disease, completely resected (regional nodes not involved: lymph node biopsy or dissection required except for head and neck lesions)
   a)Confined to muscle or organ of origin.
   b)Contiguous involvement; infiltration outside the muscle or organ of origin, as through fascial planes.

   Notation: This includes both gross inspection and *microscopic confirmation of complete resection*. Any nodes inadvertently taken with the specimen must be negative. If the latter should be involved microscopically, then the patient is placed in group IIb or c (see below).

Group II
Total gross resection with evidence of regional spread
   a)*Grossly resected tumor with microscopic residual disease*. (surgeon believes that he has removed all of the tumor, but the pathologist finds tumor at the margin of resection *and* additional resection to achieve clean margins is not feasible). No evidence of gross residual tumor. *No evidence of regional node involvement*. Once radiotherapy and/or chemotherapy have been started, reexploration and removal of the area of microscopic residual does not change the patient's group.
   b)*Regional disease with involved nodes, completely resected with no microscopic residual*

   Notation: Complete resection with microscopic confirmation of no residual disease makes this different from groups IIa and IIc. Additionally, in contrast to group IIa, regional nodes (which are completely resected, however) are involved, but the most distal node is histologically negative.
   c)*Regional disease with involved nodes, grossly resected, but with evidence of microscopic residual and/or histologic involvement of the most distal regional node (from the primary site) in the dissection*

   Notation: The presence of microscopic residual disease makes this group different from group IIb, and nodal involvement makes this group different from group IIa.

Group III
Incomplete resection with gross residual disease
   a)After biopsy only.
   b)After gross or major resection of the primary tumor ($< 50\%$).

Group IV
Distant metastatic disease present at onset (lung, liver, bones, bone marrow, brain, and distant muscle and nodes)

   Notation: The above excludes *regional* nodes and adjacent organ infiltration, which places the patient in a more favorable grouping (as noted above under group II).

or absence of distant metastases [11]. Although it is similar to the UICC classification, this TNM system uses invasiveness rather than specific size criteria in determining T stage. Using a series of 74 patients accrued over a 20-year period at Stanford University, this system does have prognostic validity [12]. Currently, the IRS is studying prospectively a variety of pretreament factors that hopefully will lead to the development of valid pretreatment classification with a firm basis.

DIAGNOSTIC EVALUATION

The purpose of the diagnostic evaluation is to determine the disease extent for staging, treatment planning, and prognosis purposes. Of course, biopsy of the tumor is the definitive diagnostic procedure. The diagnostic evaluation should be carried out preoperatively and include a complete blood count, urinalysis, chest radiograph and CT scan of the chest, bone scan and skeletal survey, and CT and/or ultrasound examination of the primary lesion. CT of the head and cerebrospinal fluid (CSF) examination are indicated if intracranial or meningeal spread is suspected by complete neurologic assessment. Abnormalities of the CSF are tumor cells, increased protein, and decreased glucose.

Lymphangiography and/or CT scan are used to assess retroperitoneal lymph node spread in patients with genitourinary lesions. Sonography is preferred over CT scan for both abdominal tumors and lymph node involvement in the thin child without much retroperitoneai fat. Bone marrow examination should be done to exclude metastasis to the marrow.

Blood chemistries should include creatinine, lactic dehydrogenase (LDH), SGOT, uric acid, bilirubin, calcium, phosphorus, and alkaline phosphatase. Chromosome studies may reveal chomosomal aberrations. Cardiac status should be evaluated before using doxorubicin. Before using cis-platin, calcium and magnesium levels should be determined, and an audiologic examination should be done.

MODE OF CLINICAL PRESENTATION

The peak age incidence is between 2 and 5 years with approximately 70% of the patients under 11 years of age at the time of presentation. The initial signs and symptoms relate either to the primary tumor or to metastases. Often times the child presents with an asymptomatic mass that is detected by the patient, parent, or physician.

Paratesticular tumors usually appear as enlarging soft tissue masses that are non-painful. They are unilateral. Tumors arising in the dome or base of the bladder and prostate may produce urinary tract symptoms and hydronephrosis. In some bladder/prostate tumors it may be difficult to determine if the tumor originated in the bladder or prostate.

Botryoid-embryonal lesions typically arise beneath a mucosal surface and appear as grape-like clusters of clear polypoid tissue protruding from the cervix of the uterus. Vaginal or vulvar tumors present as enlarging soft tissue masses. Pelvic lesions not otherwise specified may reach large proportions and cause urinary tract obstruction. Tumors of the perineum may extend to involve the bowel and bladder.

Tumor margins are generally indistinct as it spreads along fascial planes into surrounding tissues. Metastases occur through lymphatic and hematogenous spread. Regional lymph node spread occurs with increased frequency in tumors of the genitourinary system. Common sites of distant metastases are lung, bone, bone marrow, lymph nodes, brain, spinal cord, heart, and breast.

DIFFERENTIAL DIAGNOSIS

The differential diagnosis depends on the primary site of tumor origin. With any intraabdominal mass the following tumors should be considered: Wilms' tumor, neuroblastoma, hepatoma, teratoma, endodermal sinus tumor, lymphoma, carcinoma, other soft tissue sarcomas, mesenteric cyst, hydronephrotic kidney, pancreatic lesions, and intestinal duplication.

Paratesticular RMS may be confused with seminoma, embryonal carcinoma, and teratoma of the testis, and it should be distinguished from lymphoma, rare tumors of the spermatic cord, and benign tumors, including hydrococele and varicocele. Tumors to be considered in the bladder include neurofibroma, hemangioma, and, rarely, transitional cell carcinoma or leiomyosarcoma. In the vagina, a benign lesion must be excluded.

MANAGEMENT

Specific management strategies will be discussed below by primary site of tumor origin. The surgical principles of management are discussed in depth in Chapter 10. The management goal is cure without any residual effects of treatment. Cure is obtainable in a majority of patients who present with localized disease. In order to achieve the maximum benefit of therapy, coordinated team approach is required. Surgery, radiation therapy, and chemotherapy must be coordinated and integrated to derive the maximum advantage of each modality. A thorough understanding of the sites of disease spread from each specific primary site is important in developing an optimal management plan.

RADIATION THERAPY

Radiation therapy is not needed in patients with clinical group I favorable histology disease [2,13]. Surgery plus chemotherapy provide adequate therapy with survival rates of approximately 90%. For all other patients, radiation is used for the primary tumor as well as for metastases, in conjunction with chemotherapy. High-energy radiation sources should be used to achieve optimal tumor control rates. Under these circumstances local tumor control can be achieved in approximately 87% of patients. If the tumor is less than 5 cm in diameter the patient should receive a total dose of 4,000–4,500 rad. If the size is 5 cm or greater, the dose should be 4,500–5,000 rad. Patients under 6 years should receive the lower doses in each category. The daily dose rate should be approximately 180 rad. It is important to protect such vital structures as the kidney, lung, liver, etc., so that normal tissue tolerance is not exceeded. Where possible, the volume of radiation to the primary site should include a 5 cm margin around the tumor.

CHEMOTHERAPY

There is ample evidence to indicate that chemotherapy should be used for all patients with RMS as it improves the survival rate. It is most effective in eradicating microscopic foci of residual disease. It may also reduce the size of bulky disease, allowing for subsequent resection of the tumor. At present, chemotherapy alone can produce a complete clinical response in 25% of patients with gross residual after surgery. The addition of radiation therapy increases the complete response rate to 67%. An additional 15% of patients will achieve a partial response. Current chemotherapy alone will achieve a partial response. Current chemotherapy alone will be curative in less than 10% of patients.

Agents active against RMS are vincristine, actinomycin D, cyclophosphamide, doxorubicin, VP-16, cis-plastin, and imidazolecarboxamide (DTIC). Other agents that look promising include ifosfamide and melphalan. Drugs of questionable benefit are high-dose methotrexate, diglycoaldehyde, dihydroandrogalacticol, F3TDR, and mitoxanthrone. Drugs clearly inactive include VM-26, cyclocytidine, vindesine, ICRF-159, and azapicyl. Patients with positive CSF cytology respond to courses of triple intrathecal chemotherapy consisting of methotrexate, hydrocortisone, and cytosine arabinoside. Intraarterial regional chemotherapy has not been adequately studied in childhood RMS.

Currently employed chemotherapy regimens include two-to-six drug combinations of vincristine, actinomycin-D, cyclophosphamide, doxorubicin, VP-16, cis-plastin, and DITC. Less intensive therapy is used for clinical groups I and II favorable histology disease than those with unfavorable histology and clinical groups III and IV disease.

In IRS-III, which began in 1984, the following strategies are being studied.

Clinical Group I Favorable Histology: cyclic-sequential courses of actinomycin D and vincristine for 1 year. No radiation is given.

Clinical Group I Unfavorable Histology: repetitive courses of pulse VadrC (vincristine, doxorubicin, cyclophosphamide) alternating with pulse VAC (substitutes actinomycin D for doxorubicin) plus cis-platin, for 1 year. Radiation is given beginning at week 6.

Clinical Group II Favorable Histology: two regimens are being compared: cyclic-sequential courses of actinomycin-D and vincristine versus the same combination with the addition of doxorubicin, both combinations given for 1 year. Radiation is given beginning at week 6.

Clinical Group II Unfavorable Histology: same regimen as for Clinical Group I Unfavorable Histology.

Clinical Group III Any Histology, Excluding Bladder, Prostate, Vagina, Uterus, Orbit, Non-parameningeal Head: three regimens are being compared: repetitive courses of pulse VAC for 2 years, second-look surgery plus salvage chemotherapy courses of doxorubicin plus DTIC for partial responders. Radiation is given beginning at week 6; versus repetitive courses of pulse VadrC-VAC plus cis-platin and VP-16, second surgery with salvage chemotherapy courses of actinomycin-D plus DITC. Radiation is given beginning at week 6.

Clinical Group III Any Histology Bladder Dome, Vagina, Uterus: repetitive pulse courses of VadrC-VAC plus cis-platin, radiation, and/or surgery if residual disease is present after initial chemotherapy courses are completed at week 20, plus salvage chemotherapy courses of actinomycin-D plus VP-16. Chemotherapy is given for 2 years.

Clinical Group III Favorable Histology Orbit and Non-parameningeal Head: same regimen as for Clinical Group II Favorable Histology.

Clinical Group IV Any Histology: same regimens as for Clinical Group II Any Histology.

Patients with Intracranial Extension or Positive CSF Cytology: add cranial radiation plus intrathecal methotrexate, hydrocortisone, and cytosine arabinoside courses for 18–24 months to the systemic chemotherapy and radiation program.

Patients with Base of the Skull Erosion and/or Cranial Nerve Palsy: add limited field meningeal radiation plus triple-drug intrathecal chemotherapy for 18 months to the systemic chemotherapy and radiation program.

Thus, new combinations being evaluated in IRS-III are doxorubicin plus cis-platin, doxorubicin plus cis-platin plus VP-16; doxorubicin plus DTIC; single dose actinomycin-D plus DTIC; and single dose actinomycin-D plus

VP-16. The drug combinations used in IRS-III are associated with mild to severe toxicities and should be used only by experienced physicians.

Ifosfamide, given with mesna to prevent bladder toxicity, is being used in clinical trials in Europe as a substitute for cyclophosphamide. It is not known whether it improves survival. Ifosfamide in combination with VP-16 is being studied in the United States in relapsed patients.

Autologous bone marrow transplantation is being studied in poor risk clinical group IV patients. Patients must be in complete remission status before it is considered. Hemi-body or total-body radiation is given prior to transplantation. The results thus far in the few patients so treated are not encouraging.

SPECIFIC GENITOURINARY SITES

Paratesticular Lesions

Seven percent of all patients under age 21 years entered on IRS-I had primary tumors of the paratesticular region [14]. RMS of the spermatic cord and paratesticular tissues spreads by lymphatic routes to the paraaortic lymph nodes, following the course of the spermatic cord into the retroperitoneal space. Retroperitoneal lymph node involvement is seen in 28–40% of patients at diagnosis [14,15].

Ninety-six patients with paratesticular tumors were entered on IRS-I and II between 1972–1983. The median age was 11 years and age ranged from 11 months to 19 years. The median age by clinical group was 5 years for I, 14 years for II, and 15 years for III and IV. Seventy-five percent of the patients were white and 25% black. Fifty-four percent of the tumors arose on the right side of the body and the rest on the left. In over 95% of patients the histology was either totally embryonal or an admixture with botryoid elements. The tumor diameter as measured by the institutional pathologist ranged from 2–19 cm with a median of 5 cm. The distribution of these patients by clinical group was I, 59%; II, 21%; III, 4%; IV, 16%. Sites of metastases in clinical group IV patients were lung, bone marrow, bone, omentum, pleura, mesentery, and retroperitoneum.

Studies in France would tend to encourage the use of bipedal lymphangiography and to discourage retroperitoneal exploration and radiation therapy in the absence of enlarged or abnormal nodes as visualized on radiographic studies [16]. These data are limited, however, and even the larger series of patients in the IRS do not definitively address the reliability of radiographic or ultrasonographic staging procedures.

The survival rates for paratesticular RMS are excellent with the IRS recommended treatments. At 2 years, 91% of clinical group I, 88% of clinical group II, and 50% of clinical groups III and IV patients are alive and continuously free of disease. The disease-free survival rate for all groups taken together is 82% at 2 years. The recommended approach for management of the patient with a solid testicular or paratesticular mass is radical orchidectomy with high ligation of the spermatic cord. Transcrotal biopsy should not be performed. Inguinal lymphadenectomy is indicated only if there are enlarged nodes or scrotal contamination by tumor. Retroperitoneal lymph nodes can be evaluated by any or all of the imaging techniques, but there is currently no substitute for laparotomy with exploration of the retroperitoneum. Ipsilateral retroperitoneal lymph node dissection is the best way to determine whether tumor has spread beyond the local site. Other studies enumerated above should also be obtained to determine whether metastases are present.

Subsequent treatment should be guided by the clinical group of disease. Multi-agent chemotherapy should be instituted for all patients using agents described previously. Radiation therapy is reserved for patients in clinical groups II–IV and would be directed to the scrotum only when tumor contamination is documented. Radiation should be directed to the retroperitoneal nodes if they are found to contain tumor. Cure is now achievable in a large majority of patients with paratesticular lesions. Thus, accurate staging is important. The late effects of treatment in long-term survivors are being studied.

Bladder and Prostate Lesions

Approximately 5% of patients registered on the IRS studies have primary lesions of the bladder. Lesions tend to arise either in the trigone area, dome, multiple sites, or diffusely involve the bladder. These patients present with urinary tract symptoms and/or an enlarging abdominal mass. The mean age at diagnosis among males is 4.5 years, among female patients is 6.4 years. The embryonal cell type is the most common form occurring in this organ.

Primary lesions of the prostate account for 5% of the patients entered on the IRS studies. The mean age at diagnosis is 5.1 years and the predominant cell type is embryonal. In some cases it is difficult to determine whether the tumor arises in the bladder, prostate, or both.

Before effective chemotherapy was available, the treatment of bladder RMS by limited surgery, such as partial cystectomy or simple excision of the tumor, was followed by local recurrence and early development of metastases [17]. The survival rates following exenterative procedures alone were low (10–40%). Following surgery alone or surgery and local radiation, there were only a few long-term survivors of prostatic RMS, which was regarded as almost always fatal. When VAC chemotherapy was added to radiation after the exenterative procedures, rates of survival were comparable or even superior to those in RMS in other sites. For patients with primary bladder tumors entered on IRS-I, the relapse rate was 2 of 11 following pelvic exenteration (anterior, 10; total, 1); 5 of 12 following partial cystectomy or gross tumor excision; and 3 of 5 following a primary chemotherapy-radiotherapy program [17]. In patients with prostatic tumors (clinical groups I-III), relapse occurred in none of 14 patients treated by pelvic exenterations (anterior, 12; total, 2) and in 2 of 11 patients treated by a primary chemotherapy-radiotherapy program. All patients with bladder and prostate tumors received chemotherapy for 1–2 years, and other than clinical group I patients, half of whom were randomized to no radiation, all patients received postoperative radiation. The overall bladder salvage rate was 39% and the overall survival rate at 3 years approximately 70%.

In IRS-II (1978–1984) patients with primary tumors localized to the bladder, prostate, vagina, or uterus were treated with a primary chemotherapy-radiation regimen [18]. The initial management, following biopsy, consisted of monthly courses of pulse VAC chemotherapy. Radiation therapy was usually deferred until it was demonstrated that a complete response had not been achieved, or for the treatment of relapse. Surgery was employed for failure to respond or as a salvage procedure after relapse. There were 36 patients with prostatic tumors and 29 patients (17 males, 12 females) with bladder tumors followed for 1–7 years from the start of treatment. The overall survival rate was 75%. Relapses were more commonly local than distant. The bladder salvage rate was approximately 50%. Only 10% of the patients have remained on chemotherapy alone and not relapsed. All others have required the addition of radiation and/or surgery to achieve complete and sustained responses. Partial cystectomy following initial chemotherapy has been effective, but opportunities for its use are limited. The utility of prostatectomy remains uncertain. Anterior exenteration is an effective salvage procedure following any prior sequence of therapy.

The treatment program for these lesions in patients registered on IRS-III is outlined above in the section on chemotherapy. In order to try to improve survival and bladder salvage rates, more intensive chemotherapy is given for 2 years. Second and third operations to assess response and remove residual disease are included, as is salvage-chemotherapy for partial responders. Radiation therapy is given to all patients with lesions of the bladder trigone and prostate beginning at week 6, since these patients all required it eventually in IRS-II. Lesions of the dome of the bladder receive radiation only if complete response has not been achieved with the intense chemotherapy. The results of this study are not yet known.

Vagina and Uterus Lesions

Tumors of the vagina and uterus accounted for 2 and 1%, respectively, of the patients entered on the IRS. Patients may present with vaginal bleeding or discharge, the passage of tumor fragments or gross tumor protrusion. "Benign" lesions of the vagina or cervix may be confused with RMS. Occasionally, patients are treated for vaginal "polyps" by fulguration before the definitive diagnosis is made. Patients also may present with a palpable abdominopelvic mass, which may extend to the level of the umbilicus. Almost all vaginal tumors are embryonal or embryonal-botryoid histology. Uterine tumors, in addition to these cell types, sometimes show small cell sarcoma without distinguishing features.

From IRS reports, it appears that primary tumors of the vagina and uterus are two distinct groups, distinguished from each other by patient age range and prognosis as well as site [19]. The mean age of patients with vaginal tumor was 1.8 years (0–72 months) and those with uterine tumors 14.2 years (4–20 years). The distinction between vaginal and uterine sites were made by pretherapy vaginoscopy and laparotomy findings, or posttherapy vaginoscopy of remnant tumor sites or surgical procedures, or histologic studies of the specimens removed at any time.

The specific concepts of surgical management of these tumors are discussed elsewhere in this book. Primary exenteration for a vaginal tumor is no longer required to acquire cure. Primary multi-agent chemotherapy followed by total or partial vaginectomy and/or interstitial or external beam radiation therapy comprise effective therapy. Local control can be achieved in over 75% of patients treated in this manner. The overall survival rate in the IRS for localized vaginal lesions exceeded 90%.

Patients with uterine tumors described as cervical or uterine "polyps" with a stalk may be treated by simple excision of the polyp, including its base, and multi-agent chemotherapy. The primary chemotherapy-radiation therapy approach is not as effective for uterine primary tumors as it is in patients with vaginal lesions. In the IRS-I and II, three of eight patients treated relapsed and died. More intensive chemotherapy is being tried in IRS-III. Initial tumor excision, followed by chemotherapy, may be more effective in this group of patients.

REFERENCES

1. Young JL, Miller RW: Incidence of malignant tumors in U.S. children. J. Pediatr 86:254, 1975.
2. Maurer HM, Moon T, Donaldson M: The intergroup rhabdomyosarcoma study: A preliminary report. Cancer 40:2015, 1977.

3. Maurer HM: Rhabdomyosarcoma in childhood and adolescence. Curr Probl Cancer 2:, 1978, pp 1–36.
4. Li FP, Fraumeni JF: Soft tissue sarcomas, breast cancer, and other neoplasms: A familiar syndrome. Ann Intern Med 71:747, 1969.
5. Grufferman S, Wang HH, DeLong ER, et al.: Environmental factors in the etiology of childhood rhabdomyosarcoma. JNCI 68:107, 1982.
6. Ruymann FB, Maddux HR, Ragab A, et al.: Congenital anomalies associated with rhabdomyosarcoma. Med & Pediatr Oncol (in press).
7. Koufos A, Hansen M, Copeland NG, et al.: Loss of heterozygosity in three embryonal tumors suggests a common pathogenetic mechanism. Nature 316:330, 1985.
8. Palmer N, Foulkes M: Histopathy and prognosis in the second intergroup rhabdomyosarcoma study. Proc Am Soc Clin Oncol 2:229, 1983.
9. Harmer MH (ed): TNM classification of paediatric tumors. In Geneva International Union Against Cancer, Geneva: Imprimerìe de Buren S.A., 1982, pp 23–28.
10. Lawrence W, Hays DM, Beltangady M, et al.: Prognostic significance of staging factors of the UICC staging system in childhood rhabdomyosarcoma: A report from the intergroup rhabdomyosarcoma study-II. J Clin Oncol 5:46, 1987.
11. Donaldson SS, Belli JA: A rational clinical staging system for childhood rhabdomyosarcoma. J Clin Oncol 2:135, 1984.
12. Pedrick TJ, Donaldson SS, Cox RS: Rhabdomyosarcoma: The Standford experience using a TNM staging system. J Clin Oncol 4:370, 1986.
13. Maurer HM, Donaldson M, Gehan EA, et al.: The intergroup rhabdomyosarcoma study: Update, November, 1978. Natl Cancer Inst Monogr 56:61, 1981.
14. Raney RB, Hays D, Lawrence W, et al.: Paratesticular rhabdomyosarcoma in childhood. Cancer 42:729, 1978.
15. Raney RB, Tefft M, Lawrence W, et al.: Paratesticular sarcoma in childhood and adolescence. A report from the intergroup rhabdomyosarcoma studies I and II, 1972, 1983. Cancer (in press).
16. Olive D, Flamant F, Zucker JM, et al: Para-aortic lymphadenectomy is not necessary in the treatment of localized paratesticular rhabdomyosarcoma. Cancer 54:1283, 1984.
17. Hays DM, Raney RB, Lawrence W, et al.: Bladder and prostatic tumors in the intergroup rhabdomyosarcoma study (IRS-I). Cancer 50:1472, 1982.
18. Raney RB, Hays DM, Tefft M, et al.: Primary chemotherapy with or without radiation therapy, surgery, or both for children with localized sarcoma of the bladder, prostate, or vagina-uterus: Results of the intergroup rhabdomyosarcoma study-II. J Clin Oncol (submitted).
19. Hays DM, Shimada H, Raney RB, et al.: Sarcomas of the vagina and uterus: The intergroup rhabdomyosarcoma study. J Pediatr Surg 20:718, 1985.

Chapter 10
Rhabdomyosarcoma—Surgical Aspects

Walter Lawrence, Jr., and Bruce H. Broecker

Soft tissue sarcomas in infants and children are unusual tumors, as noted in Chapter 9. The most frequent histologic type of these sarcomas is rhabdomyosarcoma (RMS), accounting for approximately half of all sarcomas in childhood. In recent years a great deal of interest has centered on the marked improvement in disease control of RMS that has resulted from the combined modality treatment approach outlined in the chapter on medical aspects of this disease. As the data from the Intergroup Rhabdomyosarcoma Study (IRS) have shown, however, for optimal results operation is still required when feasible as part of the treatment plan for most primary sites (an exception is RMS arising in the orbit) [1]. This is true for those lesions arising in the genitourinary sites, which comprise 21% of the total series of patients in the first two IRS studies (I and II) carried out between 1972 and 1984. Next to primary sites in the head and neck (38% of this IRS series), genitourinary sites are the most frequent primary sites for this disease.

CLINICAL ASPECTS OF GENITOURINARY RMS

The genitourinary sites of origin for childhood RMS include paratesticular lesions and lesions arising in the bladder, prostate, vagina and uterus. Histological variations of childhood RMS do occur with embryonal tumors (including sarcoma botryoides) being the most common, as well as the most favorable prognostic histologic type. A less common histologic variety is alveolar rhabdomyosarcoma, a type also appearing to have a less desirable prognosis than embryonal rhabdomyosarcoma (Fig. 10-1) [2]. For the geni-

Pediatric Tumors of the Genitourinary Tract, pages 153–176
© 1988 Alan R. Liss, Inc.

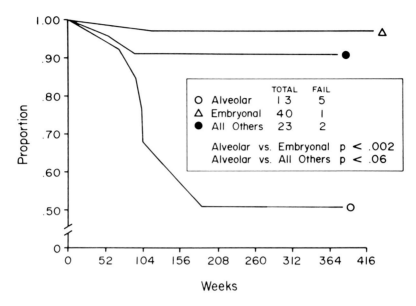

Fig. 10-1. Influence of alveolar histology of RMS on mortality in patients in IRS-I with localized and completely resectable tumors (from Reference 2).

tourinary primary sites under consideration, however, the overwhelming majority of lesions are embryonal, the alveolar type occurring in only 4% of cases. Since histologic type appears to have an influence on outcome (this is not firmly established), the genitourinary sites appear favored by the predominance of embryonal histology.

Paratesticular RMS

The clinical presentation of paratesticular rhabdomyosarcoma is similar to that of primary testicular neoplasms occurring in older patients [3,4]. The usual presenting symtom is the presence of a painless enlargement of the testis or paratesticular mass in the scrotum. The median age for patients with paratesticular lesions in the IRS was 11 years (range 11 months to 19 years), this age level being higher than that seen in children with primary epithelial (germ cell) testicular neoplasms.

General physical examination and standard radiologic studies may reveal hematogenous metastatic disease in some patients (15 of 96 patients in the IRS series 1973–1983), but the regional lymph nodes for this primary site are retroperitoneal and enlarged nodes are rarely detected on physical examination. It should be stressed that the inguinal lymph nodes are not the regional lymphatic drainage for paratesticular rhabdomyosarcoma unless there is tumor invasion of the scrotum itself. This is quite rare in these patients at the time of initial presentation. Although the incidence of proven lymphatic spread for the overall series of children with rhabdomyosarcoma in IRS-I and II was 10%, paratesticular lesions in this combined series had a 32% frequency of histologically proven lymphatic spread [5,6]. This makes lymph node assessment a factor of major importance in the staging of rhabdomyosarcoma arising in this site. Computerized tomography is more accurate than clinical examination in detecting retroperitoneal node spread from paratesticular lesions and is advocated by some as sufficient for accurate staging. However, false positive and false negative results occur, and determining the presence or absence of lymphatic metastasis is best accomplished by surgical exploration with unilateral dissection of the retroperitoneal lymph nodes.

Bladder and Prostatic RMS

Bladder RMS may present as a large lower abdominal or pelvic mass and/ or with symptoms or signs of urinary tract obstruction [7]. Hematuria, fever, constipation, the passage of urinary tumor fragments, rectal prolapse, or subacute intestinal obstruction may be other presenting symptoms and signs. In a few patients with bladder primary lesions, the tumor is relatively small and restricted to the area of the dome of the bladder. Prostatic lesions in males often present in a fashion similar to that of primary bladder RMS, and it may be difficult to distinguish the actual primary site. Others may present as a perineal mass (Fig. 10-2).

Histologically proven lymph node metastases with the primary bladder and prostate lesions occur in 10% of patients, a frequency similar to that seen in the entire IRS series [6]. However, efforts to determine the presence or absence of regional lymphatic spread in the IRS for the bladder-prostate sites has been less vigorous than for other anatomic sites due to the frequent use of non-surgical therapies as the initial treatment for these lesions.

Sarcomas of the Vagina and Uterus

Sarcomas arising from the vagina or uterus are less frequent than bladder and prostatic sites [8], only 43 patients being entered in the IRS studies between 1972 and 1984. Thirty-one patients in this series had primary lesions that were vaginal in origin and 12 originated in the uterus (including the cervix). It appears that primary tumors of the uterus are a distinct entity that can be distinguished from primary vaginal tumors by both patient age range (mean age 14 years for uterine lesions and 1.8 years for vaginal tumors) as well as prognosis.

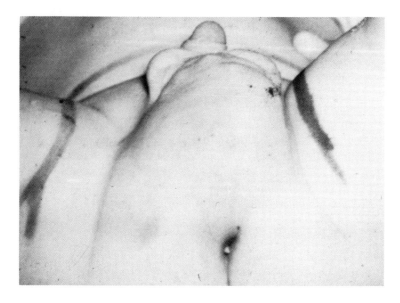

Fig. 10-2. Prostatic RMS presenting as a perineal mass.

The presenting symptoms and signs of these lesions are vaginal bleeding or discharge, the passage of tumor fragments, or gross tumor protrusion. They may appear as an edematous-appearing polypoid mass or masses at the introitus, a form of RMS known as sarcoma botryoides (Fig. 10-3). Some patients, particularly those presenting with uterine lesions, have a palpable abdominal pelvic mass at the time of initial diagnosis. Distant metastases at the time of presentation are uncommon (four of these 43 patients had disseminated disease at diagnosis) as are proven lymphatic metastases.

STAGING OF CHILDHOOD RMS—SURGICAL ASPECTS

Since the optimal treatment plan for childhood RMS involving genitourinary sites is affected by the stage of the disease at the time of diagnosis [9], a number of clinical, laboratory, and radiographic examinations are required prior to treatment (Fig. 10-4). The presence or absence of lymphatic spread is also an important factor for operative planning. Enlargement of regional lymph nodes may be appreciated on physical examination, but lymphatic spread for genitourinary sites is often more thoroughly assessed by CT examination. Histologic assessment of regional lymph nodes can be carried out most accurately for paratesticular sites by unilateral or modified unilateral

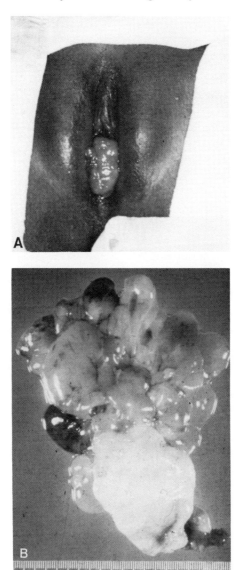

Fig. 10-3. Childhood RMS arising from vagina and presenting at introitus (A) as sarcoma botryoides (B).

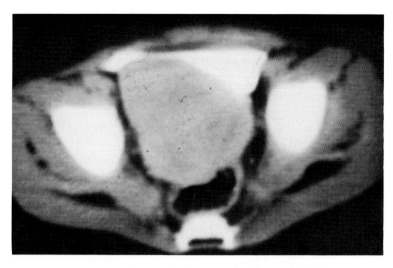

Fig. 10-4. Computerized tomography of prostatic RMS.

retroperitoneal lymph node disection. The increased frequency of lymphatic spread that has been noted for this primary site appears to warrant this approach even if clinical and radiologic studies fail to demonstrate obvious lymph node enlargement. Patients with primary lesions in the bladder, prostate, vagina, or uterus have relatively inaccessible regional lymph nodes, and pathologic evaluation of lymph nodes in these patients is usually deferred until later operative intervention since non-surgical therapies now constitute the initial treatment in most instances. Regional lymph node evaluation by biopsy is indicated in this group of patients if abdominal exploration is required for establishing the diagnosis prior to the treatment program. Diagnosis of the primary lesion is often established by less agressive operative intervention, however. When non-operative therapy is the initial treatment employed, later operation is recommended, as will be described, and regional lymphatic evaluation is accomplished at that time.

SURGICAL APPROACH TO GENITOURINARY SITES

Until the development of reasonably effective systemic chemotherapy programs for childhood RMS in the early 1960s, treatment of this disease was purely surgical unless resection was not feasible. Unfortunately, less than half the patients with childhood RMS were grossly resectable. Radiation therapy was employed in those patients who were not resectable or when there was dissatisfaction with the surgical margins of the operative resection. Under these circumstances, it became a standard of care to carry out pelvic exenteration for most patients with RMS in pelvic sites. This same principle of radical resection was applied to other anatomic sites where possible, but the overall results of therapy were not good. End results in this era of routine radical surgical resection for all anatomic primary sites (with or without radiation) were depressing. No more than a quarter of the patients undergoing resection experienced long-term control [10]. The real breakthrough in this struggle was the development of effective chemotherapy.

The striking improvement in cure rates associated with effective chemotherapy programs after surgical resection of childhood RMS led to the hope that surgery might not be necessary for many sites where resection produces major disability. It also led to the hope that the problem of incomplete resection by "debulking" could be effectively dealt with by subsequent chemotherapy programs. Data from the IRS have clearly shown, however, that end results of treatment are clearly inferior if complete gross resection of the primary lesion is not accomplished before or after the chemotherapy (the only exception to this concept is the orbital primary group) [1]. This establishes the continued importance of surgical resection, when feasible, for childhood RMS.

The approach of debulking cancers by partial resection has received considerable attention in clinical situations where the neoplasm is responsive to available chemotherapeutic agents. Appealing as this concept is in situations where there is only microscopic residual of a tumor after resection, it is unlikely that partial gross resection has any benefit for patients with childhood RMS. The procedure might even be deleterious for the patient with a lesion that is not grossly resectable since the debulking operative procedure would delay or interfere with the administration of effective nonoperative therapies. For the genitourinary sites of RMS, total gross resection of existing disease is the goal whether operation precedes or follows non-operative treatment. Since the approach to specific anatomic sites differs greatly, in terms of surgical management, they will be considered separately.

Paratesticular Mass

A solid mass adjacent to the testis or spermatic cord should be resected by inginal orchiectomy with complete resection of the spermatic cord structures to the level of the internal ring. Resection of scrotal skin is not necessary except for patients with fixation to, or involvement of the scrotal skin by the neoplasm, or unless a prior transscrotal approach for biopsy or resection has been employed. The optimal surgical approach described for both diagnosis and initial treatment of the primary site is the same as for primary epithelial tumors of the testis in adults [3,4].Unilateral retroperitoneal node dissection is, in our opinion, indicated for all patients with paratesticular sarcomas due to the frequency of lymphatic spread with this primary site and the difficulty in determining the presence or absence of lymphatic spread without such a dissection. There is not agreement on this point, and some investigators rely on lymphangiography and computed tomography as means for selecting patients for dissection [11].

The recommended approach for dissection is that of transabdominal unilateral resection of the spermatic vessels and associated node-bearing tissue along the iliac and spermatic vessels, and the aorta or vena cava from the internal ring to the level of the renal vein (Fig. 10-5) [12]. The unilateral retroperitoneal dissection of the paraaortic or perivena caval area on the side of the lesion and the intraaortocaval area stops at the lateral side of the great vessel on the contralateral side. Both renal hilar areas can be included in a modification of this unilateral dissection that deals with the concern of "cross metastasis," but this extension should not proceed caudad any further than the origin of the inferior mesenteric artery. Some surgeons favor complete bilateral retroperitoneal lymph node dissection because of crossed metastases

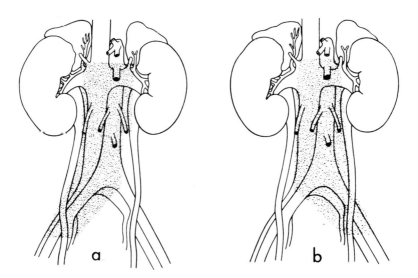

Fig. 10-5. Diagram of extent of lymph node resection with retroperitoneal lymphadenectomy for right (a) and left (b) paratesticular RMS.

[13], but this dissection has the disadvantage of the significant sequellae of bilateral sympathetic nerve resection (L1–L3) including ejaculatory impotence.

The "top" node or nodes of the dissection should be marked for special study by the pathologist as this aids in the subsequent surgical-pathological classification of the patient. In the IRS, metastatic involvement of the top node or nodes is classified as an indication of histologic involvement of the surgical margin even though all grossly detected regional lymph nodes are removed. As noted, ipsilateral inguinal lymph nodes are not a site of regional spread for patients with paratesticular RMS unless there is actually scrotal involvement, and inguinal node dissection is not indicated except under unusual circumstances.

After completion of the surgical treatment and staging procedures described for paratesticular RMS, the remainder of the treatment plan can be developed. As noted in Chapter 9, it has been considered advisable to supplement the regional operative treatment with radiation therapy, if scrotal involvement or regional lymph node spread is identified, but data from IRS-I have shown that radiation therapy is not necessary if these adverse factors have not been identified on pathological study. Systemic chemotherapy is uniformly employed, as indicated elsewhere, as this has contributed significantly to the improved prognosis that has occurred since these drug programs have been established.

In patients in whom it has been determined that postoperative regional irradiation is indicated, the contralateral testis can be transposed into a subcutaneous pocket in the ipsilateral thigh prior to this radiation. The testis is then replaced in scrotum after therapy has been completed.

The optimal initial treatment of paratesticular RMS is surgical, as described, with non-surgical therapy (chemotherapy with or without radiation) following this. However, a problem the surgeon may be faced with is a patient who has already had the diagnosis made by excision of the primary mass with histologic study showing involvement of the surgical margin at the point of transection of the spermatic cord. If the cord has been transected high in the inguinal canal, secondary resection as used for most anatomic sites is probably not feasible. In this instance, radiation therapy is required. With involvement of the margin of transection when this site is more distal, re-resection to obtain a clear margin (including hemiscrotectomy) should be considered rather than relying completely on radiation for local control.

Another surgical problem is the patient who has had an inappropriate transcrotal biopsy of a paratesticular mass proving to be RMS. When a sarcoma has been biopsied in this fashion, reoperation, including excision of the prior operative site (including hemiscrotectomy) and spermatic cord structures (to the inguinal ring) is an appropriate approach.

Surgical Management of Prostatic, Bladder, and Female Genital Sites

In IRS-I, most patients were treated initially by as complete a surgical resection as was required to totally remove the primary sarcoma (if distant metastasis was not present) [7]. For the majority of these patients, this required partial or total pelvic exenteration to achieve total removal. Because of the presence of three pelvic organs in the female, it was easier in these patients than in males to spare the bladder, in patients with posteriorly placed lesions, or the rectum, in those with anteriorly placed lesions. With the postoperative chemotherapy programs described, such radical pelvic surgery led to an excellent prognosis, but also considerable morbidy and long-term disability, particularly when total cystectomy was required.

Limited "pilot" experience in IRS-I with initial non-operative therapy followed by surgical resection, rather than initial radical resection, has led to some hope for reduced morbidity by preserving the bladder in some patients. Additional experience with primary chemotherapy for this group of lesions in IRS-II has demonstrated the worth of this approach from the standpoint of reduced treatment-associated disability [14].

At the time of clinical presentation of RMS in these special pelvic sites (bladder, prostate, and female genital tract), some form of biopsy diagnosis must be established prior to initiating the non-operative therapy that has become the standard. For primary sites in the bladder or vagina, this can be accomplished by standard biopsy techniques, either using endoscopy when feasible or laparotomy, with or without cystotomy. For patients with primary prostatic RMS, core needle biopsy can be employed, but it is usually wise to obtain several cores in order to obtain sufficient pathologic material for accurate histologic study If urinary tract obstruction is present at the time of initial clinical presentation, appropriate catheters should be employed in the bladder and/or ureter to allow control of this problem prior to the initiation of the presurgical chemotherapy program. The frequent rapid resolution of this obstruction soon after primary chemotherapy is initiated tends to encourage the use of simple intubated approaches rather than formal, non-intubated operative urinary diversion.

The purpose of an initial non-operative therapy program for this group of lesions was, hopefully, to limit the morbidity from initial radical surgery, specifically pelvic exenteration. A clinical trial was initiated in IRS-II using the primary chemotherapy approach. Careful imaging studies were employed to fully assess the extent of the primary sarcoma and to provide a baseline for evaluation of response to the chemotherapy program. Intravenous urograms, cystograms, colon contrast studies, proctosigmoidoscopy, and cystoscopy also proved helpful in this assessment. The plan that has evolved for this group of pelvic lesions is careful periodic assessment of the response to chemotherapy, with a subsequent evaluation laparotomy if it is unclear whether residual tumor is present or not. Plans for subsequent therapy are based on the findings from this operative examination and pathologic study. There is no purpose served by this approach if there is obvious residual disease *unless* it is conceivable that it can be totally resected.

It is now recommended that this evaluation laparotomy be carried out approximately 20 weeks following the initiation of the chemotherapy program, unless progression of disease is clinically apparent prior to this time. Progression would lead to earlier operation. Endoscopic procedures to evaluate response may be performed under the same anesthetic as the laparotomy. At a minimum, this operative procedure should include: 1) examination of all intraabdominal structures, 2) evaluation by biopsy of the pelvic and paraaortic lymph nodes, and 3) cystotomy for bladder or prostate lesions with biopsy of the previously involved site. If the site of origin of the prior tumor mass can be totally excised without performing exenteration, such excision should be carried out at this time. Even if the regression of the sarcoma has been grossly incomplete (partial response or PR), any indicated surgical resection less radical than pelvic exenteration should be performed at this time. This might include partial cystectomy with or without ureteral implantation for bladder tumors. For prostatic tumors, this might consist of simple prostatectomy or even a simple excision of prostatic nodules or masses. For vaginal-uterine lesions, it might include hysterectomy and/or partial or total vaginectomy. For distal vaginal lesions it might actually be possible to resect the tumor and retain the uterus. Oophorectomy is not indicated unless there is gross ovarian involvement. The purpose of this resection, if accomplished, is total removal of remaining tumor tissue without a disabling resection of normal structures.

When the procedures described above are successful in removing the remaining gross tumor mass, but "microscopic residual" remains on pathologic study, a secondary operative procedure should be seriously considered for removing the residue. In many patients, this is not feasible. In patients with either microscopic involvement of the surgical margin, or histologically positive regional lymph nodes, local irradiation should follow this limited operation in patients with primary lesions of the vagina, uterus, and dome of the bladder. In patients found to have an extent of tumor for which none of the above operative procedures is feasible, postoperative radiation therapy should be employed in most instances, rather than embarking on pelvic exenteration at this time.

For those non-resected patients in whom postoperative radiation is required for reasons mentioned above, a second evaluation laparotomy should be employed after the additional radiation therapy is administered (approximately 28 weeks). If the more limited resectional procedures described for the first evaluation laparotomy are feasible at this time, they should be accomplished, but "salvage exenteration" of some type is appropriate if this is the approach required to remove all persistent disease. Pelvic exenteration as a salvage procedure, because of progressive or persistent disease, is probably more efficacious than consideration of a secondary chemotherapy program. However, for patients with persistent lesions of the vagina or uterus, or possibly dome of the bladder, an additional intensive chemotherapy program between the 28th and 34th week can be considered before proceeding with a more extensive and disabling resection of residual disease.

Utilizing the approaches outlined and avoiding radical surgical excision as the initial therapy has not been uniformly successful in eliminating the need for subsequent total cystectomy or pelvic exenteration [14]. For patients with primary sarcomas of the bladder or prostate in IRS-II, 32% of 65 patients did retain functional bladders without significant reduction in the survival rates achieved in IRS-I by initial radical surgery. These results with primary chemotherapy with or without radiadion are somewhat disappointing, but the management approach outlined has reduced the morbidity of surgical resection to some degree. The results of this sequence of therapy for primary lesions arising in the vagina have been impressive in that all patients treated by this schedule avoided total cystectomy or complete pelvic exenteration, and there was only one tumor-related death among 24 evaluable patients [8]. In a smaller group of ten evaluable patients with primary uterine tumors, four died secondary to tumor relapse or progession, but none of these patients following this schedule subsequently underwent radical exenterative surgery. These treatment failures were due to both local extension and disseminated disease. It is apparent that the primary chemotherapy-radiotherapy approach is not effective with primary RMS of the uterus as it is in patients with vaginal primary lesions. Initial excision of the tumor, followed by a chemotherapy regimen, may be a more suitable approach for these uterine lesions based on the findings in the IRS.

Surgery for Local Recurrence and/or Metatastic Disease

Local treatment failure without distant disease after surgical resection and chemotherapy (with and without radiotherapy) has not been a common occurrence for most RMS sites. However, persistent local disease is not an infrequent problem in the group with pelvic sites treated initially by non-operative means. Pelvic exenteration can be an effective salvage procedure in this latter situation, as has been noted, but surgery has a smaller role to play in the management of later local recurrence after definitive surgical resection of RMS in this as well as most other anatomic sites. Aggressive chemotherapy with or without radiotherapy is an appropriate alternative approach to management, but this is not often effective either.

Distant metastatic disease in children with RMS is best managed by non-operative means in most instances, although resection is sometimes feasible, particularly in pulmonary sites. These treatment failures are generally associated with a short survival time despite the striking impact of non-surgical treatments on the initial treatment program.

DIVERSIONARY AND RECONSTRUCTIVE PROCEDURES FOLLOWING RESECTION IN RMS PATIENTS

As stated above, a goal of contemporary treatment of pelvic RMS from genitourinary sites is cure without resorting to exenterative surgery. While it is now apparent that some patients may achieve this goal, it is also clear that many patients cannot be cured without partial or total pelvic exenteration. This fact is of particular significance when the organ involved is the bladder or prostate where removal leads to significant morbidity. To emphasize this point the results of treatment of 33 patients with bladder neck or prostate primaries in IRS-II revealed ten patients alive with an intact bladder, three patients alive following partial cystectomy, 12 patients alive following anterior exenteration, and eight patients dead or with metastatic relapse. Only two patients were successfully treated with chemotherapy alone [15]. Thus, many children with pelvic RMS will require diversionary or reconstructive procedures of the urinary tract as part of their surgical management. The following section outlines the currently available procedures for these situations.

Reconstruction Following Limited Surgical Resection

Tumors restricted to the fundus or dome of the bladder may generally be removed with minimal impairment of bladder function. Following partial cystectomy the normal bladder gradually expands until it resumes a normal capacity. However, when high dose radiotherapy has been employed, sufficient fibrosis may result, leaving the bladder functionally contracted, non-complaint, and unable to expand following partial cystectomy. Chemotherapy alone will not produce this effect. In the patient who is left with a small contracted bladder following initial treatment, augmentation of bladder capacity may be accomplished using an intestinal segment. Techniques of bladder augmentation, pioneered by Hendren, have evolved from reconstruction of those children with congenital urologic malformations and congenital neuropathic bladders who had formerly been managed with temporary or "permanent" cutaneous urinary diversion [16]. Small and large bowel are both useful for this purpose though large bowel will tend to have more mucus production and uninhibited high pressure tonic contractions than small bowel [17,18]. With either type of segment, a sufficient length of bowel is carefully isolated on its vascular pedicle, opened along its antimesenteric border, rotated 90°, and approximated to the open bladder as a cap (Fig. 10-6). It is important to remember that if the bladder has been irradiated (as will generally be the case), healing will be impaired. A two layer anastomosis using absorbable suture, prolonged catheter drainage during healing, and a cystogram prior to catheter removal to confirm healing are recommended.

Occasionally, tumor resection may encompass the trigonal area unilaterally. While the features of the above discussion may also apply to this situation, one must additionally deal with the ureter that has been detached from the bladder. This may be accomplished either with transureteroureterostomy or psoas hitch ureteroneocystostomy.

Five of 33 patients in IRS-II with prostate primaries were treated surgically by radical prostatectomy with preservation of the bladder. The technique is similar to that described for localized adult prostatic carcinoma and will not be described here. The morbidity of this procedure is chiefly related to removal of the bladder neck sphincteric continence mechanism and destruction of the nervi erigentes essential for normal erectile function. Continence following this procedure depends on successful construction of an internal sphincter from a tubularized flap of anterior detrusor muscle as well as normal function of the striated muscle of the pelvic diaphragm (external sphincter). Urinary incontinence rates following this procedure in adults range from 2 to 57% [19–25]. Impotence, formerly occurring in virtually 100% of patients following standard radical prostatectomy, is now reported to occur in only 30% of adults with the nerve-sparing radical prostatectomy described by Walsh [26]. This procedure has not yet been adapted for the pediatric patient with prostatic RMS.

Urinary Diversion and Reconstruction Following Exenteration

As demonstrated by IRS-II data, many patients with prostatic primaries are curable with anterior exenteration as the surgical arm of multimodel therapy

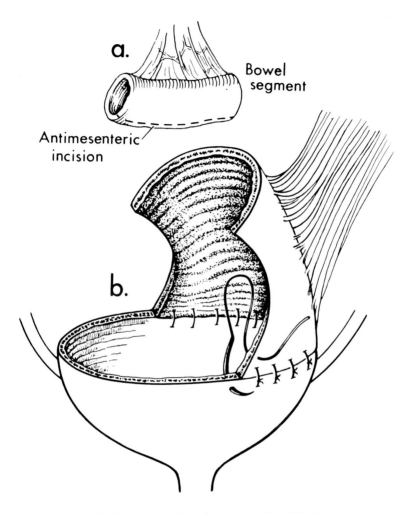

Fig. 10-6. Patch enterocystoplasty for augmentation of bladder capacity.

[15]. There may also be a small number of patients who are cured of a pelvic primary by chemotherapy and radiotherapy alone, but subsequently develop a contracted, functionally useless bladder and can be managed successfully only with cystectomy. These patients will then need a diversionary or reconstructive procedure to rehabilitate their urinary tract. Those patients with heavily irradiated pelves are probably better served by urinary diversion

(using less irradiated bowel from the upper abdomen) than by bladder reconstruction.

Urinary Diversion

Changing the flow of urine from its normal collection and expulsion by the bladder to cutaneous stomal drainage may be classified as either continent or incontinent urinary diversion. Incontinent stomas requiring a collection bag are historically more established, but recent years have brought a surge of interest in developing continent diversions in which a cutaneous stoma may be intermittently catheterized to drain urine from a surgically constructed reservoir. This has significant aesthetic appeal to the patient and has spawned a number of innovative and sometimes challenging surgical procedures. Although long term followup, a particularly important consideration with regard to pediatric diversionary procedures, is lacking with most of the continent forms of diversion, they offer the promise of an improved quality of life for those patients in whom cystectomy is necessary for survival.

Incontinent Urinary Diversion

The permanent forms of incontinent urinary diversion include the ileal conduit, colon conduit, and ileocecal conduit.

Ileal conduit.   Although ureterointestinal cutaneous diversion was described as early as 1908 by Verhoogen [27], the early half of the 20th century saw little use of this procedure due to high mortality rates and the greater popularity of internalized ureterosigmoid diversion. Credit for improvement and popularization of the ureteroileal conduit goes to Bricker who described the procedure in patients following total pelvic exenteration [28]. Since that time it has become the predominant form of urinary diversion following total cystectomy and the standard by which all other diversionary procedures must be measured. Details of the technique are standard in numerous textbooks and will not be described here. Followup studies of the ileal conduit are longer than for any other procedure with the exception of ureterosigmoidostomy and despite its remarkable success, the long term complications as well as the lack of aesthetic appeal have stimulated a continuing search for alternative methods. Late complications of intestinal obstruction, pyelonephritis, renal deterioration, ureteroileal obstruction, stomal stenosis, and renal calculi have been described by several authors with rates ranging from 28 to 81% [29–35]. Complication rates are related to length of followup. Its continued use is primarily in adult bladder cancer patients, where a more limited life span following diversion may be anticipated.

Colon conduit. The impetus for the development and popularization of the colon conduit has been the belief that the free reflux of urine through the ureteroileal anastomosis is responsible for many of the long-term complications of ileal conduit diversion. The thicker muscular wall of the colon compared to the ileum allows a tunnelled anti-reflux anastomosis between the ureter and colon (Fig. 10-7). The anticipated protection of the upper tracts afforded by the anti-reflux anastomosis has proved to be a reality. Variations in the long-term complication rates following colonic conduit diversion are primarily related to the success (or lack of success) of the anti-reflux anastomosis. Followup studies comparing the upper tract complications in those with and without reflux demonstrate a significantly lower rate in those without reflux [36].

Ileocecal conduit. The concept of ileocecal conduit is to take advantage of the reinforced or unreinforced ileocecal valve as an anti-reflux mechanism. As an incontinent system, this has been less popular than the colon conduit. However, it may be adapted to a continent system, as will be described below, and is gaining popularity in this regard.

Continent Urinary Diversion

The permanent forms of continent urinary diversion include ureterosigmoidostomy, the rectal bladder, and the continent abdominal wall stoma (Koch pouch and continent ileocecal reservoir).

Ureterosigmoidostomy. Ureterosigmoidostomy is the oldest form of urinary diversion for patients following cystectomy. First described by Simon in 1852 in a patient with exstrophy of the bladder, it has gone through a

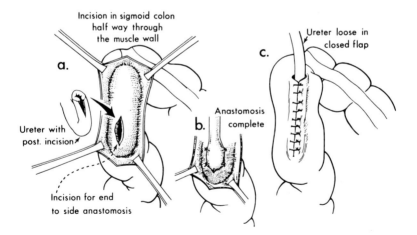

Fig. 10-7. Technique for creating an anti-refluxing ureterocolonic anastomosis.

number of modifications in the method of creating the ureterosigmoid anastomosis [37–41]. The original technique involved creation of a ureterointestinal fistula by means of a strangulating approximation of the distal ureter and sigmoid colon. Though this proved initially successful, the patient ultimately succumbed 12 months later with peritonitis. Autopsy revealed the fistulae to be patent but stenotic and obstructed by calculi. The subsequent modifications developed over the next century culminated in the present technique of Leadbetter (1950) and Goodwin (1953) incorporating the techniques described by Smith (direct mucosa-to-mucosa anastomosis, 1879) and Coffey (submucosal tunnel, 1911). Though it continues to be one of the most popular forms of urinary diversion due to its simplicity, continence, and lack of a cutaneous stoma, it has been associated with complication rates equal to or greater than those of any other forms of diversion. The list of complications includes pyelonephritis, metabolic acidosis, renal deterioration, incontinence, and colonic neoplasia. A major complication is reported to occur in up to 65% of patients [42]. While the upper tract complications are ameliorated somewhat by creation of an anti-reflux anastomosis, and the metabolic complications by alkalinizing medications and frequent bowel evacuation, the specter of later colonic neoplasia remains a major disadvantage of this form of diversion in the pediatric patient. Neoplasms are thought to occur due to conversion of urinary nitrate to nitrosamine, a known carcinogen, by the action of colonic bacteria. It characteristically occurs at the anastomatic suture line with a lag period of 10–46 years (mean 25 years). The increased risk of colon neoplasia is estimated to be 100- to 500-fold [43]. In those patients who do have ureterosigmoidostomy, a yearly coloniscopic examination beginning 10 years after diversion is recommended.

Rectal bladder. Several techniques have been described by which an intestinal urinary reservoir is excluded from the fecal stream but utilizes the anal sphincter as a continence mechanism. Monclaire (1895) was the first to report this by means of a proximal end colostomy and rectal urinary reservoir [44]. Gersuny (1898) utilized the rectum as a urinary reservoir and brought the proximal end of a divided colon to the anal verge between the rectal stump and anal sphincter (anterior to the rectum) [45]. Heitz-Boyer (1912) described a similar technique, bringing the colon posterior to the rectum [46]. None of these procedures have gained widespread acceptance. The technically easier Monclaire procedure suffers the major disadvantage of exchanging a urinary stoma for a fecal stoma. The Gersuny and Heitz-Boyer procedures are technically more difficult, associated with pyelonephritis and renal deterioration and have the potential to damage the anal sphincter, resulting in both urinary and fecal incontinence.

Continent abdominal wall stoma. Koch in 1969 described a continent ileal reservoir in patients having had a proctocolectomy for ulcerative colitis [47]. Leisinger (1976) was the first to report the adaptation of this procedure for use as a continent urinary reservoir [48]. Continence and reflux prevention both depend on an intussuscepted segment of ileum producing a nipple valve. The procedure is difficult, lengthy, and prone to complications. Another major drawback is the eventual failure, in some cases, of pouch continence and/or anti-reflux nipple due to chronic pressure from a full reservoir on the intussuscepted segment [49]. However, it has been responsible for renewed interest in continent diversion with this and other procedures (vida infra).

Ileocecal reservoir. The ileocecal segment is well suited for use as a continent reservoir. Though first described by Gilchrist in 1950, it received less initial enthusiasm than the Bricker ileal conduit described in the same year [50]. The renewed interest in continent diversion in recent years has increased its popularity. The reinforced (intussuscepted) or unreinforced ileocecal valve functions as the continent stoma, and the ureters are anastomosed to the cecum (Fig. 10-8). Since the reservoir pressures may reach

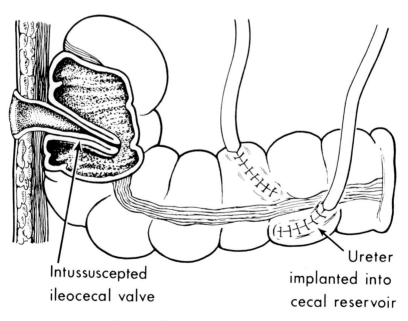

Intussuscepted
ileocecal valve

Ureter
implanted into
cecal reservoir

Fig. 10-8. Continent ileocecal reservoir.

high levels, it is essential to create an anti-reflux ureterocolonic anastomosis. As with the intussuscepted nipple of the Koch pouch, eventual failure of the continence mechanism is a cause for some concern. Both of these reservoirs are emptied by periodic catheterization.

Bladder Substitution

Although bladder substitution is not new, interest has been rekindled among urologists as an alternative for adult patients following cystectomy for malignant disease. Couvelaire (1951) first reported use of the ileum as a bladder substitute with direct anastomosis between the ileum and urethra [51]. Camey developed this concept, beginning in 1958 with the procedure that now bears his name (Fig. 10-9). He has recently published results for patients having this procedure over the previous 25 years and remains enthusiastic about this alternative to stomal or sigmoid diversion in selected patients [52]. Patients have been able to effectively empty their reservoir by a valsalva maneuver and remain acceptably dry if voiding is performed every 2–3 hours. Continence is maintained by the tonus of the external urethral sphincter. Others have built on this concept with the adaptation of other bowel segments for use as the reservoir and an artificial sphincter as a continence mechanism [53,54]. Experience with these various modifications

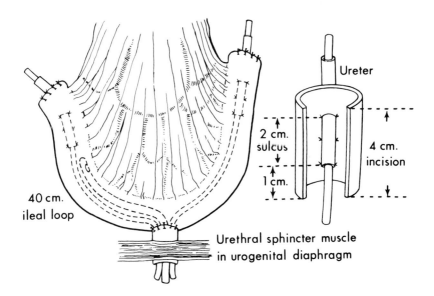

Fig. 10-9. Camey procedure.

is quite limited and none have sufficient followup to warrant critical evaluation at this time. It is important to remember that experience with these procedures has been primarily in the adult population with transitional cell carcinoma and may not be as easily adapted to the pediatric patient following cystectomy for RMS. This is particularly true with the prostatic primary lesion where sufficient urethra and external sphincter may not be available following removal of the tumor for adequate urethral anastomosis and continence. Finally, experimental efforts have been made by several investigators to develop an artificial bladder of biocompatible synthetic material [55]. These efforts remain experimental and to date no long-term success has been achieved either clinically or experimentally.

SUMMARY

The contemporary chemotherapeutic agents for RMS are incapable of curing all children with genitourinary primaries. As such, surgery remains an integral arm of multimodal therapy as both a diagnostic and therapeutic procedure. It is also clear that recurrent disease fares poorly, and the best chance of cure is with the first attempt at therapy. While this does not require initial radical surgical removal of all tumors, it does require surgical removal of all tumor when there has been less than a complete response to chemotherapy and radiotherapy. How long to treat and wait for a partial response to become a complete response before resorting to exenterative surgery remains an area of continued investigation.

The fact that total cystectomy remains a necessity for cure for some patients with RMS mandates that the surgeon also continues to explore ways of making urinary diversion and reconstruction safer and more socially acceptable. In line with this, techniques of continent abdominal wall stomas, bladder substitution, and artificial urinary sphincters hold the promise of a better quality of life and deserve continuing investigation.

REFERENCES

1. Lawrence W, Jr., Hays DM: Surgical lessons from the Intergroup Rhabdomyosarcoma Study. Natl Cancer Inst Monogr 56:159, 1981.
2. Hays DM, Newton W, Jr., Soule EH, et al.: Mortality among children with rhabdomyosarcoma of the alveolar histologic subtypes. J Pediatr Surg 18:412, 1983.
3. Raney RB, Hays D, Lawrence W, et al.: Paratesticular rhabdomyosarcoma in childhood. Cancer 42:729, 1978.
4. Raney RB, Tefft M, Lawrence W, et al.: Paratesticular sarcoma in childhood and adolescence: A report from the Intergroup Rhabdomyosarcoma Studies I and II, 1973–1983 (in preparation).

5. Lawrence W, Hays DM, Moon TE: Lymphatic metastasis with childhood rhabdomyosarcoma. Cancer 39:556, 1977.
6. Lawrence W, Jr., Hays D, Heyn R, et al.: Lymphatic metastases in childhood rhabdomyosarcoma (RMS): Intergroup Rhabdomyosarcoma Study (IRS) I and II. Cancer 60:910–915, 1987.
7. Hays DM, Raney RB, Lawrence W, et al: Bladder and prostatic tumors in the Intergroup Rhabdomyosarcoma Study (IRS-I). Cancer 50:1472, 1982.
8. Hays DM, Shimada H, Raney RB, et al.: Sarcomas of the vagina and uterus: The Intergroup Rhabdomyosarcoma Study. J Pediatr Surg 20:718, 1985.
9. Lawrence W, Jr, Hays DM, Beltangady M, et al.: Prognostic significance of staging factors of the UICC staging system in childhood rhabdomyosarcoma: A report from the Intergroup Rhabdomyosarcoma Study-II. J Clin Oncol (in press).
10. Lawrence W, Jr., Jegge G, Foote FW, Jr.: Embryonal rhabdomyosarcoma. A clinicopathological study. Cancer 17:361, 1964.
11. Olive D, Flamant F, Zucker JM, et al: Para-aortic lymphadenectomy is not necessry in the treatment of localized paratesticular rhabdomyosarcoma. Cancer 54:1283, 1984.
12. Ray B, Hajdu SI, Whitmore WF, et al.: Distribution of retroperitoneal lymph node metastases in testicular germinal tumors. Cancer 33:340, 1974.
13. Staubitz WJ, Magoss IV, Oberkircher OJ, et al.: Management of testicular tumors in children. J Urol 94:683, 1965.
14. Raney RB, Hays DM, Tefft M, et al.: Primary chemotherapy with or without radiation therapy, surgery, or both for children with localized sarcoma of the bladder, prostate, or vagina-uterus: Results of the Intergroup Rhabdomyosarcoma Study-II (in preparation).
15. Hays DM: Rhabdomyosarcoma and other soft tissue sarcomas. In Hays DM (ed): Pediatric Surgical Oncology. Orlando, Fla: Grune and Stratton, 1986, p 102.
16. Hendren WH: Reconstruction of previously diverted urinary tracts in children. J Pediatr Surg 8:135, 1973.
17. Light JK, Engleman UH: Reconstruction of the lower urinary tract: Observations on bowel dynamics and the artificial urinary sphincter. J Urol 133:594, 1985.
18. Hradec EA: Bladder substitution: Indications and results in 114 operations. J Urol 94:406, 1965.
19. Culp OS: Radical perineal prostatectomy: Its past, present and possible future. J Urol 98:618, 1968.
20. Jewett JH, Bridge RW, Gray GF, Jr., et al.: The palpable nodule of prostatic cancer. Results 15 years after radical excision. JAMA 203:115, 1968.
21. Kopecky AA, Lasdowshi TL, Schott R, Jr.: Radical retropubic prostatectomy in the treatment of prostatic carcinoma. J Urol 103:641, 1970.
22. Boxer RJ, Kaufman JJ, Goodwin WE: Radical prostatectomy for carcinoma of the prostate 1951–1976. A review of 329 patients. J Urol 103:641, 1970.
23. Nichols RT, Barry JM, Hodges CV: The morbidity of radical prostatectomy for multifocal stage 1 prostatic adenocarcinomas. J Urol 117:83, 1977.
24. Bass RB Jr, Barret DM: Radical retropubic prostatectomy after transurethral prostatic resection. J Urol 139:1007, 1983.
25. Linder A, Dekernion JB, Smith RB, et al.: Risk of urinary incontinence following radical prostatectomy. J Urol 129:1007, 1983.
26. Eggleston JC, Walsh PC: Radical prostatectomy with preservation of sexual function: Pathologic findings in the first 100 cases. J Urol: 134:1146, 1985.
27. Verhoogen J, de Graeuve A: La cystectomie totale. Folia Urol 3:629, 1909.

28. Bricker EM: Bladder substitution after pelvic evisceration. Surg Clin North Am 30:1511, 1950.
29. Jaffe BM, Bricker EM, Butcher HR: Surgical complications of ileal segment urinary diversion. Ann Surg 167:367, 1968.
30. Schmidt JD, Hawtry CE, Flocks RII, et al.: Complications, results and problems of ureteroileals. J Urol 109:210, 1972.
31. Remigailo RV, Lewis EL, Woodard JR, et al.: Ileal conduit urinary diversion: Ten-year review. Urology 7:343, 1976.
32. Pitts WR, Muecke EC: A 20-year experience with ileal conduit: The fate of the kidneys. J Urol 122:154, 1979.
33. Sullivan JW, Grabstald H, Whitmore WF: Complications of ureteroileal conduit with radical cystectomy: Review of 336 cases. J Urol 124:797, 1980.
34. Heath AL, Eckstein HB: Ileal conduit urinary diversion in children: A long term follow-up. J Urol (Paris) 90:91, 1984.
35. Shapiro Sr, Lebowitz R, Colodny AH: Fate of 90 children with ileal conduit urinary diversion a decade later: Analysis of complications, pyelography, renal function and bacteriology. J Urol 114:289, 1975.
36. Elder DD, Moisey CU, Rees RWA: A long-term follow-up of the colonic conduit operation in children. Br. J Urol 51:462, 1979.
37. Simon J: Ectopia vesicae (absence of the anterior walls of the bladder and pubic abdominal porietes): Operation for directing the orifices of the ureters into the rectum; temporary success; subsequent death; autopsy. Cancer 2:568, 1852.
38. Smith T: An account of an unsuccessful attempt to treat extraversion of the bladder by a new operation. St Barth Hosp Rep 15:29, 1879.
39. Coffey RC: Physiologic implantation of the severed ureter or common bile duct into the intestine. JAMA 56:397, 1911.
40. Goodwin WE, Harris AP, Kauffman JJ, et al.: Open transcolonic ureterointestinal anastomosis: A new approach. Surg Gynecol Obstet 97:295, 1953.
41. Leadbetter WF: Consideration of problems, incident to performance of ureteroenterostomy: Report of a technique. Trans Am Assoc Genitourin Surg 42:39, 1950.
42. Spirnak PJ, Caldamone AA: Ureterosigmoidostomy. Urol Clin North Am 13:285, 1986.
43. Gilles R: Carcinogenesis in ureterosigmoidostomy. Urol Clin North Am 13:201, 1986.
44. Mauclaire M: De quelques essais de chirurgie experimentale applicables au traitement de l'existrophie de la vessie et des anus coutre natur complexes. Ann Mal Org Génito-urin 13:1080–1089.
45. Gersuny R: Cited by Foges: Officielles protokoll der kk. gesellschaft der aertze in Wien. Wien Klin Wschr 11:989, 1898.
46. Heitz-Boyer M, Hovelacque A: Creation d'une nouvelle vessie et un nouvel uretre. J Urol Nephrol 1:237, 1912.
47. Koch N: Intra-abdominal "reservoir" in patients with ileostomy. Arch Surg 99:223, 1969.
48. Leisinger HJ, Sauberli H, Schauweker H, et al.: Continent ileal bladder: First clinical experience. Eur Urol 2:8, 1976.
49. Skinner DG, Boyd SD, Lieskovsky G: Clinical experience with Koch continent ileal reservoir for urinary diversion. J Urol 132:1101, 1984.
50. Gilchrest RK, Merricks JW, Hamlin MH, et al.: Construction of a substitute bladder and urethra. Surg Gynecol Obstet 90:752, 1950.
51. Couvelaire R: Le reservoir ileal de substitution apres la cystectomie totale chez l'homme. J Urol 57:408, 1951.

52. Lilien O, Camey M: 25-year experience with replacement of the human bladder (Camey procedure). J Urol 132:886, 1984.
53. Perinetti EP: Total bladder reconstruction after cystectomy. J Urol 135:135, 1986.
54. Light JK, Scott FB: Total reconstruction of the lower urinary tract using bowel and the artificial urinary sphincter. J Urol 131:953, 1984.
55. Kaleli A, Ansell JS: The artificial bladder: A historical review. Urology 24:423, 1984.

Chapter 11
Unusual Bladder Tumors in Children

Frederick A. Klein

Neoplasms of the lower urinary tract in the first two decades of life (either benign or malignant) are unusual. Malignant tumors are more common and in contrast to those tumors found in adults, are predominantly mesenchymal rather than epithelial in origin. Due to ever-increasing experience with these neoplasms, there is resulting improvement in survival and a better under-standing of the natural history of an individual type of lesion. This chapter will deal with bladder neoplasms other than rhabdomyosarcoma.

EPITHELIAL BLADDER TUMORS

Epithelial tumors of the bladder in the first two decades of life are uncom-mon, with only 114 cases reported [1–28]. The age distribution of these cases is shown in Figure 11-1. Only 19 cases have been reported under the age of 10 years with the majority of the cases occurring in the late teens. The usual male predominance is evident with a ratio of approximately 6:1 in those cases where the sex was reported. The most common presenting symptom is gross hematuria; however, irritative symptoms including frequency, dysuria, and suprapubic pain also frequently occur.

The cell type is predominantly transitional; however, there are rare reports of squamous cell and adenocarcinoma [4]. Intravenous pyelograms and/or cystourethrography may show abnormal filling defects in the bladder in up to 50% of cases, but the best procedure for diagnosis remains cystoscopy. Urinary cytology, although in general a sensitive and specific diagnostic tool, is notoriously poor for papilloma and low grade carcinomas, with recognition

Pediatric Tumors of the Genitourinary Tract, pages 177–186
© 1988 Alan R. Liss, Inc.

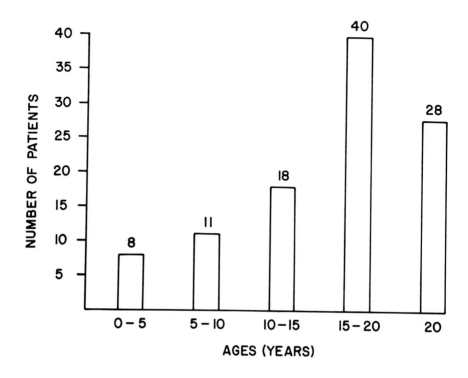

Fig. 11-1. Age distribution in children with epithelial bladder tumors.

of tumor in only about 22% of cases [29]. Since the majority of these lesions in children are papillomas or grade I carcinomas, this procedure is unreliable. The role of flow cytometric determination of DNA and RNA content in these lesions has not been determined but may be useful, as results in adults revealed that up to 83% of papillomas could be recognized with this technique [30]. A disadvantage, however, is that a bladder irrigation specimen which requires bladder catheterization is necessary.

The primary treatment for these lesions is transurethral resection, fulguration, or photocoagulation with the Neodymium Yag laser. The lesions are generally solitary, involving the trigone or lateral walls. Multiple tumors at initial diagnosis were only present in four cases (3.5%) [4,14,22,28]. In addition, recurrence is uncommon, ranging from 2.5–5% [4,22]. For these reasons additional treatment with intravesical chemotherapy has been unnecessary except in the two cases reported by Kroovand and associates [28].

Only two patients have died of metastatic disease, both within 6 months of diagnosis; no other deaths have been reported [22].

Since transitional cell tumors of the bladder are uniformly low grade, non-invasive, and rarely recurrent, specific followup recommendations are not as well agreed on as are recommendations for followup in adults. Certainly, periodic roentgenographic, cytologic, and flow cytometric evaluations are necessary. The frequency of cystoscopy should be determined by the presence of solitary or multiple tumors at initial diagnosis and the presence of positive cytology or flow cytometry. In those unusual instances where multiple and/or high grade tumors are present, followup should be identical to that used for adults.

OTHER MALIGNANT BLADDER TUMORS

Although leiomyosarcoma of the bladder is most commonly seen in the fifth and sixth decades of life, approximately 30% have been reported in the first two decades of life [24]. Signs and symptoms are usually non-specific including frequency, dysuria, and hematuria; boys are affected about twice as often as girls. Unlike rhabdomyosarcoma, it usually arises in portions of the bladder other than the trigone and tends to infiltrate and recur locally [30–36]. If distant metastases do occur, they generally involve the lungs, liver, and bowel [32,34,35]. The preferred treatment is partial cystectomy if the size and location of the tumor are amenable to this procedure. If the lesion is more extensive, radical cystectomy may be necessary. For those lesions originally presenting with metastases, a combination of radiotherapy and chemotherapy may be potentially curative [24].

There have been occasional case reports of malignant tumors involving the urachus. Two have been sarcomas and another an undifferentiated tumor, in contrast to adults where adenocarcinoma is the most common type [37,38]. These lesions have been universally fatal, probably secondary to late diagnosis. The treatment of choice remains radical surgical extirpation and urinary diversion.

BENIGN BLADDER TUMORS

Benign bladder tumors in children are rare lesions in the urinary tract. In general, they are only discussed in isolated case reports; however, they may be of clinical importance because of significant hemorrhage or obstruction of the bladder outlet or ureters. Identified tumors in decreasing order of frequency include hemangiomas, neurofibromas, fibromas, fibromatous polyps, leiomyomas, pheochromocytomas, nephrogenic adenomas, inverted papillomas, myxomas, and dermoid cysts [39]. In addition, clinicians should be aware that other benign inflammatory proliferative mucosal changes may be mistaken for tumors of the bladder. Varsona and associates reported two male children, one 3.5 months old and one 6 years old, who had bladder filling defects on cystography and what appeared to be tumor on cystoscopy [40]. In each case, histologic sections revealed inflammatory tissue with hyperplasia of the transitional cell epithelium. In addition, the latter case had changes consistent with cystitis glandularis. In neither case were malignant cells present. Harris and associates reported three children, 2,8, and 12 years old, with bulbous bladder mucosal lesions histologically interpreted as cystitis cystica [41]. The cystogram in one of these cases had persistent filling defects giving the radiographic impression of neurofibromatosis and rhabdomyosarcoma. Kaplan and King reported proliferative bladder lesions (cystitis cystica, cystitis follicularis, and von Brunn's nest) present in 18 of 763 patients having cystoscopy for urinary tract infections [42]. In no patient was there evidence of neoplasm. Kroovand and associates reported similar proliferative and metaplastic changes to be present in three patients with chronic infection and reflux who underwent ureteral reimplantation [28]. Two of these cases, however, were recurrent transitional cell papillomas. Therefore, it should be emphasized that these proliferative and metaplastic glandular changes may have been erroneously diagnosed as carcinoma, but they have also been associated with the presence and development of carcinoma [43,44]. Histologic confirmation of these lesions as well as careful long-term followup is a necessity.

Hemangioma

Hemangiomas of the bladder are vascular lesions that Ganem and Ainsworth considered the most common benign connective tissue neoplasm arising from this organ [17]. Approximately 32 cases have been reported in the first two decades of life [45]. The cardinal symptom is gross hematuria, which may be intermittent but profuse enough in some cases to lead to marked anemia. The diagnosis is made on cystoscopic examination where the hemangioma appears blue or pink in color, is covered by intact epithelium, and may be pedunculated or sessile, lobulated or flattened. Of those patients reported to be evaluated by intravenous pyelography, only half had an abnormal bladder outline [45].

In approximately two-thirds of the cases, the lesion is solitary, well defined, and involves the upper portion of the bladder. Many of these lesions may be extensive (larger than 3 cm) with two-thirds involving the muscle or perivesical fat and one-third involving only the superficial bladder wall [46]. The most common histologic type is cavernous, but lymphangiomatous and capillary elements have been seen in a small number of patients. In addition, about one-third have hemangiomatous lesions elsewhere on their body. Treatment depends on the extent of the lesion. Transurethral resection or fulguration is limited to small superficial lesions. Although there has been one report by Liang of successful resolution with radiotherapy in two patients [47], Hamer and Mertz did not report any beneficial results from radiotherapy in their patients [48]. The primary treatment of this lesion, therefore, continues to be partial cystectomy. Because of no recorded involvement of the bladder neck or ureteral orifices, ureteral reimplantation has not been necessary. The overall success rate has been excellent with no recorded deaths, and only an occasional patient has required repeated fulguration.

Neurofibroma

Since the first case of neurofibromatosis involving the bladder of a child was reported by Kass in 1932 [49], there have been only 22 additional reports in children from birth to 13 years of age in the English language literature [39]. This entity is two to three times more common in males than females and approximately 75% have generalized stigmata of von Recklinghausen's disease (café-au-lait spots and cutaneous neurofibromas). Approximately 25% of the patients have a family history of neurofibromatosis [46].

Although the bladder is the most commonly involved site within the urinary tract, neurofibromas can also be found in the prostate, urethra, penis, spermatic cord, and testes [39]. These lesions may be asymptomatic and found incidentally during abdominal or pelvic surgery for other conditions or they may produce symptoms of urinary tract obstruction. The symptoms of frequency and urinary retention may be due to true obstruction from the tumor or due to neurologic dysfunction. In about 50% of the patients, a nodular suprapubic mass may be palpable [39]. On cystoscopic examination, there may be solitary or multiple grayish-white nodules or a diffuse swelling that is not readily distinguishable from the bladder wall. The mucosa overlying the lesion is generally intact [24].

Diagnosis is made by transurethral biopsy or occasionally open exploration. Treatment may be by transurethral resection, local excision, or segmental resection for small or moderate-sized symptomatic nodules. Large lesions with diffuse bladder involvement and those that involve adjacent viscera usually require total cystectomy. Small asymptomatic lesions discovered incidentally should be locally excised for diagnosis and prevention of future problems [24]. Although most of these lesions are histologically benign, they may invade locally and cause vesical outlet obstruction. Malignant degeneration has been reported in 5-16% of cases of neurofibromatosis [24]; however, only once has such a change been reported in the bladder [50]. In the two patients with neurogenic sarcoma of the bladder reported by Mintz, neither had a history of preexisting neurofibroma [51]. In general, the prognosis with bladder neurofibroma is good with appropriate therapy administered at an early date. Therefore, it is important to evaluate thoroughly any urinary symptoms in children with neurofibromatosis.

Miscellaneous Benign Bladder Tumors

Fibromas and benign fibrous polyps of the bladder have been reported 15 times in case reports [39]. Symptoms are primarily hematuria or obstruction. Treatment is simple excision, either open or transurethral.

Since the original description of a nephrogenic adenoma of the bladder by Friedman and Kuhlenbeck in 1950 [52], numerous cases have been reported by others [53-59]. Of these, nine have involved children aged 5-16. In one instance, this lesion occurred in two siblings in a single family [59]. Nephrogenic adenoma is characterized histologically by the formation of tubular structures in the lamina propria resembling the loop of Henle, distal convoluted tubule, or collecting tubule of the kidney. The clinical features of nephrogenic adenoma range from gross hematuria to bladder irritative symptoms such as dysuria, frequency, and urgency. Most patients have a history of chronic infection or inflammation or trauma (surgical or otherwise). Lesions have been found incidentally in specimens removed for carcinoma as well as diverticulae of the bladder or urethra [55,60,61]. In addition, there has been one report of this lesion found in association with malakoplakia [56].

The most important concern in regard to nephrogenic adenoma is the question of neoplastic potential, as it has been found in association with carcinoma [62]. Its development into frank carcinoma, however, has not been documented. Because of concern over the natural history, the lesion should be surgically treated. This usually consists of endoscopic fulguration and/or resection. Occasionally, because of a large lesion, partial cystectomy with possible augmentation might be necessary. In addition, periodic followup cystoscopic and cytologic examination are recommended [58].

Inverted papillomas of the bladder have been reported in children [63-65]. The presenting sign in all cases has been gross hematuria. The lesion is more common in boys than girls and is found either on the trigone or bladder base. Simple transurethral resection is the treatment of choice.

Pheochromocytoma of the urinary bladder is manifested by a distinct symptom complex including headache, fainting, palpitations, and dizziness frequently brought on by voiding. In addition, hypertension is present (usually sustained) as well as hematuria. Approximately 42 cases have been reported in children, of which nine have been malignant [66]. The appropriate preoperative diagnosis should be made by biochemical means and with cystography, pelvic angiography, and cystoscopy. Appropriate surgical treatment depends on the location and extent of the tumor. When feasible, segmental cystectomy is adequate; otherwise cystectomy and urinary diversions are necessary. Followup periodic monitoring of urinary catecholamine levels, as well as blood pressure, are essential to identify local recurrences or the development of metastases.

CONCLUSIONS

Despite their rarity, bladder neoplasms should be considered in the differential diagnosis of hematuria in the first two decades of life. Although in general, cystoscopic examination of a child is not necessary, this procedure still is the most accurate method of diagnosing or confirming the presence of a bladder neoplasm. Non-epithelial tumors are more common than epithelial tumors, with rhabdomyosarcomas being the most prevalent. Of the epithelial tumors, low grade papillary transitional cell neoplasms are the most common. In general, these lesions are solitary and do not recur. Other tumors including hemangioma, neurofibroma, fibroma, fibromatous polyps, leiomyoma, pheochromocytoma, nephrongenic adenoma, inverted papilloma, and myoma are rarely encountered and are usually only the subject of individual case reports. The most common presenting symptom is hematuria, usually gross, followed by obstruction with malignant tumors and irritative symptoms of frequency and dysuria with other tumors.

REFERENCES

1. Deming CL: Primary bladder tumors in the first decade of life. Surg Gynecol Obstet 39:432, 1924.
2. Ash JE: Epithelial tumors of the bladder. J Urol 44:135, 1940.
3. Miller A, Mitchell JP, Brown MD: The Bristol bladder tumor registry. Br J Urol 41:7(suppl), 1969.
4. Javadpour N, Mostofi FK: Primary epithelial tumors of the bladder in the first two decades of life. J Urol 101:706, 1969.
5. Li R, Kim K, Brendler H: Multiple and recurrent epithelial tumors of the bladder in a child. J Urol 108:644, 1972.
6. Siegel WH, Pincus MB: Epithelial bladder tumors in children. J Urol 101:55, 1969.
7. Melicow MM: Tumors of the urinary bladder. J Urol 74:498, 1955.
8. Rossi MB, Wogalter H, Spatz M: Papillary transitional cell tumor of the bladder in a 5 year old boy. J Urol 97:88, 1967.

9. Firstatter M, Heyman I, Lowenthal M: Bladder papilloma in a child: Case report. J Urol 101:57, 1969.
10. Fitch LB, Rubenstone A: Carcinoma of the bladder in childhood. J Urol 87:549, 1962.
11. Johnson AJ, Taylor JN: Papillary tumor of the bladder in a twelve year old boy. J Urol 87:869, 1962.
12. Kohler FP: Carcinoma of the bladder in the second decade. J Urol 85:284, 1961.
13. Benton B, Henderson BE: Environmental exposure and bladder cancer in young males. JNCI 51:269, 1974.
14. Waller JI, Roll WA: Bladder carcinoma in a teen-aged girl. J Urol 78:764, 1957.
15. Lowry EC, Soanes WA, Forbes KA: Carcinoma of the bladder in children: Case report. J Urol 73:307, 1955.
16. Franzblau AH: Bladder carcinoma in the young. Rocky Mtn Med J 65:54, 1968.
17. Ganem EJ, Ainsworth LB: Benign neoplasms of the urinary bladder in children: Review of the literature and report of a case. J Urol 73:1021, 1955.
18. Castellanos RD, Wakefield PB, Evans AT: Carcinoma of the bladder in children. J Urol 113:261, 1975.
19. Brumskine W, Dragan P, Sanvee L: Transitional cell carcinoma and schistosomiasis in a 5-year old boy. Br J Urol 49:540, 1977.
20. Chandy PCX, Pai MG, Budihal MR, et al.: Carcinoma of the bladder in young children: Report of 2 cases. J Urol 113:264, 1975.
21. Campbell M: Tumors of the urogenital tract. In Campbell M (ed): Clinical Pediatric Urology. Philadelphia: WB Saunders, 1951, pp 713–720.
22. McGuire EJ, Weiss RM, Baskin AM: Neoplasms of transitional cell origin in first twenty years of life. Urology 1:57, 1973.
23. McCarthy JP, Gavrell GJ, LeBlanc GA: Transitional cell carcinoma of the bladder in patients under thirty years of age. Urology 13:487, 1979.
24. Ray B, Grabstald H, Exelby PR, et al.: Bladder tumors in children. Urology 2:426, 1973.
25. Benson RC, Jr., Tomera KM, Kelalis PP: Transitional cell carcinoma of the bladder in children and adolescents. J Urol 130:54, 1983.
26. Fitzpatrick JM, Reda M: Bladder carcinoma in patients 40 years old or less. J Urol 135:53, 1986.
27. Kretschmer HL, Barringer BS, Braasch WF, et al.: Cancer of the bladder. A study based on 902 epithelial tumors of the bladder in the Carcinoma Registry of the American Urological Association. J Urol 31:423, 1934.
28. Kroovand RL, Chang CC, Broecker BH, et al.: Epithelial lesions of bladder mucosa following ureteral reimplantation. J Urol 126:822, 1981.
29. Farrow GM: Pathologists' role in bladder cancer. Semin Oncol 6:198, 1979.
30. Klein FA, Melamed MR, Whitmore WF, Jr., et al.: Characterization of bladder papilloma by two-parameter DNA-RNA flow cytometry. Cancer Res 42:1094, 1982.
31. Weitzner S: Leiomyosarcoma of urinary bladder in children. Urology 12:450, 1978.
32. Silbar JD, Silbar SJ: Leiomyosarcoma of bladder: Three case reports and a review of the literature. J Urol 73:102, 1955.
33. Brown HE: Leiomyosarcoma of the bladder: Follow-up report of two cases with 4 and 10 years survival. J Urol 94:247, 1965.
34. Ramey WB, Ashburn LL, Grabstald H, et al.: Myosarcoma of the urinary bladder. J Urol 70:906, 1953.
35. Uehling D, Frable WJ: Myosarcoma of the bladder: Report of two cases. J Urol 91:354, 1964.

36. Laurenti C, DeDominicis C, Dal Forno S, et al.: Leiomyosarcoma of the bladder in a girl. Eur Urol 8:185, 1982.

37. Cornil C, Reynolds CT, Kickham CJE: Carcinoma of the urachus. J Urol 98:93, 1967.

38. Oriana S, Zingo L, Cogliati I, et al.: Topography and clinical characteristics of malignant tumors of the urachus. Tumori 65:497, 1979.

39. Smithson WA, Benson RC, Jr.: Lower genitourinary tract. In Kelalis PP, King LR, Belman AB (eds): Clinical Pediatric Urology. Philadelphia: WB Saunders, 1985, p 1189.

40. Varsano I, Savir A, Brunebaum M, et al.: Inflammatory processes mimicking bladder tumors in children. J Pediar Surg 10:909, 1975.

41. Harris VJ, Javadpour N, Fizzotti G: Cystitis cystica masquerading as a bladder tumor. AJR 120:410, 1974.

42. Kaplan GW, King LR: Cystitis cystica in childhood. J Urol 103:657, 1970.

43. Lin JI, Tseng CH, Marsidi PS, et al.: Diffuse cystitis glandularis associated with adenocarcinomatous change. Urology 15:411, 1980.

44. Koss LG: Tumors of the urinary bladder. In Atlas of Tumor Pathology, 2nd Series. Washington, D.C.: Armed Forces Institute of Pathology, FASC 11, 1975.

45. Hendry WF, Vinnicombe J: Hemangioma of bladder in children and young adults. Br J Urol 43:309, 1971.

46. Sarma KP: Tumors of the Urinary Bladder. London: Appleton-Century-Crofts, 1969, pp 90–111.

47. Liang DS: Hemangioma of the bladder. J Urol 79:956, 1958.

48. Hamer HG, Mertz HO: Angioma of the bladder. Surg Gynecol Obstet 51:541, 1930.

49. Kass IH: Neurofibromatosis of the bladder. Am J Dis Child 44:1040, 1932.

50. Ross JA: Case of sarcoma of urinary bladder in von Recklinghausen's disease. Br J Urol 29:121, 1957.

51. Mintz ER: Pedunculated neurofibroma of the bladder. J Urol 43:268, 1940.

52. Friedman NB, Kuhlenbeck H: Adenomatoid tumors of the bladder reproducing renal strictures (nephrogenic adenomas). J Urol 64:657, 1950.

53. Ritchey ML, Novicki DE, Schultenover SJ: Nephrogenic adenoma of bladder: A report of 8 cases. J Urol 131:537, 1984.

54. Leonard SA, Silverman AJ, Langstron JW, et al.: Postoperative nephrogenic adenoma of the bladder. Urology 7:327, 1976.

55. Berger BW, Bhagavan SBS, Reiner W, et al.: Nephrogenic adenoma: Clinical features and therapeutic considerations. J Urol 126:824, 1981.

56. Raghavaiah NW, Noe HN, Parham DM, et al.: Nephrogenic adenoma of urinary bladder associated with malakoplakia. Urology 15:190, 1980.

57. Kaloor GJ, Shaw RE: Nephrogenic adenoma of the bladder. Br J Urol 46:91, 1974.

58. Kay R, Lattanzi C: Nephrogenic adenoma in children. J Urol 133:99, 1985.

59. Billia A, Lima ACL, Queiroz LS, et al.: Adenoma of bladder in siblings with renal dysplasia. Urology 16:299, 1980.

60. Peterson LJ, Matsumoto LM: Nephrogenic adenoma in urethral diverticulum. Urology 11:193, 1978.

61. Mostofi FK: Potentialities of bladder epithelium. J Urol 71:705, 1954.

62. Skor AB, Warren MW: Mesonephric adenocarcinoma of the bladder. Urology 10:64, 1977.

63. Francis RR: Inverted papilloma in a 14 year old male. Br J Urol 51:327, 1979.

64. Lorentzen M, Rohr N: Urinary bladder tumors in children: Case report of inverted papilloma. Scand J Urol Nephrol 13:323, 1979.
65. Theoret G, Paguin F, Schick E, et al.: Inverted papilloma of urinary tract. Urology 16:149, 1980.
66. Meyer JJ, Sane SM, Drake RM: Malignant paraganglioma (pheochromocytoma) of the urinary bladder: Report of a case and review of the literature. Pediatrics 63:879, 1979.

Chapter 12
Testicular Tumors in Children

J. Pritchard and C.D. Mitchell

Testicular tumors are rare in childhood, accounting for only 1–2% of solid tumors [1,2]. There has been, however, a well-documented increase in the overall incidence of testicular cancer, so that it is now the most common malignancy in the 25–40-year age range [3] and may come to assume a position of greater importance in pediatric practice. The single most important "risk factor" is the presence of an undescended testis [4]. Pediatricians and pediatric surgeons are in a unique position to recognize this anomaly and to ensure that appropriate treatment and advice are given.

EPIDEMIOLOGY

The lifetime risk of developing a testicular tumor is now about 1 in 500, in both white males in the United States and in males in the United Kingdom [5,6]. There are, however, geographic and racial variations in incidence. The risk for U.S. blacks is only one-fourth that of U.S. whites; the incidence is low in Finland, yet high in Denmark [3,5]. These differences suggest an interplay between environmental and genetic factors in the etiology of testicular tumors.

Although there was little change in the age-specific mortality due to testicular tumors in the 40 years from 1936–1976, there was a 100% increase in absolute mortality in the 15–19-year age group during the same period [3], probably reflecting the population increase within this age range. There is also good evidence to suggest that the overall incidence of malignant testicular tumors is rising [3,7]. The peak incidence is in the 25–40-year age range,

Pediatric Tumors of the Genitourinary Tract, pages 187–206
© 1988 Alan R. Liss, Inc.

with a slightly later peak for seminomas and a slightly earlier peak for other germ cell tumors. Thus, testicular tumors primarily occur in young men and are relatively rare in pediatric practice, where they contribute only 1–2% of all solid tumors seen [3].

The histologic spectrum of testicular tumors in childhood differs from that found in adults. The proportion of non-germinal tumors is higher in childhood. Seminoma, the most common testicular neoplasm in adults, is hardly ever seen before puberty, correlating with findings in animal models that this tumor is only found after sexual maturation [2]. The yolk sac tumor (YST), also known by a variety of synonyms (Table 12-1), is by far the most common type of childhood germ-cell tumor. In a review of the world literature, Weissbach et al. found that YST represented 70.8% of all childhood germinal tumors. With an overall incidence of germinal tumors of 50% YST is also, therefore, the most common pediatric testicular tumor. Over 75% are seen in the first 2 years of life [2].

PREDISPOSING FACTORS

The most important predisposing factor for testicular malignancy is the presence of an undescended testis (UDT). This association was first noted by Le Conte in 1851 [8]. In two very large series of germ cell tumors, 9.5–9.8% occurred in UDT [9,10]. The incidence of UDT in the general population is in the range of 0.23–0.28%. Thus, the risk that malignancy will arise in a UDT is 35 times greater than in one that has descended normally.

The location of the UDT is also important. About 15% of all UDTs are located in the abdomen, yet up to 48.5% of tumors in UDT patients are found in this small group [9]. The risk of malignancy for an abdominally located testis appears to be about 6 times greater than for an inguinally located testis. About 10–25% of all patients with UDTs will have bilateral cryptorchidism; these patients frequently have intraabdominal testes. Should such a patient develop a germ cell tumor, there is a 25% risk of developing a tumor in the contralateral testis. Ninety-five percent of malignant germ cell tumors developing in patients with a unilateral UDT will develop in that

TABLE 12-1. Synonyms for Yolk Sac Tumor of Testis

Clear cell adenocarcinoma

Orchioblastoma

Embryonal carcinoma, juvenile type

Endodermal sinus tumor

testis. That 5% of tumors develop in the scrotal testis is, however, still an excess risk compared to men with bilaterally normal descended testes [11].

The precise reason for the association between non-descent and malignancy is not known. The excess of malignancy in "opposite" scrotal testes supports the suggestion that both testes are intrinsically abnormal, and that both this and their position contribute to the predisposition. Germ cells from maldescended testes have been shown to contain hyperdiploid amounts of DNA and to have larger nuclei than normal testes [12]. Unfortunately this study did not include information on the cell size and DNA content of the normal contralateral testes; similar findings in the latter would have provided strong support for the theory of "intrinsic abnormality."

Early operation for UDT is becoming more common. Hospital Inpatient Enquiry data for England and Wales shows that the orchidopexy rate at ages 0–4 years in 1981 was 10 times greater than in 1962 [13]. The reasons for early operation are beliefs that fertility will be enhanced and that the risk of cancer may be reduced. Data from the Royal Marsden Hospital, however, suggests that the age of orchidopexy has no influence on the subsequent incidence of cancer. The incidence of the various histological types of tumors are similar in both normally descended and undescended testes [10].

By comparison with UDT, gonadal dysgenesis—as in Klinefelter's syndrome, Swyer's syndrome, and Sohval's syndrome—is a much rarer cause of predisposition to the development of testicular tumors, particularly gonadoblastoma [14]. Patients with these syndromes all carry a Y chromosome, and the mechanism whereby normal testicular organization and differentiation are impaired is unclear [15], but may relate to H-Y antigen density. The H-Y antigen appears important in normal male differentiation. There is some evidence that, when expression of H-Y antigen in individuals with dysgenetic gonads is in the normal male range, the risk of a testicular tumor is higher than when antigen expression is within the female range [16].

HISTOGENESIS AND PATHOLOGICAL CLASSIFICATIONS

Knowledge of the embryological origins of testicular components provides a basis for the understanding of testicular pathology, but the area is beset by a confusing multiplicity of classifications.

Germ cells do not arise in the gonad but migrate there from the yolk sac. In early somite embryos, about 100 germ cells are found among the endodermal cells of the yolk sac, close to the allantois. These cells become ameboid and, dividing as they travel, migrate via the dorsal mesentery to the intermediate mesoderm, there to await the development of the gonad. During the fifth week the coelomic surface epithelium of the intermediate mesoderm thickens to become the germinal epithelium, so-called because it was once believed to give rise to the germ cells. From this epithelium, strands of cells grow down into the underlying mesoderm to form the sex cords. Germ cells migrate along the sex cords and come to form the outer (cortical) and inner (medullary) layers of the gonad.

The gonads are indifferent until the seventh week of gestation, but thereafter the male gonad differentiates rapidly. The cortical germ cells and sex cords degenerate during the seventh and eighth weeks, while the medullary sex cords become more prominent, forming the primitive seminiferous tubules. These tubules consist of strands of androgen-secreting cells (of Leydig) and primordial male germ cells (spermatogonia). The spermatogonia lie dormant until the tenth postnatal year, when the tubules acquire a lumen and the germ cells initiate spermatogenesis. The Leydig cells increase in number to a maximum at 24 weeks. The Sertoli cells provide nutritive support for the spermatogonia; the former, together with the tubuli recti and the rete testes, arise from the coelomic epithelium [17].

A critical distinction in all pathological classifications is that between tumors of germ-cell origin and those of gonadal/stromal origin. Germ-cell tumors may either be unipotential, giving rise to a seminoma, or multipotential, giving rise to embryonal carcinoma. Multipotential germ cells can follow either embryonal or extraembryonal pathways of differentiation [18,19]. Cells of germinal origin that have followed an embryonic pathway will form teratomas, containing various cellular or organoid components reminiscent of more than one germ layer. Three basic variants can be recognized; benign cystic teratomas, mature solid teratomas, and immature solid teratomas. The mature solid teratoma is usually malignant, and the immature form is invariably so. Cells following an extraembryonal pathway of differentiation can give rise either to yolk sac tumors or to choriocarcinoma. Testicular tumors may also exhibit more than one histological pattern, so that there may be combinations of embryonal carcinoma with teratoma (teratocarcinoma), or a combination of teratoma with seminoma (teratoseminoma).

Tumors of the gonadal stroma include Leydig and Sertoli cell tumors. Androgen production by Leydig cell tumors causes precocious puberty in the prepubertal boy; gynecomastia may also be occasionally noted [20]. They may also secrete estrogens and corticosteroids.

Tumors composed of a mixture of germ cells and sex cord stromal derivatives have only been recognized over the last 30 years [21]. It has become evident that two specific types of tumor, gonadoblastoma and mixed germ cell sex cord stromal tumors, may be distinguished. These two entities differ from each other in a number of respects. Gonadoblastoma, so-called because it appears to recapitulate normal gonadal development [22], is the more common. It is seen only in patients with gonadal dysgenesis. Ninety-six percent of such patients carry a Y chromosome. About 80% are phenotypic females, more than half of them virilized. The remaining 20% are male pseudohermaphrodites. The affected gonad, when not indeterminate, is a streak or a testis. The tumor is usually small and will be bilateral in 50% of cases. Overgrowth by other neoplastic germ cell elements is frequent. Mixed germ cell/sex cord stromal tumors occur in somatically and genetically normal female infants and children in the first decade of life. The tumors may be large and are usually unilateral. Metastases have not been described, and admixture with other neoplastic germ cell elements is rare [21].

Tumors may also arise in the paratesticular tissues. Although their precise mesodermal structure of origin is unknown [23,24], by far the most common is the rhabdomyosarcoma.

Metastatic tumors may occur; usually due to infiltration by lymphoblastic leukemia and lymphoma [25]. Infiltration by neuroblastoma has also been reported but is very rare [26].

It is worth noting that in the British classification, embryonal carcinoma is referred to as malignant teratoma, undifferentiated; choriocarcinoma as malignant teratoma, trophoblastic; and teratocarcinoma as malignant teratoma, intermediate [27].

TUMOR MARKERS

Serum tumor markers are extremely useful in the management of malignant testicular tumors. Over three-quarters of adults with non-seminomatous germ cell tumors have elevated serum levels of alpha feto-protein (AFP) and/or beta human chorionic gonadotrophin (hCG) at the time of diagnosis [28,29]. Since the marker level in serum is an accurate reflection of tumor burden, measurements are useful in diagnosis, staging, and prognosis, monitoring the effect of treatment, and subsequent followup.

hCG is a glycoprotein hormone composed of two different subunits. The alpha subunit is similar to that of other glycoprotein hormones such as follicle stimulating hormone (FSH), thyroid stimulating hormone (TSH), and luteinizing hormone (LH). The beta subunit is specific for HCG [30]. More recently, a pregnancy-specific beta-1 glycoprotein, SP1, has been identified in the same syncytiotrophoblastic giant cells that are a feature of gestational trophoblastic tumors and choriocarcinoma of the testis [32], but it is not yet clear that measurement of SP1 offers any advantage over the longer-established BhCG assay [33].

AFP is synthesized in cells of the primitive endoderm and the fetal liver from about the sixth week of gestation, reaching its highest serum level at about the thirteenth week, and falling to undetectable levels by the age of 1 year [34]. In testicular tumors, the protein may be identified within the mononuclear cells of embryonal carcinoma or yolk sac tumors [32]. Raised levels in serum therefore correlate with the presence within the tumor of cells derived from the endodermal sinus region [35].

Serum lactate dehydrogenase (LDH) levels are elevated in patients with non-seminomatous germ cell tumors at about the same frequency as AFP and BhCG [36]. Elevations of LDH do not, however, correlate with a particular histological type of tumor, nor do elevations of LDH necessarily correspond to elevations of AFP or BhCG[35]. In occasional patients with normal AFP and BhCG, elevated levels can, however, be of value in monitoring the effect of treatment and in detecting relapse [35].

Some knowledge of the kinetics of clearance of these markers is important for a correct interpretation of data. BhCG has a serum half life of only 30 hours, so a fairly rapid fall can be anticipated following complete surgical resection. AFP, by contrast, has a much longer half life of some 5 days, so serum levels decline more slowly, and the unwary may be deceived into believing that undected disease is present [37]. LDH also has a prolonged half life [38].

In postpubertal patients, a mild but persistent elevation of BhCG may be seen during therapy. This is due to cross-reaction with LH in patients who have been rendered hypogonadal by therapy. The point can be proved by demonstrating suppression with testosterone [37]. Difficulties with interpretation of serum AFP levels may occur in infants, in whom there is physiological persistence of AFP synthesis, albeit at a declining rate, during the first year of life [34]. Persistent low level elevations of AFP in patients without other evidence of relapse should provoke a search for liver disease [39].

A large multicenter study has demonstrated the prognostic value of serum marker measurements at the time of diagnosis in adults. An initial serum AFP level of greater than 50 kU/L generally indicates a large or very large volume of disease and is an independent adverse prognostic factor (1kU/L = 1.09 μg/L). Serum levels of BhCG greater than 1,000 IU/L tend to occur with large or very large volume disease and, again, provide independent prognostic information [40]. Though a similar correlation has not yet been proven in children, it would be surprising if the same trends were not evident.

A favorable response to treatment for postsurgical residual or metastatic disease is accompanied by falling serum levels of AFP, BhCG, and/or LDH. As testicular tumors may have doubling times of less than 2 weeks, it seems reasonable to check marker levels at least weekly during the initial stages of treatment, but less frequently later [41]. Following cessation of treatment, marker levels provide a ready assessment of the presence of residual disease and early detection of recurrence. Sometimes, however, the marker pattern at relapse may differ from that seen at diagnosis. Patients with raised levels of serum AFP and BhCG at diagnosis may relapse with only one or the other, or neither marker elevated. This presumably represents the selection of one or more chemoresistant subpopulation(s) of cells during therapy.

CLINICAL FEATURES

As in adults, the major clinical feature of testicular tumors in childhood is the presence of a slowly enlarging testicular mass. Unless there is a complication such as infarction or torsion, pain is not usually a feature [42]. The presence of transillumination does not rule out the diagnosis of a tumor since about 25% of testicular tumors are associated with a hydrocoele [1]. The differential diagnosis also includes hernia, hematocoele, and infarction following torsion. Careful questioning of the parents or patient about a history of undescended testes, the length of the history of a mass, recent trauma, and the presence of pain will help exclude some of these possibilities.

Physical examination reveals the presence of a smooth, firm, non-tender testicular mass. The presence of scars from an orchidopexy or herniorrhaphy should be noted. The ability to "get above" the mass will enable differentiation from a hernia although the two conditions may co-exist. Inguinal lymphadenopathy does not occur unless the scrotum has been involved by direct extension [43]. The lungs are the most common site for hematogenous metastases [44], but pulmonary involvement is asymptomatic unless secondaries are very large and pleural fluid is present. Signs of precocious puberty suggest a stromal (Leydig cell) tumor [20]. Rarely, children may present with symptoms of metastatic disease such as fever, anemia, bone pain, and weight loss. It is therefore important that examination of the testes should be included as part of the routine physical examination of any child with suspected cancer.

Specific features of individual tumors are described below.

STAGING AND OTHER INVESTIGATIONS

Staging investigations should be tailored to the natural history of each tumor type. Testicular and paratesticular malignancy tends to spread to the paraortic lymph nodes in the retroperitoneum, and then to the chest and neck. The main site of hematogenous spread is to the lungs. More rarely there may be spread to bone or bone marrow, peritoneum, brain and meninges, and liver.

Imaging should include a two-view chest radiograph, abdominal ultrasonography, and a bone scan. Computerized tomographic (CT) scanning is undoubtedly a more sensitive method of searching for occult pulmonary disease, and scanning the abdomen will delineate any hepatic or retroperitoneal abnormality. There is general agreement, however, that lymphangiography is unnecessary because of 1) the invasive nature of the procedure, including the need for two surgical incisions; 2) the difficulty of cannulating pedal lymphatics in infants; 3) the most likely positive nodes (renal hilum) are not usually filled by dye injected into the feet; and 4) the unlikelihood of therapeutic benefit. Bone marrow aspiration may be indicated on occasion if there is unexplained thrombocytopenia, neutropenia, or anemia.

Initial investigations should include a full blood count, serum biochemistry including liver function tests, and AFP and hCG. These two tumor markers may help confirm a diagnosis preoperatively and, if possible, will provide an indication of tumor burden.

If the patient is to receive chemotherapy, other investigations are indicated so that toxicity may be anticipated and minimized. Patients receiving cisplatinum should have serial audiological assessments and measurements of glomerular filtration rate, preferably using chrome[51] EDTA filtration [45], while those receiving bleomycin should have pulmonary function monitored regularly, preferably by spirometric methods, including total lung volume and compliance.

SURGICAL CONSIDERATIONS
Primary Tumor

The affected testis should be approached through an inguinal, not a scrotal, incision. The external oblique fascia should be opened, and the spermatic cord should be isolated up to the internal ring. The cord should then be secured using a vascular clamp to prevent egress of tumor cells before the testis is delivered into the wound. Inspection of the testis usually enables a diagnosis to be made. In doubt, orchidectomy is preferable to an open biopsy [46]. Any fluid aspirated from a hydrocoele should be sent for cytological examination but there is no published data on the cytology of pediatric testicular tumors. Needle biopsy of testicular masses is not indicated since all such lesions will require surgical removal. In addition, there is the risk of seeding the tumor along the needle track, thereby potentially "upstaging" the tumor by opening new routes for lymphatic spread.

Retroperitoneal Lymph Node Dissection

As previously noted, testicular tumors predictably metastasize to the paraaortic lymph nodes, especially those just inferior to the renal hila. About 40% of adult patients with pure seminoma and about 66% of patients with non-seminomatous germ cell tumors (NSGCT) will have nodal metastases at the time of presentation [47]. In the past, patients with stage I NSGCT (i.e., disease-free after radical orchidectomy) were treated with radical retroperitoneal node dissection (RPND) or radiotherapy. Either form of treatment combined with immediate or deferred chemotherapy will cure all but a few patients.

RPND has consistently been recommended by urologists in the United Stages in the management of adults with NSGCT. Although early studies showed that even with assiduously careful surgery, more than 25% of retroperitoneal lymph nodes were left behind following a therapeutic dissection [48], reports during the 1970s suggested that improvements in surgical techniques allowed more effective surgical control of early metastatic disease [49].

Staging has, however, improved considerably since RPND was introduced, particularly since the introduction of CT scanning. In addition, a number of studies have demonstrated an improved understanding of prognostic factors in stage I NSGCT, including histology, spermatic cord involvement by tumor, and changes in tumor markers following orchidectomy [40]. The development of cis-platinum-based chemotherapy has provided the means whereby patients relapsing after primary surgical treatment can be "rescued" [50].

RPND has always been less popular in Europe than in the United States. Studies from the Royal Marsden Hospital suggest that relapse in Stage I patients is no more common in those treated by orchidectomy alone when compared with those treated with adjuvant radiotherapy [51]. The few patients who do relapse will probably be retrievable with chemotherapy.

SPECIFIC TUMOR TYPES

Germ Cell Tumors

These include pure yolk sac tumors and embryonal carcinoma.

Yolk sac tumor (orchioblastoma). These usually have pure yolk sac histology, though in some there are embryonal carcinoma elements [53]. At diagnosis, the serum AFP is correspondingly elevated in the range 100–100,000 μg/l. So long as the patient's age is taken into account, especially in the case of infants, elevated serum AFP is virutally diagnostic of orchioblastoma when a testicular mass is present.

There is no universally accepted staging system, but that of Brodeur is straightforward and effective [53]. Since over 75% of children are cured by orchiectomy alone and nearly all of the remainder by surgery plus chemotherapy, there are two schools of thought as to which staging investigations are necessary. In one view, staging procedures should be limited to those that are non-invasive—PA and lateral chest x-rays and abdominal ultrasound—while, according to the second, a more aggressive approach, including CAT scanning of chest and abdomen and bone scanning are advocated in addition. Proponents of the former policy point out that CAT scanning is expensive and that, in infants, a general anesthetic is required; they also point out that, because of the exquisite sensitivity of the tumor to chemotherapy, it is almost certainly unnecessary to detect very small volume disease.

Management of stage I tumors. Patients with stage I disease should receive no treatment after orchidectomy. Careful monitoring of serum AFP levels is sufficient. Weekly samples should be taken until the level falls into the normal range (in most laboratories <5 ug/l or <5 ng%). Thereafter, tests can be repeated monthly for 1 year and bi-monthly to complete 2 years' followup. Although recurrence without elevation of serum AFP is probably exceedingly rare, most centers also monitor with chest x-rays and ultrasounds every 4 months, at least for the first 12 months after surgery.

Management of advanced tumors. Children with stage II–IV disease should receive adjuvant chemotherapy. Vincristine-actinomycin D-cyclophosphamide (VAC) or VAC-adriamycin combination chemotherapy is moderately successful in the treatment of low volume disease [54], but the advent of more effective regimens in adults has led to a reappraisal [55]. There is no doubt that cis-platinum, vinblastine, and etoposide (VP16), together with bleomycin, are the most active agents in testicular cancer and have been crucial to the dramatic improvement in prognosis for men with advanced disease. There has been some reluctance to introduce these regimens into pediatric practice partly because of the rarity of orchioblastoma and other malignant germ cell tumors in children (which means that experience develops slowly), but also because of concerns about the long-term toxicity of cis-platinum and bleomycin. The best-known cis-platinum-containing regimes are PVB (Cis-platinum-vinblastine-bleomycin) and BEP (bleomycin-etoposide-cis-platinum); variants have also been described. In the largest reported series of children treated with PVB or BEP, including four patients with advanced orchioblastoma, Pinkerton et al. reported a complete response rate of 93% (13 of 14 patients) and identical long-term survival [56]. In their series, BEP was better tolerated than PVB because the abdominal symptoms associated with high-dose vinblastine administration (abdominal pain and constipation) were avoided. The series now includes 22 patients, with no further relapses, giving a probable cure rate of >90%. The fact that a median of only five courses (range 4–7) of chemotherapy is needed, given over 3–6 months, makes these regimens particularly suitable for pediatric use and, though the oto- and nephrotoxicity of cis-platinum and pulmonary toxicity of bleomycin are of concern, the regimens are likely to leave patients with normal or near-normal fertility. By contrast, alkylating agent-containing regimens such as VAC or Vac-adriamycin are not only more protracted but are more likely to lead to infertility and can be leukemogenic. Randomized trials are needed to prove the superiority of cis-platinum-containing regimens, but the rarity of the tumors will probably make this impossible. The only tumors unlikely to be cured by BEP/PVB are those with very bulky disease. In these cases the regimen pioneered by the Charing Cross Hospital, U.K. (so-called POMB-ACE) may be more effective [57].

The major chemotherapy issues at present are 1) is bleomycin necessary, i.e., is EP as effective as BEP, and 2) are the newer, less toxic platinum derivatives, which can be given in the out-patient setting because no diuresis is needed, as effective as cis-platinum? If so, there would be no case for the continued use of regimens containing alkylating agents.

Given such effective chemotherapy for orchioblastoma, the role of surgery is limited, but there may be a case for delayed laparotomy or thoracotomy in patients with normal AFP levels but radiologically residual mass disease in the abdomen or lung. Anecdotal evidence in children suggests that surgery in these circumstances will yield similar results to those in adults, i.e., 60–70% of masses will consist of fibrosis or scar only, 10–15% will contain benign teratoma, and 10–15% residual malignant teratoma. Thus, though further data in children are needed, surgery may improve the complete response (CR) rate by 10–20%. Radiation therapy is necessary only in the very rare instance where local recurrence follows an adequate course of a cis-platinum-containing chemotherapy regimen. Pulmonary irradiation is not indicated and may be extremely dangerous if the patient has received bleomycin.

Monitoring of these patients, off treatment, is similar to that used for stage I disease. It is doubtful whether, given the high cure rates with modern chemotherapy, more invasive procedures (e.g., CAT scanning) can be justified.

Recurrence is so rare after 2 years off chemotherapy that parents can be told their child is "almost certainly cured" and that the trauma of finger pricking for serum AFP measurement can be avoided. Obviously, any worrisome symptoms should lead to immediate reinvestigation.

Stromal Tumors

Sertoli cell tumors. These are usually diagnosed in infancy, noted by parental observations when the tumor is small and is causing no symptoms. Androgens or estrogens may be secreted, though rarely in sufficient quantities to cause clinically evident masculinization or feminization. Although several have occurred in adults, only one case of a malignant Sertoli cell tumor has been reported in childhood [58]. A simple orchidectomy is usually curative. In view of the improbability of malignancy it seems that clinical follow-up only is needed if the typical histological features of a Sertoli cell tumor are seen.

Leydig cell tumors. Symptoms and signs of sexual precocity are the usual mode of presentation. The sexual precocity, is, strictly speaking, precocious pseudopuberty since the process is not driven by pituitary gonadotropins [59]. Gynecomastia may be present and is secondary to increased levels of estrogen and progesterone. As in most causes of precocious puberty or precocious pseudopuberty, bone age tends to be advanced. In occasional patients a small intratesticular tumor may cause a local androgenic effect with enlargement of both the affected testis and the epididymis, thus concealing the presence of the tumor [60].

Testicular tumors may occur in association with congenital adrenal hyperplasia (CAH). Most such tumors are adrenal cell rests and are dependent on ACTH for growth and secretion. These tumors are seen in boys with incomplete suppression of ACTH. In some boys, LH secretion may also be elevated, and the distinction from Leydig cell tumors then becomes difficult.

A significantly elevated urinary 17-ketosteroid level favors the diagnosis of CAH, particularly those with 21-hydroxylase deficiency. Administration of corticosteroids will reduce urinary 17-ketosteroid excretion and diminish the testicular swelling associated with CAH [61].

Leydig cell tumors in childhood are benign, in contradistinction to those seen in adults. Simple orchidectomy is adequate treatment. Urinary 17-ketosteroid excretion will fall to normal after excision. If it does not or if the level subsequently rises, then bilateral tumors associated with CAH should be suspected [62,63].

Gonadoblastoma. Most patients with gonadoblastoma are phenotypic females and about half have some degree of virilization. About 20% are male pseudohermaphrodites. The vast majority have a Y chromosome, with either a 46XY karyotype or various forms of mosaicism. Presentation is usually during the second decade, with a history of primary amenorrhea followed by the development of a lower abdominal mass. The histological picture is rarely pure, but is usually associated with seminomatous elements. In a further 10% of cases, malignant germ cell elements such as embryonal carcinoma, yolk sac tumor or choriocarcinoma are admixed [21].

Treatment should be bilateral orchidectomy, as both gonads are intrinsically abnormal even though malignancy may not have developed in the contralateral gonad [21].

Subsequent treatment should be dictated by the histological features of the resected tumor and the results of staging investigations, as in any other cases of malignant germ cell tumor.

Paratesticular Rhabdomyosarcoma

Only 7% of all rhabdomyosarcomas arise in the paratesticular region, compared with 36% in the head and neck including orbit, 23% in the trunk and limbs, and 10–12% in other genitourinary sites of both sexes [64]. So, although it is the most frequently occurring paratesticular tumor of childhood, rhabdomyosarcoma is actually rare with only 25–40 new cases per year in the United States. Nevertheless, the principles of management are similar to those of rhabdomyosarcoma at other sites and are now well established thanks to large multi-center trials, especially those in the United States (Intergroup Rhabdomyosarcoma Study, IRS) and, more recently, in Europe (Société Internationale d'Oncologie Pediatrique, SIOP).

The histogenesis of these tumors, and the occasionally recorded paratesticular fibrosarcoma and leiomyosarcoma, is presumed to be from the supporting stromal tissue of the spermatic cord. The swelling may be testicular but often arises above the testis and, rarely, in the inguinal region. Inguinal node enlargement is very uncommon but can occur when the scrotal or inguinal skin has been invaded or previously biopsied. In the case of high intrascrotal tumors, differential diagnosis includes irreducible inguinal hernia, hydrocele of the cord, and epididymal cyst.

Stage, size of primary tumor, and histological subtype are generally regarded as the most important prognostic variables for patients with rhabdomyosarcoma. Most paratesticular primaries, because they are accessible to examination, are relatively small when diagnosed and since the vast majority are of embryonal subtype [65] (generally regarded as prognostically the most "favorable" variety), tumor stage assumes great importance. The staging system of the IRS is summarized in Table 12-2 [64]. Tumor spread is most commonly to lymph nodes, lungs, and bones, while bone marrow, liver, and other sites are only very rarely involved. Given this pattern of spread, chest x-rays/CT lung scans, isotope bone scans, and bone marrow examination are mandatory for all patients. However, especially in the absence of useful tumor markers, the choice of investigations to seek possible retroperitoneal

TABLE 12-2. Intergroup Rhabdomyosarcoma Study's
Classifications (Simplified)

Stage I	Localized tumor, completely resected
Stage II	Residual local microscopic disease; and/ or regional, involved nodes (resected); and/or extension into contiguous structure (resected with or without residual microscopic disease)
Stage III	Gross residual disease
Stage IV	Distant metastases

node involvement is more controversial. From 19–40% of patients with paratesticular rhabdomyosarcoma are said to have retroperitoneal lymph node metastases [65,66], indicating a greater propensity to lymphatic spread from primaries at this anatomic site compared with those at other locations. However, the accessibility of retroperitoneal nodes to imaging and dissection may mean that the relative incidence has been exaggerated. Given that microscopic disease at other sites can usually be effectively controlled by chemotherapy alone, the need for lymphangiography (despite the fact that this procedure may be more feasible in patients that are, on average, older than those with orchioblastoma) is questionable. In principle, the same argument applies to the use of retroperitoneal node dissection in patients whose abdominal CT scan is normal [67].

Because rhabdomyosarcoma is a chemoresponsive tumor and because it is not possible to distinguish between stage I patients with and without micrometastases, it is now conventional to give chemotherapy to all these patients [64,65,68,69]. Though newer agents, such as cis-platinum and the epipodophyllotoxins (VM26 and VP16) are under evaluation in the third IRS study, current treatment programs are still based on the VAC (vincristine, actinomycin D, cyclophosphamide) or VAC-adriamycin schedules. Most paratesticular primary tumors are clinically and radiologically stage I. These children should receive adjuvant chemotherapy with vincristine and actinomycin D (VA) but not cyclophosphamide. The cure rate is high (>80%) whether or not the alkylating agent is included [65] and the risk of infertility and secondary leukemia is reduced or negated. Similarly, regional irradiation [64] and retroperitoneal node dissection [67] have been shown to be of no therapeutic value in this group of patients. Management of children with stage II and III disease is more controversial. Those patients who have stage II disease by virtue of local extension into scrotal or inguinal skin should have wide excision of the involved area and, probably, even if the surgical margins appear clear, local radiotherapy (35–45 Gy). When disease is classed as stage II by virtue of involved (excised) paraaortic nodes, patients can be treated either with intensive chemotherapy(VAC) without radiotherapy or ipselateral paraaortic irradiation with a less intensive chemotherapy program (e.g., VA). The rare patients with stage III (unresectable local and/or nodal tumor) and stage IV disease should be treated initially with intensive chemotherapy (VAC, VAC-adriamycin, or the more complex schedule used in IRS-III) followed by surgery and irradiation to sites of initial bulk disease. The duration of chemotherapy is still under study. Although 6 months of treatment is almost certainly sufficient for patients with stage I disease, children with more advanced tumors are usually treated for 12-18 months.

Novel approaches to improvement of prognosis for stage III and IV patients include 1) the addition of new agents to VAC-adriamycin in induction chemotherapy (as in IRS-IV) and 2) the use of high-dose chemotherapy consolidation (using melphalan, cyclophosphamide, and busulphan with additional total body irradiation in selected patients with disseminated disease). This kind of approach has been shown to prolong remission in patients with stage IV neuroblastoma, but preliminary results in rhabdomyosarcoma are disappointing, indicating that chemoresistance, even to high doses of drugs, has developed early stage during treatment.

Fortunately, most boys with paratesticular rhabdomyosarcomas have early stage disease and a good prognosis. In the largest series published to date, most patients had stage I or stage II disease [65,67] and for the majority neither irradiation or alkylating agents are necessary. It is essential that treatment for patients with rhabdomyosarcoma is individually tailored, not only to maximize the chance of cure but also to reduce morbidity. These days, planning and supervision of treatment is invariably from a pediatric oncology center [68], and most patients are now entered into national study protocols. Hopefully these investigations will soon provide further information useful in the management of these rare tumors.

Metastatic Tumors

Secondary infiltration of the testis in childhood is most commonly due to acute lymphoblastic leukemia (ALL) or lymphoblastic non-Hodgkin's lymphoma (NHL). Evidence for the presence of a blood-testis barrier is not as strong as that for a blood-brain barrier, but the testis (which is affected much more commonly than the ovary) is usually regarded as a sanctuary site. Occasionally, unilateral or bilateral testicular swelling is the presenting manifestation of ALL or NHL, but more commonly the diagnosis will have been made some time beforehand and the development of a testicular mass will represent disease relapse.

Some patients with ALL, usually those with adverse prognostic factors at the time of diagnosis, may develop overt testicular relapse while still on chemotherapy. The majority of testicular relapses, however, occur within the first 2 years after the cessation of therapy [70]. Although bone marrow and CSF are often normal in children relapsing during this time, more extensive staging investigations, including lymphangiography and laparotomy may reveal involvement of paraaortic lymphnodes in some [71].

In the recent past, many groups adopted the policy of elective testicular biopsies in an attempt to detect early disease and possibly to reduce the incidence of associated marrow relapse. Biopsy during therapy has not proved to be of benefit [72]; there is also a significant incidence of false negative biopsies for those performed at the end of therapy [73,74]. Attempts to improve diagnostic precision using immunofluorescent techniques to detect the enzyme terminal deoxynucleotidyl transferase (Tdt) have not been helpful [75,76]. Testicular biopsies have been abandoned in the current UKALL trial because of the apparent lack of benefit and the high false negative rate.

Isolated testicular disease in ALL requires both local radiotherapy and systemic chemotherapy. The use of local measures alone is insufficient, since this will inevitably result in a systemic or CNS relapse at some time in the near future. Effective local control of testicular leukemia may be achieved with either orchidectomy or radiotherapy. Current recommendations are for both testes and their spermatic cords as far as the internal ring to receive 2,400 cGy; chemotherapy to be resumed; and some form of CNS-directed treatment to be given, usually in the form of intrathecal methotrexate [77]. It is obviously essential that all of these patients are managed in association with a pediatric oncologist and radiotherapist.

Testicular relapse in neuroblastoma is extremely rare and is either a manifestation of a sanctuary site or a rare random occurrence. There will usually be evidence of relapsed disease at other sites, and so it would seem prudent that such patients receive systemic therapy in addition to local treatment [78].

CONCLUSIONS

Advances in the management of testicular cancer in adults have led to major improvements in the prognosis of children with these tumors. Major factors are 1) an improved understanding of their natural history, 2) the use of serum tumor markers, 3) improved chemotherapy, and 4) genuine interdisciplinary management by a team including chemotherapist, radiotherapist, and surgeon. Pediatric tumor therapists are all too aware of the unwanted side effects of their treatment. Where, as in the case of most children with testicular or paratesticular malignancy, the prognosis is excellent, the treatment team is obliged to develop and implement protocols that are less toxic but as effective. Examples include the omission of cyclophosphamide from the treatment of patients with stage I rhabdomyosarcoma so that fertility is maintained and the risk of secondary leukemia decreased, and modifications in the BEP/PVB regimens for malignant germ cell tumors aimed at reducing their nephro- and ototoxicity. Rather than "cure at any cost," the objective should be "cure at least cost."

With modern therapy, the main cause of treatment failure is the presence at diagnosis of advanced, bulky disease. It has been shown that diagnostic delay is correlated with advancing disease stage [79,80]. Education of the general public, particularly teenage boys, about the risks of testicular cancer and the benefits of early diagnosis via testicular self-examination [81], might lead to a further improvement in the overall prognosis for patients with this group of tumors.

REFERENCES

1. Li FP, Fraumeni JF, Jr.: Testicular cancers in children: Epidemiologic characteristics. JNCI 48:1575, 1972.
2. Weissbach L, Allwein JE, Steins R: Germinal testicular tumours in childhood. Eur Urol 10:73, 1984.
3. Schottenfeld D, Warshauer ME, Sherlock S, et al.: The epidemiology of testicular cancer in young adults. Am J Epidemiol 112:232, 1980.
4. Martin DC: Malignancy in the cryptorchid testis. Urol Clin North Am 9:371, 1982.
5. Jones WG: Tumours of the testes. Aetiology, epidemiology and animal models. Ett Maj Int Sci Ser Life Sci 18:41, 1985.
6. Davies JM: Testicular cancer in England and Wales: Some epidemiological aspects. Lancet 1:928, 1981.
7. Nethersell AB, Drake LK, Sikora K: The increasing incidence of testicular cancer in East Anglia. Br J Cancer 50:377, 1984.
8. Quoted in: Johnson DC, Woodhead DM, Poll DR: Cryptorchidism and testicular tumour-igenesis. Surgery 63:919, 1968.
9. Campbell HE: Incidence of malignant growth in the undescended testicle. Arch Surg 44:353, 1942.
10. Pike MC, Chilvers C, Peckham MJ: Effect of age at orchidopexy on risk of testicular cancer. Lancet 1:1246, 1986.
11. Gilbert JB, Hamilton JF: Incidence and nature of tumours in ectopic testes. Surg Gynecol Obstet 71:731, 1940.
12. Muller J, Skakkeback NE: Abnormal germ cells in maldescended testes: A study of cell density, nuclear size and DNA content in testicular biopsies from 50 boys. J Urol 131:730, 1984.
13. Chilvers C, Pike MC, Forman D, et al.: Apparent doubling of the frequency of undescended testis in England and Wales 1962–1981. Lancet 2:330, 1984.

14. Mulvihall JJ, Wade WW, Miller RW: Gonadoblastoma in dysgenetic gonads with a Y chromosome. Lancet 1:863, 1975.

15. Schellhas HF: Malignant potential of the dysgenetic gonad. Obstel Gynecol 44:298, 1974.

16. Amice VA, Amice J, Bercovici JP, et al.: Gonadal tumour and H-Y antigen in 46XY pure gonadal dysgenesis. Cancer 57:1313, 1986.

17. Fitzgerald MJT: Human Embryology: A Regional Approach. London: Harper and Row, 1978.

18. Mostofi FK: Classification of tumours of testis. Ann Clin Lab Sci 9:455, 1979.

19. Dehner LP: Gonadal and extragonadal germ cell neoplasia of childhood. Hum Pathol 14:493, 1983.

20. Johnstone G: Prepubertal gynaecomastia in association with an interstitial-cell tumour of the testis. Br J Urol 39:211, 1967.

21. Talerman A: The pathology of gonadal neoplasms composed of germ cells and sex cord stroma derivatives. Pathol Res Pract 170:24, 1980.

22. Scully RE: Gonadoblastoma. A gonadal tumour related to dysgerminoma (seminoma) and capable of sex hormone production. Cancer 6:455, 1953.

23. El-Badawi AA, Al Ghorab MM: Tumours of the spermatic cord: A review of the literature and a report of a case of lymphangioma. J Urol 94:445, 1965.

24. Raney RB, Jr., Hays DM, Lawrence W, Jr., et al.: Paratesticular rhabdomyosarcoma in childhood. Cancer 42:729, 1978.

25. Wong KY, Ballard ET, Strayer FH, et al.: Clinical and occult testicular leukaemia in long term survivors of acute lymphoblastic leukaemia. J Pediatr 96:569, 1980.

26. Voute PA: Neuroblastoma. In Sutow WW, Fernbach DJ, Vietti TJ (eds): Clinical Pediatric Oncology. St. Louis: C.V. Mosby, 1984, p 559.

27. Pugh RCB: Pathology of the Testis. London: Blackwell Scientific Publications, 1976.

28. Javadpour N: The value of biologic markers in diagnosis and treatment of testicular cancer. Semin Oncol 6:37, 1979.

29. Norgaard-Pedersen B, Schultz HP, Arends J, et al.: Tumour markers in testicular germ cell tumours. Five year experience from the DATECA study 1976–1980. Acta Radiol (Oncol) 23:287, 1984.

30. Swaninatham N, Bahl OP: Dissociation and recombination of the subunits of human chorionic gonadotropin. Biochem Biophys Res Commun 40:422, 1970.

31. Tatarinov YS, Masyukevich VN: Immunological identification of a new beta-1-globulin in the blood serum of pregnant women. Bull Exp Biol Med USSR 69:666, 1970.

32. Furumoto M: Cellular localization of AFP, hCG and its free subunits, and SP1 in embryonal carcinoma of the testis and ovary. Pathol Res Pract 173:12, 1981.

33. DeBruijn HWA, Sleijfer DT, Koops HS, et al.: Significance of human chorionic gonadotropin alpha-fetoprotein, and pregnancy specific beta-1-glycoprotein in the detection of tumour relapse and partial remission in 126 patients with non-seminomatous testicular germ cell tumours. Cancer 55:829, 1985.

34. Wu JT, Book L, Sudar K: Serum alpha fetoprotein levels in normal infants. Pediatr Res 15:50, 1981.

35. Bosl GJ, Lange PH, Nochomovitz LE, et al.: Tumour markers in advanced non seminomatous testicular cancer. Cancer 47:572, 1981.

36. Lippert MC, Javadpour N: Lactic dehydrogenase in the monitoring and prognosis of testicular cancer. Cancer 48:2274, 1981.

37. Hamsworth JD, Greco FA: Testicular germ cell neoplasms. Am J Med 75:817, 1983.

38. Zilva JF, Pannell PR: Clinical Chemistry in Diagnosis and Treatment. London: Lloyd Luke, 1984.

39. Grem JL, Trump DL: Reversible increase in serum alpha fetoprotein content associated with hepatic dysfunction during chemotherapy for seminoma. J Clin Oncol 4:41, 1986.

40. The Medical Research Council Working Party on Testicular Tumours: Prognostic factors in advanced non-seminomatous germ cell tumours: Results of a multicentre study. Lancet 1:8, 1985.

41. Rustin GJS: Tumour markers in germ cell tumours. Br Med J 292:713, 1986.

42. Exelby PR: Testicular cancer in children. Cancer 45:1803, 1980.

43. Ray B, Hahdu SI, Whitmore WF: Distribution of retroperitoneal lymph node metastases in testicular germinal tumours. Cancer 33:340, 1974.

44. Peckham MJ: Investigation and staging: General aspects and staging classification. In Peckham MJ (ed): The Management of Testicular Tumours. London: Edward Arnold, 1981.

45. Womer RB, Pritchard J, Barratt TM: Renal toxicity of cisplatin in children. J Pediatr 106:659, 1985.

46. Duckett JW: Surgical aspects of testis tumours in children. In Hayes DM (ed): Pediatric Surgical Oncology. New York: Grune and Stratton, pp. 189–204, 1986.

47. Taylor RE, Duncan W: The management of germ-cell testicualr tumours. J Roy Coll Surg Edinburgh 32:1, 1987.

48. Tavel FR, Osius TG, Parker JW, et al.: Retroperitoneal lymph node dissection. J Urol 89:241, 1963.

49. Skinner DG, Scardino PT: Relevance of biochemical tumour markers and lymphadenectomy in management of non-seminomatous testis tumours: Current perspective. J Urol 123:378, 1980.

50. Peckham MJ, Barrett A, Liew KH, et al.: The treatment of metastatic germ-cell testicular tumours with bleomycin, etoposide and cis-platinum (BEP). Br J Cancer 47:613, 1983.

51. Peckman MJ, Barrett A, Husband JE, et al.: Orchidectomy alone in stage 1 non-seminomatous germ-cell tumours. Lancet 2:678, 1982.

52. Gonzalez-Crussi F: The human yolk-sac and yolk-sac tumours. A review. Perspect Paediatr Pathol: 179, 1979.

53. Brodeur GM, Howarth CB, Pratt CB, et al.: Malignant germ-cell tumour in 57 children and adolescents. Cancer 48:1890, 1981.

54. Cangir A, Smith J, Van Eys J: Improved prognosis in children with ovarian cancers following modified VAC (vincristine sulphate, dactinomycin and cyclophosphamide) chemotherapy. Cancer 42:1234, 1978.

55. Einhorn LH: Testicular cancer as a model for a curable neoplasm. Cancer Res 41:3275, 1981.

56. Pinkerton CR, Pritchard J, Spitz L: High complete response rate in children with advanced germ-cell tumours using cis-platin containing combination chemotherapy. J Clin Oncol 4:194, 1986.

57. Newlands E, Rustin GJS, Begent RHJ, et al.: Further advances in the management of malignant teratomas of the testis and other sites. Lancet 1:948, 1983.

58. Rosvell RV, Woodward JR: Malignant Sertoli cell tumour of the testis. Cancer 22:8, 1968.

59. Aynsley-Green A: Growth. In Godfrey S, Baum JD (eds): Clinical Paediatric Physiology. London: Blackwell Scientific Publications, 1979, p 434–468.

60. Gittes RF, Smith G, Conn CA, et al.: Local androgenic effect of interstitial cell tumour of the testis. J Urol 104:774, 1970.

61. Newell ME, Lippe BM, Ehrlich RM: Testis tumours associated with congenital adrenal hyperplasia: A continuing diagnostic and therapeutic dilemma. J Urol 117:256, 1977.

62. Grem JL, Robins HI, Wilson KS, et al.: Metastatic Leydig cell tumour of the testis. Report of three cases and review of the literature. Cancer 58:2116, 1986.
63. Brosman SA: Testicular tumours in prepubertal children. Urology 13:581, 1979.
64. Maurer HM, Moon TM, Donaldson M, et al.: The Intergroup Rhabdomyosarcoma Study. Cancer 40:2015, 1977.
65. Raney RB, Hayes DM, Lawrence W, et al.: Paratesticular rhabdomyosarcoma in childhood. Cancer 42:729, 1978.
66. Lawrence W, Hays, DM, Moon TE: Lymphatic metastasis with childhood rhabdomyosarcoma. Cancer 39:556, 1977.
67. Olive D, Flamant F, Zucker JM, et al.: Paraaortic lymphadenectomy is not necessary in the treatment of localized paratesticular rhabdomyosarcoma. Cancer 54:1283, 1984.
68. Cromie WJ, Raney RB, Duckett JW: Paratesticular rhabdomyosarcoma in children. J Urol 122:80, 1979.
69. Flamant F, Hill C: The improvement in survival associated with combined chemotherapy in childhood rhabdomyosarcoma. A historical comparison of 345 patients at the same centre. Cancer 53:2417, 1984.
70. Medical Research Council: Testicular disease in acute lymphoblastic leukaemia in childhood. Br Med J 1:334, 1978.
71. Baum E, Nesbit M, Tilford D, et al.: Extent of disease in pediatric patients with acute lymphoblastic leukaemia experiencing an apparent isolated testicular relapse. Proc Am Assoc Cancer Res Am Soc Clin Oncol 20:435, 1979.
72. Pui CH, Bowman PW, Abromovitch M, et al.: Elective testicular biopsy during chemotherapy for childhood leukaemia is of no clinical value. Lancet 2:410, 1985.
73. Tiedemann K, Chessells JM, Sandland RM: Isolated testicular relapse in boys with acute lymphoblastic leukaemia: Treatment and outcome Br Med J 285:1614, 1982.
74. Chessells JM, Durrant J, Hardy RM, et al.: Medical Research Council Leukaemia Trial—UKALL V: An attempt to reduce the immunosuppressive effects of therapy in childhood acute lymphoblastic leukaemia. J Clin Oncol 4:1758, 1986.
75. Thomas JA, Janossy G, Eden OB, et al.: Nuclear terminal deoxynucleotidyl transferase in leukaemic infiltrates of testicular tissue. Br J Cancer 45:709, 1982.
76. Chessells JM, Pincott J, Janossy G: TdT+ cells in routine testicular biopsy: Significance and relation to histology and clinical outcome. Br J Haematol 58:184, 1984.
77. Chessells JM: Acute leukaemia in children. Clin Haematol 15:727, 1986.
78. Kellie SJ, Waters KW: Testicular neuroblastoma. J Surg Oncol 29:201, 1985.
79. Oliver RTD: Factors contributing to the delay in diagnosis of testicular tumours. Br Med J 290:356, 1985.
80. Bosl GJ, Goldman A, Lange PH, et al.: Impact of delay in diagnosis on clinical stage of testicular cancer. Lancet 2:970, 1981.
81. Marty PJ, McDermott RJ: Teaching about testicular cancer and testicular self examination. J Occup School Health 53:351, 1983.

Chapter 13
Tumors of the Female Genital Tract in Children

John C. Adkins and Ronald Jaffe

Malignant tumors of the reproductive organs are uncommon in girls. The most common of these, ovarian tumors, account for only about 1% of childhood malignancies [1]. Most of these childhood neoplasms are composed of immature tissues. The common adult malignancies are quite rare in children, yet virtually all have been found in girls under the age of 16 years.

Preservation of reproductive capacity and endocrine function are important considerations in these patients. In many cases, radical surgery, as practiced in adults, may be avoided. Modern combination chemotherapy has greatly improved the prognosis for many patients and often makes a more limited surgical resection possible. Accurate surgical staging and histological classification of the tumor, combined with an understanding of its behavior allows the surgeon to provide optimal care for each patient.

OVARIAN TUMORS

Although most ovarian masses occurring in children are benign (such as dermoid cysts or mature teratomas), a significant percentage will be malignant. In the review by Breen and Maxson, 35% of 1,309 tumors were malignant [2]. These malignancies have a poor prognosis because of their rapid recurrence and resistance to therapy [3–5]. Specific treatment modalities including extent of operation, administration of chemotherapy, and use of radiation therapy are governed by the extent or stage of the disease at diagnosis, its histologic type, and the response to chosen therapy.

Pediatric Tumors of the Genitourinary Tract, pages 207–228
© 1988 Alan R. Liss, Inc.

Staging

Adult ovarian cancers have been relatively predictable according to the stage of the tumor. Historically, the pediatric malignant ovarian neoplasms have been rapidly lethal even when initial involvement appeared to be limited. Staging of childhood ovarian malignancies has been of little prognostic value. Brodeur, however, reported a series of 57 girls with ovarian germ cell malignancies, and the most important indicator of prognosis was the stage of the tumor at the time of diagnosis [6].

Wolner et al. [7] have given an excellent discussion of the staging systems proposed by the International Federation of Gynecology and Obstetrics (FIGO) [8] and by Munell et al. [9], and have proposed the first staging system for pediatric ovarian malignances. More recently, the Children's Cancer Study Group (CCSG) has adopted a staging system we feel is most satisfactory for these tumors (Table 13-1). Meticulous complete staging

TABLE 13–1. Staging of Ovarian Tumors (CCSG)[1]

Stage I	Ovarian involvement only
	Disease limited to one or both ovaries.
	Capsule intact.
	Peritoneal fluid negative for malignant cells.
	a. Limited to one ovary
	b. Bilateral ovarian tumors
Stage II	Ovarian and limited contiguous involvement
	Disease including or beyond the ovarian capsule with local pelvic extension. Retroperitoneal nodes and peritoneal fluid negative for malignant cells.
	a. Disease limited to one ovary with local extension
	b. Bilateral ovarian tumors with unilateral or bilateral pelvic extension
Stage III	Extensive abdominal involvement
	Ovarian tumor with positive retroperitoneal nodes and/or malignant cells in the peritoneal fluid and/or abdominal extension
	a. Peritoneal fluid positive in patients with otherwise group I or II disease
	b. Unilateral or bilateral ovarian tumors with positive retroperitoneal nodes. Local extension present or absent.
	c. Tumor extension to abdominal organs, peritoneal implants, liver, etc.
	d. Any combination of a, b, or c
Stage IV	Extraabdominal (distant) dissemination

[1]R after the stage indicates recurrent disease.

should be assessed in these patients at the time of the first operation. These tumors may be found at the time of an emergency laparotomy, and the surgeon must include staging of the tumor with its removal. The operating surgeon must evaluate both ovaries, the uterus and its adnexae, the omentum, and all (especially diaphragmatic) peritoneal surfaces. Pelvic, iliac, and paraaortic lymph nodes, if enlarged, should be biopsied.

Histology

Classification of ovarian tumors has been a source of confusion. The classification scheme adopted by the World Health Organization is now generally accepted for use by both adult and pediatric pathologists. Table 31-2 gives a modification of that classification that lists the tumors of importance in the pediatric age group.

TABLE 13–2. World Health Organization Classification of Ovarian Tumors[1]

Common epithelial tumors
  Serous
  Mucinous
  Other

Sex cord-stromal tumors
  Granulosa-stromal cell tumors
    Granulosa cell tumor
    Thecoma-fibroma tumors
  Androblastomas: Sertoli-Leydig cell tumors

Lipid cell tumors[2]

Gonadoblastomas[2]

Germ cell tumors
  Dysgerminoma
  Anaplastic dysgerminoma[3]
  Endodermal sinus tumor
  Embryonal carcinoma[4]
  Polyembryoma[2]
  Choriocarcinoma
  Teratomas
    Immature teratoma
    Mature teratoma
  Mixed forms

Metastatic tumors[2]

[1]Adapted from Reference 2.
[2]Not discussed in the text because of infrequent occurrence.
[3]Not listed by WHO; suggested in Reference 23.
[4]Not listed by WHO; suggested in Reference 5.

Norris reported the Armed Forces Institute of Pathology (AFIP) series of 353 primary ovarian neoplasms in patients below the age of 20 years [10]. One hundred fifty patients were less than 15 years old, and 71% of their tumors were of germ cell origin. Eighty percent of the germ cell tumors in this series were malignant. Almost 10% of the tumors were of epithelial origin. Most of these occurred in the late teens, and most were benign. Twenty percent of these tumors were of stromal origin.

The spectrum and incidence of pediatric ovarian neoplasms have been studied by La Vecchia et al. [11] (Table 13-3). Interestingly, only 5% of patients in this study were found to have Stage II or Stage IV disease. The remainder were evenly divided between stages I and III.

Classification

Ovarian tumors can be classified into three major types: epithelial, sex cord-stromal, and germ cell tumors.

Epithelial tumors. The low incidence of epithelial tumors in children and adolescents is shown in Table 13-3. They are ususally seen in the older girl. Their behavior and histology (Fig. 13-1) is similar to that seen in adults. Treatment is based on regimens developed for the adult patient. In the pediatric age group, these tumors tend to be well differentiated, and Copeland recommends fertility-sparing surgery for stage Ia tumors [12]. For further information regarding treatment of these tumors, the surgeon is referred to the gynecologic literature.

Sex cord-stromal tumors. Despite the rarity of these tumors, their occasional spectacular hormonal activity stimulates great interest. About half are accompanied by such activity, and early discovery is often made during an evaluation for precocious puberty. Fox has recently reviewed this group of tumors, adding several subtypes to the classification [13]. Newly appreciated neoplasms in the group are particularly well described. Young reported an association between some of these tumors and the Peutz-Jeghers syndrome, indicating a possible hereditary influence on the etiology [14].

Roth et al. have reported a good prognosis in patients with Sertoli-Leydig cell tumors [15]. This is despite the poor differentiation in those occurring in younger patients. Virtually all of these tumors are associated with virilization.

The histology of two of these tumors is illustrated in Figures 13-2 and 13-3. The histopathologic assessment of malignancy may be impossible in the sex cord-stromal tumors. Fortunately, the clinical behavior is usually benign. Surgical treatment is limited to removal of the involved ovary and tube. Partial removal or tumor spill is often followed by recurrence. Followup is facilitated by assay for the elaborated hormones. The rare recurrence follow-

TABLE 13-3. Histologic Distribution of 522 Cases of Malignant Ovarian Tumors

Pt. age (yr)	Epithelial carcinoma	Sex cord/stromal tumor			Germ cell tumor						
	All types	Granulosa cell	Sertoli-Leydig cell	Un-classi-fied	Dysgermi-noma	Malig. teratoma	Endodermal sinus tumor	Embryonal carcinoma	Chorio-carcinoma	Mixed germ cell	Others
<5	—	—	—	1	3	4	2	—	—	—	1
5-9	—	1	2	1	5	11	9	—	—	5	2
10-14	13	2	1	1	46	21	15	4	2	15	5
Total[1]	13	3	3	3	54	36	26	4	2	20	8
(%)	(7.5)	(1.7)	(1.7)	(1.7)	(31.4)	(20.9)	(15.1)	(2.3)	(1.2)	(11.6)	(4.6)
<20											
Total[2]	22	10	3	8	111	74	57		6	39	20
(%)	(6.3)	(2.9)	(0.9)	(2.3)	(31.7)	(21.1)	(16.3)		(1.7)	(11.1)	(5.7)

[1]From Reference 11 (172 cases).
[2]From Reference 2 (350 cases).

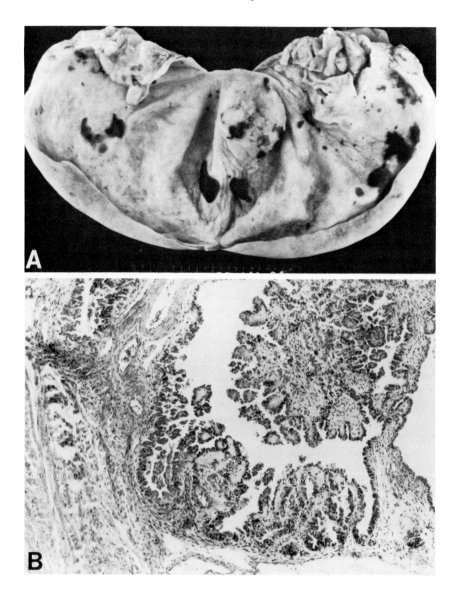

Fig. 13-1. Serous cystadenocarcinoma. A 12-year-old girl had an iliac node metastasis at the time of presentation with this 20-cm cystic tumor of the right ovary. **A:** Opened, the tumor is revealed to be thin-walled with smooth and some papillary areas (with dark hemorrhage). **B:** Microscopy reveals a serous papillary cystadenocarcinoma with solid undifferentiated areas (not shown). She died within a year with widespread metastases of the undifferentiated elements. H&E ×95.

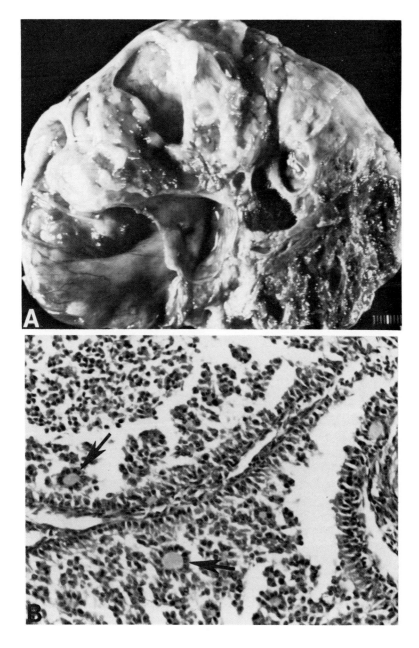

Fig. 13–2. Juvenile granulosa cell tumor. This 1.5-year-old girl had a unilateral ovarian tumor 12 cm in diameter. **A:** extensive cystification with few solid areas. **B:** The juvenile granulosa tumor may be cystic and have papillary-like growth. More solid areas with the characteristic Call-Exner growth pattern are typical (arrows). H&E ×260.

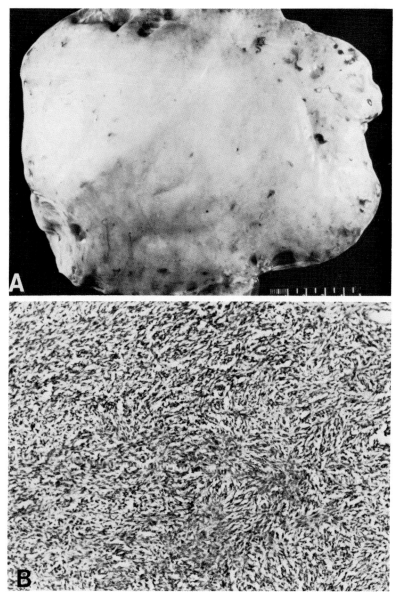

Fig. 13–3. Thecoma. **A:** 15-year-old girl had this 30-cm (1,800 gram) solid fibrous tumor of the right ovary. **B:** Sections highlight the interwoven whorling pattern of a thecoma. H&E ×95.

ing complete removal is usually preceded by the clinically evident hormonal effects. Patients with granulosa cell and theca tumors have been found to be at increased risk of subsequently developing a variety of malignant neoplasms, particularly breast cancer and malignant lymphoma [16].

Germ cell tumors. For many years these tumors were poorly understood because of the variety of histologic forms they may take and the multiplicity of primary tumor sites. Witschi, in his excellent embryologic studies, determined the origin of the primordial germ cells to be in the yolk sac [17]. Their circuitous path to the embryonic gonads may leave deposits of these cells in the retroperitoneum, which may later develop into benign or malignant neoplasms. This work and that by Teilum [18] supported a common histogenesis of the tumors now collectively termed "germ cell tumors." Figure 13-4 is an illustration of their interrelationship, as suggested by Teilum. These neoplasms often occur as mixed tumors, containing several cell types. Dysgerminoma and low-grade immature teratoma have characteristic natural histories. Despite histologic dissimilarity, the other germ cell neoplasms usually follow clinically similar courses, and their treatment is fairly uniform.

Dysgerminoma (germinoma) is the ovarian counterpart of seminoma of the testis, and is its histologic and embryologic equivalent. The gross and microscopic appearance of the dysgerminoma is illustrated in Figure 13-5. Like other malignant germ cell tumors, dysgerminoma is often found in combination with other germ cell types. Nodal metastases are common. They are

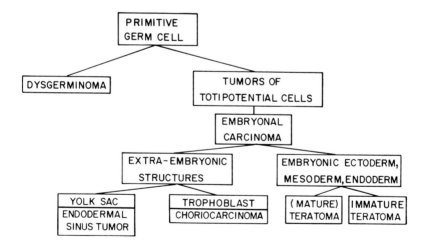

Fig. 13–4. Histogenesis of germ cell tumors. Adapted from Reference 18.

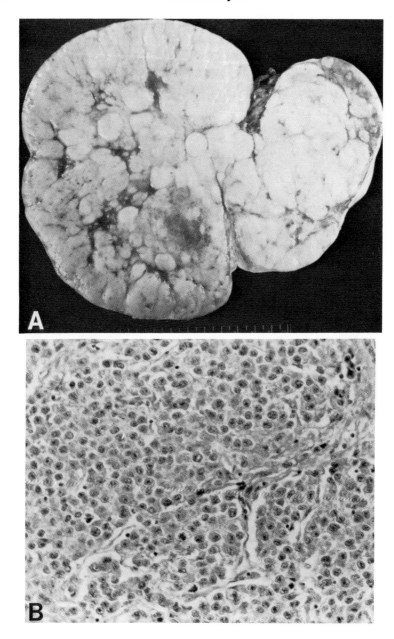

Fig. 13–5. Dysgerminoma. A 10-year-old girl with precocious puberty had a 28-cm left ovarian tumor weighing 2,240 grams. **A:** Fairly homogeneous fleshy tumor nodules with some areas of hemorrhage. **B:** Microscopy characterized by compartmentalized growth of sheets of large cells. H&E ×260.

exquisitely radiosensitive, though the mixed varieties usually follow the behavior pattern of the most malignant component.

Although many patients are found to have an abdominal mass, most present with abdominal pain related to torsion of the involved ovary [19]. The tumor in its pure form is not hormonally active, but the presence of stromal or teratomatous elements will often cause hormonal effects and bring such girls to medical attention with smaller lesions. Bilateral ovarian involvement, unusual in the other malignant germ cell tumors, occurs in 10% of these patients, necessitating evaluation of the opposite ovary in all cases [20]. As might be expected, the best prognosis is found in patients having stage Ia tumors, unruptured and unbiopsied, with pure dysgerminoma histology [19]. Burkons found that 25% of these patients had metastatic disease at the time of diagnosis [21]. If blood-borne metastases are found, the tumor is rarely pure dysgerminoma, and the metastases are usually of another cell type.

If disease is limited to one ovary, it is possible and desirable to preserve the fertility of the patient. Primary surgery consists of unilateral oophorectomy, cytology of peritoneal washings, and adequate biopsy of the apparently uninvolved ovary. Radiotherapy is not given. If the remaining ovary proves to have tumor on biopsy, or if the washings are positive, radiation is given. The field should cover the entire abdomen. Stage Ib (bilateral) tumors require bilateral salpingo-oophorectomy and hysterectomy. Although some treat stage Ib tumors with radiotherapy, it is generally recommended only for patients with recurrent or more extensive disease.

Asadourian reported a series of patients with *anaplastic dysgerminoma* in whom there was a survival of 77% if there were > 8 mitoses/5 hpf, compared to a 90% survival with less mitotic activity [22]. Creasman et al., based on Asadourian's report, proposed the classification of anaplastic dysgerminoma for those patients with > 3 mitoses/hpf [23]. Because of the poorer prognosis associated with the tumors of this category, he recommended the use of methotrexate, actinomycin-D, and chlorambucil as an adjunct to the standard treatment of dysgerminoma. For these particular tumors, we would recommend treatment as for the more resistant germ cell malignancies outlined below.

Endodermal sinus tumor (EST) (yolk sac tumor) has also been called mesonephroma and mesoblastoma. Teilum coined the currently used term because of the histologic similarity to the endodermal sinus of the rat placenta [18]. The tumor is illustrated in Figure 13-6. He separated this tumor from embryonal carcinoma (EC) with which it was previously included and from which it is probably derived. Originally thought to be quite rare, the diagnosis has increased in frequency as pathologists have become more familiar with

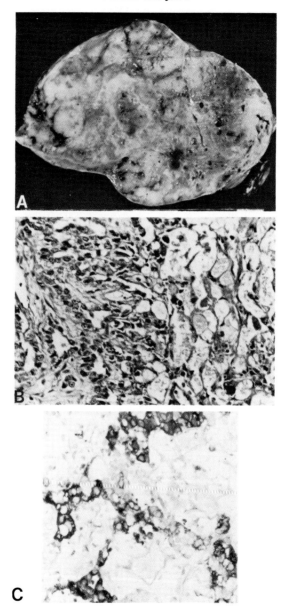

Fig. 13–6. Endodermal sinus (yolk sac) tumor. A 10-year-old girl had this 20-cm tumor confined to the right ovary. The child died of widespread metastases within a year. **A:** Microcystic changes in a solid and heterogeneous-appearing tumor. **B:** Histology varies enormously even within a single tumor. The loose reticular and more solid epithelial patterns are among the more common ones. H&E ×260. **C:** Alpha fetoprotein can be identified in the cytoplasm of tumor cells. DAB-peroxidase ×260.

the classification. EST is usually the malignant component of teratocarcinoma and may also appear with dysgerminoma or embryonal carcinoma in mixed germ cell tumors.

It is an aggressive malignancy that metastasizes early and rapidly invades abdominal and pelvic structures. Kurman reported the AFIP series of 71 ovarian EST cases accumulated over a 30-year period [4]. Of these, 43 occurred in patients under 20 years of age, most in their teens. Of 49 patients in the overall series with stage I (FIGO) tumors, only 8 (16%) survived. In Kurman's autopsy series, all 26 patients were found to have liver, abdominal, and pelvic peritoneal metastases. Retroperitoneal node involvement was noted in 62% of patients. Slightly less than half showed bowel and lung metastases. The uterus and residual ovary were found to be involved in 27% of these patients. Initial treatment had been unilateral salpingo-oophorectomy. Any autopsy series tends to reflect extensive end-stage disease, but this series emphasizes the propensity of EST for abdominal metastasis. "Prophylactic" exenteration or panhysterectomy offers little for this tumor whose area of risk is so broad.

After the work by Teilum, the classification of *embryonal carcinoma* entered a period of disuse until revived by Kurman and Norris in 1976 [5]. Its histologic similarity to EC of the adult testis was emphasized. Ten of the 15 cases in their report occurred in patients under 18 years of age. Of these ten, five were stage I, three stage II, and two stage III. Only three of the ten pediatric cases survived. Half of the tumors were hormonally active. All patients tested for human chorionic gonadotropin (hCG) were found to have elevated levels, and half of the patients were found to have an elevated assay for alpha fetoprotein (AFP). These assays emphasize the distinction from EST, which always produces AFP, but rarely elaborates hCG.

The 50% survival rate in stage I tumors reported by Kurman is better than expected for EST, but, because of its similar response to chemotherapy, the same surgical and chemotherapeutic approach is recommended.

Immature teratomas (IT) differ from mature ones by the presence of immature or embryonal tissues (Fig. 13-7). They consist of tissue derived from two or more germ cell layers (ectoderm, endoderm, and mesoderm). Immature teratomas are graded from grade 0 to grade 3, depending on the amount of immature neuroepithelium present [24]. Those with higher histologic grade behave more aggressively.

The cut tumors may resemble mature teratomas (Figs. 13-8 and 13-9), with the presence of well-organized tissues such as bone, hair, or teeth. They are often found to have cysts and areas of hemorrhage and necrosis. These tumors grow rapidly, and particularly those of high grade histology, may

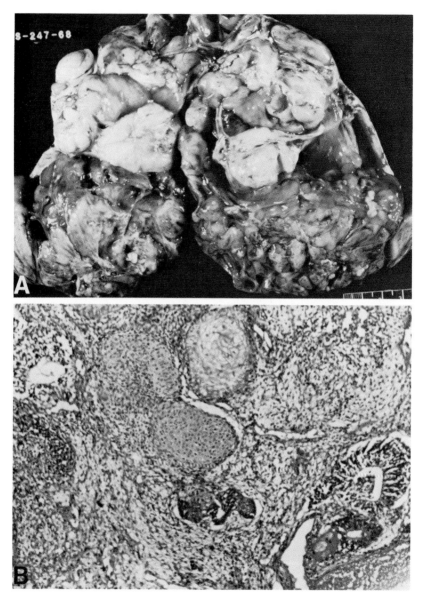

Fig. 13–7. Immature teratoma. **A:** Section of a 13-cm left ovarian tumor in a 1-year-old girl reveals the marked heterogeneity of a solid teratoma. Solid, cystic, neural, bony, and epidermoid elements are found. **B:** The immature teratoma contains elements seen in the developing fetus, but by definition, it contains no recognizable malignant elements after extensive search and sampling. H&E ×95.

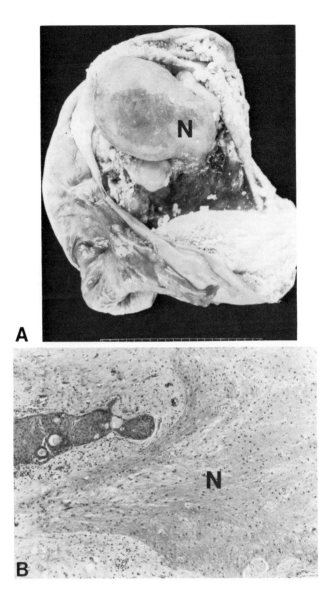

Fig. 13–8. Mature teratoma. This 27-cm cystic tumor from a 15-year-old girl weighed 3,790 grams. **A:** Cut surface shows the variety of organized tissues. This tumor contained skin, its appendages, bone, teeth, eye, central nervous system, choroid, and a variety of intestinal epithelia. A nodule of brain tissue is present (N). **B:** The predominant elements are skin and its appendages, as well as neuroglial tissue (N). H&E ×95.

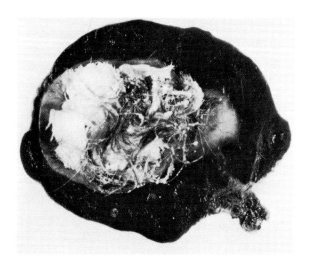

Fig. 13–9. Mature cystic teratoma (dermoid). Components are restricted to dermal elements, such as hair, teeth, and keratinizing squamous epithelium; 10% of such tumors occur bilaterally.

penetrate the capsule. A frequent finding is widespread peritoneal studding by neuroglial implants. Kosloske reported five children with grade 2 IT treated with unilateral salpingo-oophorectomy [25]. Those with peritoneal implants were also given vincristine, actinomycin-D, and cyclophosphamide. All survived. Interestingly, "retroconversion" or reduction of grade of peritoneal implants has been reported in patients with [26] and without [27] treatment with chemotherapy.

Treatment recommendations consist of surgical removal of as much tumor as possible, including large peritoneal implants. Exenteration is not recommended. High grade (2 or 3) tumors should undergo chemotherapy as proposed for EST and ECT, as should patients who have nodal or hematogenous metastases. These tumors are resistant to radiation therapy.

Primary ovarian *choriocarcinoma* may occur in a pure form or mixed with other germ cell elements. Unlike gestational trophoblastic disease, it is not highly sensitive to chemotherapy. The tumor secretes hCG, which is of value in establishing the diagnosis and following the course of the disease. Although methotrexate is of little value when used alone, Gerbie et al. reported its use with vincristine and actinomycin-D in achieving cure in three pediatric cases having pure choriocarcinoma [28]. More recently, treatment of this germ cell malignancy has been the same as recommended for EST.

Clinical Presentation

The most common presenting complaint of children with ovarian tumors is abdominal pain [3]. Often this acute onset of the pain mimics appendicitis. This acute onset is usually the result of torsion of the pendulous ovarian tumor, though rupture of a necrotic area may also precipitate symptoms. Other girls are brought to medical attention because of abdominal enlargement or parental appreciation of a mass. Precocious puberty, vaginal bleeding, or virilization may signal the presence of hormonally active tumors. Occasional difficulty in voiding or urinary retention, may be the presenting complaint [29]. Once symptoms or signs are apparent, about half are brought to medical care within a week, and about 25% will be admitted within 24 hours [30]. There can be a delay of several months in the remaining patients, though the fulminant nature of these tumors tends to abbreviate the time between symptom appearance and diagnosis.

Evaluation

Most patients will have a palpable mass. Sonography and computed tomography are of value in determining the nature and extent of disease. However, they are imprecise in determining whether a mass is benign or malignant. Tumors of either type may be solid or contain cysts or calcification. Peritoneal lesions may be benign glial implants of teratoma. The role of magnetic resonance imaging has yet to be determined. Gross lymphadenopathy or extraabdominal disease, detected by any modality, indicates malignant disjease. Blood should be collected for biochemical marker assay (AFP and hCG). These may be of value in following the patient, but surgery for the tumor should not be delayed awaiting the results. Complete preoperative workup should be expeditious and take no more than 24 hours due to the danger of sudden rupture of these tumors.

Treatment

Chemotherapy. Samuel's 1970 report of the activity of vinblastine for the treatment of testicular germ cell neoplasms offered hope in the treatment of ovarian germ cell tumors [31]. Blum et al. [32] and Higby et al. [33] showed activity for bleomycin and diaminodichloroplatinum (cis-platinum), respectively, against certain germ cell tumors. In 1976, Wolner et al. utilized a multidrug regimen as an adjunct to aggressive surgery for the treatment of ovarian malignancies in children [7]. They gave vincristine, actinomycin-D, cyclophosphamide, and adriamycin to nine patients with advanced disease. Five survived. Slayton et al. reported similar results using only three of these agents [34].

Einhorn and Donohue reported the use of vinblastine, bleomycin, and cis-platinum with and without adriamycin for metastatic testicular germ cell tumors [35]. Significant activity was shown against these tumors that have histologic, biochemical, and immunologic features similar to ovarian germ cell tumors. CCSG had previously adopted a six-drug protocol employing bleomycin, vinblastine, cis-platinum, cyclophosphamide, and adriamycin for the treatment of germ cell neoplasms excluding dysgerminomas. Ablin et al. in 1982 reported a complete response to this regimen in 19 of 20 patients [36]. Four of these 19 subsequently developed fatal recurrence. Toxicity of the regimen itself was minimal. In 1985, Taylor et al. reported 14 patients, treated with vinblastine, bleomycin, and cis-platinum [37]. All 14, ten of whom had stage IjII or IV disease, showed a complete response, and 13 survived. The single death was due to bleomycin pulmonary toxicity.

Surgery. Surgery for these neoplasms has undergone a similar evolution during the past two decades. Initially, reflecting treatment recommendations for adult gynecologic malignancies, aggressive operations were commonplace. Harris and Boles, however, favored a limited operation in recommending thorough exploration and staging, but eliminating exenteration for the more extensive local tumors [38]. Limited surgery and adjuvant chemotherapy consisting of vincristine, actinomycin-D, and cyclophosphamide were shown to be effective by Cangir et al. [39]. Twenty-one girls were treated with removal of as much tumor as possible, but salvage of the opposite ovary and uterus when uninvolved with tumor. Nine patients with FIGO stage I or II tumors all survived as did seven of eight patients with stage III tumors. One of the five stage IV patients survived.

If an ovarian mass is discovered at the time of surgery for another condition, the incision should be enlarged or altered to allow tumor resection and adequate staging including collection of peritoneal washing for cytology. If there is a question of operative violation of the capsule of the tumor, washings may also be collected at the end of the procedure. Such specimens, however, may be difficult to interpret because of heavy contamination by red cells. Postoperatively, blood should be collected and sent for assay of AFP and hCG [40]. Maximum tumor removal and accurate staging are the goals of the surgical procedure. The choice of an incision is important. The Pfannenstiel incision, though cosmetically appealing, is usually unsatisfactory for the removal of large tumors and for necessary staging. We have found the midline incision most advantageous, although "smile" incisions are equally satisfactory in girls under the age of 2 or 3 years. The staging should be complete and detailed explicitly in the operative note: inspection of the pelvic organs; evaluation of pelvic and retroperitoneal nodes; inspection and palpation of peritoneal surfaces, including that of the diaphragm. Peritoneal washings for cytology should be obtained at the beginning of the procedure. The opposite ovary should be carefully inspected and biopsied (if dysgerminoma is a possibility, the opposite ovary should be bivalved and biopsied generously). Stage Ia tumors are treated by unilateral salpingo-oophorectomy only. Internal genitalia involved by tumor should be removed. The uterus and opposite ovary, if uninvolved, should be left in place. If the omentum is attached to the tumor, omentectomy should be performed. We do not recommend debulking procedures that leave behind gross residual tumor. Exenteration is not recommended.

TUMORS OF THE UTERUS, CERVIX, AND VAGINA

Tumors of the lower genital tract are rare in children. Those that do occur nearly always fall into one of three categories: rhabdomyosarcomas, germ cell tumors, and genital clear cell adenocarcinomas. An occasional report of another tumor cell type will be seen, such as Bell's case of a cervical Wilms' tumor [41], but these rarities will not be considered here. The most frequent malignancy of the area in adults, squamous cell carcinoma, does not occur in childhood.

Regardless of the histology of the tumor involved, nearly all come to medical attention because of abnormal vaginal bleeding or passage of tumor fragments. Vaginal bleeding is such an uncommon occurrence in the prepubertal girl that it deserves a full workup at first appearance. Protrusion of a mass through the introitus may also signal the presence of tumor. This may at first be confused with a urethral cyst or other benign lesion, but even casual inspection should reveal the true nature of the lesion.

The workup of these patients is expeditious. Pelvic sonogram is of value, and computed tomography or magnetic resonance imaging are helpful in establishing preoperatively the extent of the lesion. Prior to definitive surgery, examination under anesthesia, including vaginoscopy and cystoscopy, should be done. Bimanual rectal (in older girls, vaginal) examination and punch biopsy or fine needle aspiration of accessible tumor should be performed. Rarely, benign vaginal polyps occur that can resemble malignancy [42]. Blood should be drawn preoperatively for biochemical tumor markers (AFP and hCG).

Endodermal Sinus Tumor

Vaginal or cervical EST presents like other malignancies of these structures in children [43,44]. Bleeding or protrusion of a mass brings these infants (usually under 3 years of age) to medical attention. Although Anderson et al. have suggested primary chemotherapy for treatment [44], we prefer resection, as recommended for genital RMS, followed by chemotherapy specific for EST. Exenteration would be reserved for pelvic recurrence.

Other Tumors

Other tumors of the lower genital tract are very unusual. However, special mention should be made of genital clear cell adenocarcinoma. In 1971, Herbst et al. reported the occurrence of this previously very rare tumor in children exposed in utero to diethylstilbestrol [45]. Since that time, the use of this drug has been stopped, and females at risk are passing beyond the pediatric age range. The reports by Johnston and Jones [46] and Emens [47] are excellent starting points for those interested in this problem.

REFERENCES

1. Young JL, Miller RW: Incidence of malignant tumors in U.S. children. J Pediatr 8:254–258, 1975.
2. Breen JL, Maxon WS: Ovarian tumors in children and adolescents. Clin Obst Gynecol 20:607–623, 1977.
3. Ein SH: Malignant ovarian tumors in children. J Pediatr Surg 8:539–542, 1973.
4. Kurman RJ, Norris HJ: Endodermal sinus tumor of the ovary—a clinical and pathologic analysis of 71 cases. Cancer 38:2404–2419, 1976.
5. Kurman RJ, Norris, HJ: Embryonal carcinoma of the ovary—A clinocopathologic entity distinct from endodermal sinus tumor resembling embryonal carcinoma of the adult testis. Cancer 38:2420–2433, 1976.
6. Brodeur GM, Howarth CB, Pratt CB, et al.: Malignant germ cell tumors in 57 children and adolescents. Cancer 48: 1890–1898, 1981.
7. Wolner N, Exelby P, Woodruff JM, et al.: Malignant ovarian tumors in childhood. Prognosis in relation to initial therapy. Cancer 37: 1953–1964, 1976.
8. Kottmeier HL: Classification and staging of malignant tumors in the female pelvis. Int J Gynecol Obstet 9:172–180, 1971.
9. Munell EW, Jacox HW, Taylor HC Jr.. Treatment and prognosis in cancer of the ovary. Am J Obstet Gynecol 74:1187–1200, 1957.
10. Norris HJ, Jensen RD: Relative frequency of ovarian neoplasms in children and adolescents. Cancer 30:713–719, 1972.
11. La Vecchia C, Morris HB, Draper GJ: Malignant ovarian tumours in childhood in Britain, 1962. Br J Cancer 48:363–374, 1983.
12. Copeland LJ: Malignant gynecologic tumors. In Sutton WW (ed): Clinical Pediatric Oncology, St. Louis: C.V. Mosby, 1984.
13. Fox, H: Sex cord-stromal tumours of the ovary. J Pathol 145:127–148, 1985.
14. Young RH, Dickersin GR, Scully RE: A distinctive ovarian sex cord-stromal tumor causing sexual precocity in the Peutz-Jeghers syndrome. Am Surg Pathol 7:233–243, 1983.
15. Roth LM, Anderson MC, Govan ADT, et al.: Sertoli-Leydig cell tumors: A clinicopathologic study of 34 cases. Cancer 48:187–197, 1981.

16. Bjorkholm E: Granulosa and theca cell tumors—an epidemiological and clinocopatholog- ical study. Acta Radiol 3:1–18, 1980.

17. Witschi E: Migration of the germ cells of human embryos from the yolk sac to the primitive gonadal folds. Carnegie Contrib Embryol 32:67–80, 1948.

18. Teilum G: Classification of endodermal sinus tumor (Meioblastoma vitellinum) and so called embryonal carcinoma of the ovary. Acta Pathol Microbiol Scand 64:407, 1965.

19. Linton EB: Dysgerminoma of the ovary. J Reprod Med 26:255–260, 1981.

20. Kurman RJ, Norris HJ: Malignant germ cell tumors of the ovary. Hum Pathol 8:551– 564, 1977.

21. Burkons DM, Hart WR: Ovarian germinomas (dysgerminomas). Obstet Gynecol 51:221– 224, 1978.

22. Asadourian LA, Taylor HB: Dysgerminoma. An analysis of 105 cases. Obstet Gynecol 33:370–379, 1979.

23. Creasman WT, Fetter BF, Hammond CB, et al.: Germ cell malignancies of the ovary. Obstet Gynecol 53:226–230, 1979.

24. Norris HJ, Zirkin HJ, Benson WI: Immature (malignant) teratoma of the ovary. A clinical and pathologic study of 58 cases. Cancer 37:2359–2372, 1976.

25. Kosloske AM, Favara BE, Hays T, et al.: Management of immature teratoma of the ovary in children by conservative resection and chemotherapy. J Pediatr Surg, 11:839–846, 1976.

26. Aronowitz J, Estrada R, Lynch R, et al.: Retroconversion of malignant immature terato- mas of the ovary after chemotherapy. Gynecol Oncol 16:414–421, 1983.

27. Favara BE, Franciosi RA: Ovarian teratoma and neuroglial implants on the peritoneum. Cancer 31:678–681, 1979.

28. Gerbie MV, Brewer JI, Tamimi H: Primary choriocarcinoma of the ovary. Obstet Gynecol 46:720–723, 1975.

29. Bosio M, Ballerini G, Cattaneo A: Acute urinary retention: A rare onset sign of ovarian cystic teratoma. Int J Pediatr Nephrol 4:263–265, 1983.

30. Orr PS, Gibson A, Young DG: Ovarian tumours in childhood: A 27-year review. Br Jr Surg 63:367–370, 1976.

31. Samuels ML, Howe CD: Vinblastine in the management of testicular cancer. Cancer 25:1009–1017, 1970.

32. Blum RH, Carter S, Agre K: A clinical review of bleomycin—a new antineoplastic agent. Cancer 31:903–914, 1973.

33. Higby DJ, Wallace HJ, Albert D, et al.: Diaminodichloro-platinum in chemotherapy of testicular tumors. J Urol 112:100–104, 1974.

34. Slayton RE, Hreshchyshyn MM, Silverberg SG, et al.: Treatment of malignant ovarian germ cell tumors, response to vincristine, dactinomycin, and cyclophosphamide (prelim- inary report). Cancer 42:390–398, 1978.

35. Einhorn LH, Donohue JP: Combination chemotherapy in disseminated testicular cancer. Semin Oncol 6:87–93, 1979.

36. Ablin A, Ramsay N, Krailo M, et al.: Effective therapy for malignant germ cell tumors in children: A study by the Children's Cancer Study Group. Proc ASCO, p 108, 1982.

37. Taylor MH, DePetrillo AD, Turner AR: Vinblastine, bleomycin, and cisplatin in malig- nant germ cell tumors of the ovary. Cancer 56:1341–1349, 1985.

38. Harris BH, Boles ET: Rational surgery for tumors of the ovary in children. J Pediatr Surg 9:289–293, 1974.

39. Cangir A, Smith J, van Eys J: Improved prognosis in children with ovarian cancers following modified VAC (vincristine sulfate, dactinomycin, and cyclophosphamide) chemotherapy. Cancer 42:1234–1238, 1978.

40. Tsuchida Y: Markers in childhood solid tumors. In Hays DM (ed): Pediatric Surgical Oncology. Orlando: Grune & Stratton, pp 47–62, 1986.

41. Bell DA, Shimm DS, Gang DL: Wilms' tumor of the endocervix. Arch Pathol Lab Med 109:371–373, 1985.

42. Norris HJ, Taylor HB: Polyps of the vagina. Cancer 19:227–231, 1966.

43. Young RH, Scully RE: Endodermal sinus tumor of the vagina: A report of nine cases and review of the literature. Gynecol Oncol 18:380–392, 1984.

44. Anderson WA, Sabio H, Durso N, et al.: Endodermal sinus tumor of the vagina: The role of primary chemotherapy. Cancer 56:1025–1027, 1985.

45. Herbst AL, Ulfelder H, Postanzer UC: Adenocarcinoma of the vagina. N Engl J Med 284:878–881, 1971.

46. Johnston GA, Jr, Jones HA: Genital clear cell adenocarcinoma. Int Surg 68:257–261, 1983.

47. Emens M: Vaginal adenosis and diethylstilbestrol. Brit J Hosp Med, 31:42–48, 1984.

Chapter 14
Tumors Associated With Disorders of Sexual Differentiation

Mark F. Bellinger

The relationship between both gonadal and extragonadal neoplasia and disorders of sexual differentiation is well documented but poorly understood. It is known that several categories of intersex carry a higher risk for the development of neoplasia than others and that certain tumors are likely to occur in these patients. By surveying available histologic and epidemiologic data, it is possible to identify a population at risk and to outline a plan for the management of gonadal tissue in the patient with anomalous sexual differentiation.

NORMAL VERSUS ABNORMAL SEXUAL DIFFERENTIATION

The establishment of gender identity is a complex phenomenon involving genetic, gonadal, and local factors, some of which are poorly understood. In the past, the Y chromosome was considered to be the male factor necessary for transformation of the indifferent gonad into a testis [1]. In the absence of this genetic influence, an ovary was formed. However, the occurrence of XX individuals with ovotestes was poorly explained. In 1955, Eichwald and Silmser discovered the H-Y (histocompatibility-Y) antigen in mice [2]. Subsequent studies have confirmed the presence of this male-specific antigen in heterogametes of all species [3]. Wachtel et al. have proposed that this antigen is a product of the testis-organizing gene and is responsible for testicular organogenesis [4]. Clinical evidence to support this postulate in-

Pediatric Tumors of the Genitourinary Tract, pages 229–240

cludes the presence of H-Y antigen in the testicular component of ovotestes, XX sex-reversed males, and XX true hermaphrodites [3,5]. It thus appears that the critical factor in testicular development is not the Y chromosome, but the expression of H-Y antigen. Whether a tendency toward gonadal neoplasia in intersex conditions is similarly linked to genetic influence is currently debated, but the relationship between gonadal histology and genotype cannot be dismissed as coincidence.

Within the complex mechanisms that result in the determination of genetic sex and its translation into phenotype, there are several pathways by which sexual ambiguity may result. Since the risk of gonadal and extragonadal neoplasia is tremendously variable within the constellation of intersex, it is necessary to study not only the histological manifestations of neoplasia, but its distribution among the clinical categories of anomalous sexual differentiation. A broad generalization of intersex states based on gonadal histology is found in Table 14-1.

FEMALE PSEUDOHERMAPHRODISM

Female pseudohermaphrodism secondary to virilization of the external genitalia by endogenous androgens (congenital adrenal hyperplasia, adrenogenital syndrome) is the most common anomaly of sexual differentiation [6]. Fetal virilization from exogenous sources (maternal androgen ingestion or androgen-secreting tumors) is very rare [7]. In affected females, normal ovaries and mullerian elements are present, while variable degrees of masculinization of the external genitalia, urogenital sinus, and prostatic anlage

TABLE 14-1. Classification of Disorders of Sexual Differentiation

Female pseudohermaphrodism
  Congenital adrenal hyperplasia (endogenous)
  Secondary to maternal androgens (exogenous)
Male pseudohermaphrodism
  Congenital adrenal hyperplasia (defective testosterone synthesis)
  Complete and incomplete testicular feminization (defective end-organ sensitivity)
  Persistent mullerian duct syndrome or hernia uteri inguinalis (deficient mullerian regression factor)
  Pseudovaginal perineoscrotal hypospadias (deficiency of 5-alpha reductase)
Disorders of gonadal differentiation
  True hermaphrodism
  Seminiferous tubule dysgenesis (Klinefelter's syndrome)
  Gonadal dysgenesis (Turner's syndrome, variants)
  Mixed gonadal dysgenesis
Miscellaneous

(tissues containing 5-alpha reductase and exquisitely sensitive to androgens during embryogenesis) occur. In spite of the tremendous excesses of both ACTH and androgens in these patients, there is no evidence for increased risk of neoplasia, an indication that hormonal excesses are not oncogenic [8].

MALE PSEUDOHERMAPHRODISM

Male pseudohermaphrodism defines a heterogeneous group of genetic males with testes and variable degrees of incomplete masculinization of the external genitalia. Most commonly, genital ambiguity results from defective testosterone synthesis (congenital adrenal hyperplasia) [9] or end-organ insensitivity to androgen (complete testicular feminization syndrome [10] or its incomplete variants: the Lubs [11], Reifenstein's [12], or Gilbert-Dreyfus [13] syndromes). Also included in this category are normal men with defects in mullerian regression factor (MRF) [14] and persistence of mullerian structures (upper vagina, uterus, fallopian tube), and individuals with 5-alpha reductase deficiency and inadequate virilization of the external genitalia (pseudovaginal perineoscrotal hypospadias) [15]. Because of the heterogeneity of this group, the risk of neoplasia will be considered separately for each subclass. The category of gonadal dysgenesis termed dysgenetic male pseudohermaphrodism will be considered under disorders of gonadal differentiation.

Congenital Adrenal Hyperplasia

Incomplete virilization may result from defects in 20,22-desmolase, 20-alpha hydroxylase, 3-beta-ol dehydrogenase, 17-alpha-hydroxylase, 17,20-desmolase, or 17-ketosteroid reductase activity during steroidogenesis [9]. All disorders are rare and none have been associated with increased risk of neoplasia.

Complete Testicular Feminization Syndrome

Complete testicular feminization describes a distinctive X-linked syndrome of 46, XY, H-Y antigen-positive males who are phenotypically female and develop normal female secondary sex characteristics at puberty, but do not menstruate [16]. A blind-ending vagina is present, together with abdominal testes. Lack of virilization results from end-organ androgen insensitivity caused by defective receptors for both testosterone and dihydrotestosterone [17]. Testicular estradiol production and peripheral conversion of testosterone to estradiol cause feminization at puberty. The prepubertal gonads of patients with testicular feminization are histologically identical to cryptorchid tests. After puberty, atrophic seminiferous tubules with absent spermatogenesis are combined with Leydig cell hyperplasia [18].

Morris and Mahesh reviewed the risk of gonadal neoplasia in 187 patients with testicular feminization. They found an increased risk of tumor (22% over the age of 30 years, but a low risk under this age) [10]. Other authors have confirmed these data. Simpson and Photopulos consider 2–5% a reasonable estimate for the risk of gonadal neoplasia in the group as a whole, slightly higher than the risk for cryptorchid testes in normal males [8]. The most common neoplasm found is seminoma, but the range of histologic patterns parallels the findings in patients with cryptorchidism. As in the cryptorchid male, it remains to be determined whether neoplasia represents an inherent tendency of the gonad or the effect of an intraabdominal environment. The increased incidence of gonadal neoplasia in testicular feminization has led most authors to concur that these patients should be allowed to feminize naturally at puberty and undergo elective bilateral gonadectomy soon thereafter, before reaching the age of increased risk [10]. Extragonadal neoplasia is uncommon.

Incomplete Testicular Feminization

All patients with testicular feminization have bilateral testes, lack of mullerian structures, and pubertal breast development. Those with incomplete feminization may display inguinal or labial testes and variable degrees of clitoromegaly with labial fusion, evidence for incomplete androgen sensitivity [19]. A specific subset of patients described by Reifenstein has small scrotal testes, a normal-sized but hypospadiac phallus, and lack of pubertal virilization [12]. Lubs et al. [11] described a less virilized group with labioscrotal fusion, and the patients of Gilbert-Dreyfus were similarly ambiguous [13]. Gonadal neoplasia in these incomplete forms of testicular feminization is less common than in the complete syndrome, likely due to the extraabdominal location of the testes or because less abnormal gonads are more likely to undergo partial descent [15]. Extragonadal neoplasia is uncommon.

Persistent Mullerian Duct Syndrome

This rare disorder is discovered in a normal XY male when mullerian structures are found incidentally at laparotomy performed for unrelated reasons or at inguinal exploration for a cryptorchid testis or hernia [14]. Presumably, a local defect in MRF production or utilization is causative [17].

Although gonadal neoplasia in this group is generally felt to be rare and related to the abdominal location of the testis, Snow and colleagues found 11 cases of testicular tumor (five seminoma, two embryonal carcinoma, one choricarcinoma, two teratoma, one yolk sac tumor) in 80 patients with this syndrome, an incidence of 14% [20]. All testes except one were cryptorchid. Presumably, the incidence of testicular tumor in persistent mullerian duct syndrome is at least equal to the incidence of tumor in the cryptorchid testis. Clearly, abdominal testes of these patients should be removed or undergo orchiopexy at the time of discovery. Extragonadal tumors are rare.

Pseudovaginal Perineoscrotal Hypospadias

This autosomal recessive form of male pseudohermaphrodism results from a defect in 5-alpha reductase and a resulting block in the conversion of testosterone to dihydrotestosterone [21]. Inadequate virilization of the fetus results in an infant with a small hypospadiac phallus, bifid scrotum, and a urogenital sinus that opens onto the perineum. Testes are inguinal or labio-scrotal in location. At puberty, evidence of virilization includes increased muscle mass, phallic enlargement, scrotal rugation, and testicular descent [22]. The risk of neoplasia in these gonads is identical to that of the cryptor-chid testis [8].

DISORDERS OF GONADAL DIFFERENTIATION

True Hermaphrodism

By definition, true hermaphrodism denotes the presence of both testicular and ovarian tissue, distributed in the same or separate gonads. Histologically, the ovarian component is usually better differentiated, while testicular tissue is commonly atrophic with hyalinized tubules [23]. Karyotype is 46,XX in the majority of cases, with the remainder being mosaic (46,XX/46,XY or 46,XX/47,XXY) or rarely 46,XY [24,25]. In concert with the variable genotype, phenotype has a wide variety of presentation. Gonadal neoplasia in the true hermaphrodite is uncommon. Testicular tumors are most common secondary to both the lack of differentiation and the cryptorchid location of the gonads. Nichter postulated that H-Y antigen might predispose to malig-nant degeneration [26], but the cytogenetic complement of most patients with tumors is unknown. Seminoma, gonadoblastoma, dysgerminoma, yolk sac carcinoma, and Sertoli cell tumors have been reported [27–30]. It is recom-mended that intraabdominal gonads inappropriate to the sex of rearing be removed, appropriate gonads be preserved, and cryptorchid testes be re-moved or brought to a scrotal position for continued observation [17].

Breast carcinoma has been reported in three patients with true hermaphrodism, two of whom carried a 46,XX karyotype [31]. Periodic screening and breast self-examination is warranted.

Seminiferous Tubule Dysgenesis

Males with seminiferous tubule dysgenesis (Klinefelter's syndrome) have one Y chromosome and two or more X chromosomes. Since the first description of this syndrome in 1949, many variants have been recognized, including XY/XXY mosaicism and XX sex-reversed males [17]. Clinically, these individuals have small firm testes, azoospermia, and a male phenotype. Gynecomastia, eunechoidism, and poor muscular development become evident in adolescence [32]. Mental retardation is more common in the XXY pattern. Klinefelter's syndrome is one of the most common causes of hypogonadism and infertility in males. Testicular tumors are uncommon although seminoma, embryonal carcinoma, and teratoma have been reported [33]. No gonadal tumors have been reported in 46,XX males. Extragonadal germ cell tumors have occurred in the mediastinum, pineal gland, and retroperitoneum [33].

Breast carcinoma has an increased incidence in patients with the Klinefelter's syndrome, particularly in those with a 47,XXY karyotype [34,35]. Approximately 4% of males with breast carcinoma have a Klinefelter karyotype, an incidence 18 times greater than that of the normal male population [36].

Gonadal Dysgenesis and Mixed Gonadal Dysgenesis

Clinically, the syndrome of gonadal dysgenesis encompasses Turner's syndrome and its variants, a group of phenotypically female but sexually infantile individuals with bilateral streak gonads composed of connective tissue without ovocytes [17]. Study of this interesting group has provided a great deal of information about abnormal cytogenetics and neoplasia. In general, it appears that the risk of gonadal neoplasia is extremely low in those individuals lacking a Y chromosome [37]. Individuals with 45,XO karyotype are usually easily recognized clinically and have a low risk of gonadal neoplasia. Extragonadal tumors including skin and gastrointestinal, however, have been reported [38]. Patients with the XX variant of gonadal dysgenesis may be diagnosed at puberty because of failure to develop normal secondary sex characteristics. Mild virilization may occur. Laparotomy or laparoscopy may be indicated to confirm the status of the gonads and internal duct structures. Streak or dysgenetic gonads may be removed to confirm the diagnosis. Gonadal neoplasia is uncommon.

The XY variant of gonadal dysgenesis may also present at puberty. The striking feature of this cytogenetic variant is the associated, increased risk of gonadal malignancy [39]. Histologically, the streak gonads are indistinguishable from those of the 45,XO or 46,XX variants, but 20–30% of patients with the XY variant develop gonadal tumors. These tumors most commonly are gonadoblastomas or dysgerminomas occurring during the first decade of life [40–42]. Gonadectomy is appropriate in these patients upon diagnosis.

Mixed gonadal dysgenesis was described by Sovhal in 1963 to describe individuals with both a testis and a streak gonad [43]. As a form of gonadal dysgenesis, this category has been broadened to include some patients with bilateral streaks or bilateral dysgenetic testes [44]. Individuals with mixed gonadal dysgenesis represent one of the largest groups of intersex patients. External genitalia vary in the degree of masculinization, and either sex of rearing may adopted. Mullerian structures are usually present. Karyotype is mosaic, most commonly 45,XO/46,XY, but 45,XO/46,XY/47,XXY and others have been reported [45]. The risk of gonadal malignancy in mixed gonadal dysgenesis is estimated to be 10–15% [8]. Most gonads with tumors have been undescended. Dysgenetic or abdominal testes in this group of patients should be removed. If a cryptorchid testis in a child with male sex of rearing can be brought into the scrotum, orchidopexy should be combined with long-term followup. Although extragonadal neoplasia in patients with mixed gonadal dysgenesis is not increased, endometrial carcinoma has been reported, most likely related to estrogen replacement therapy.

SPECIAL ASSOCIATION: WILMS' TUMOR, INTERSEX, NEPHRITIS

Wilms' tumor is known to have an association with a variety of congenital anomalies including aniridia, hemihypertrophy, hypospadias, and anomalies of the external genitalia [46]. Drash et al. were the first to note the frequent association between Wilms' tumor, nephritis, and male pseudohermaphrodism and to suggest that these abnormalities constitute a syndrome [47]. Subsequent reports have noted various combinations of at least two of the components of this clinical syndrome [48]. Rajfer reported on ten patients with intersex who subsequently developed Wilms' tumor [49]. Five had an XY karyotype, ambiguous genitalia, a testis and a streak gonad; one had a 46,XX/XY karyotype with a unilateral testis; and four had an unknown karyotype and variable gonadal histology. Beheshti et al. reviewed 188 patients with Wilms' tumor and six with mesoblastic nephroma [50]. External genital anomalies were present in 27% of patients with bilateral tumors and 2.3% of patients with unilateral tumors. One patient had mixed gonadal dysgenesis and three had male pseudohermaphrodism. It has been proposed that the frequent occurrence of this pattern of congenital anomaly represents the end result of a common genetic and/or teratogenic insult to the urogenital ridge early in gestation [49]. Recent recognition of the presence of chromosomal anomalies in many patients with Wilms' tumor and the genetic tendencies of other neoplasms have confirmed the need for further research into the etiologies not only of Wilms' tumor but also of the relationship between chromosomal anomalies, anomalies of sexual differentiation, and gonadal neoplasia.

GONADAL NEOPLASIA AND INTERSEX: A SUMMARY

Malignant germ cell tumors have been reported in approximately 25% (0–30%) of patients with forms of gonadal dysgenesis and a karyotype including a Y chromosome. It is well documented that XY gonadal dysgenesis and mixed gonadal dysgenesis carry the highest risk for gonadal neoplasia of all intersex groups. Manuel et al. estimated the tumor risk in gonadal dysgenesis to be 4% at 10 years, 10% at 15 years, 73% at 30 years, and 80% at 40 years [51]. In mixed gonadal dysgenesis, the risk is 3% at 10 years, 10% at 13 years, 20% at 15 years, and 74.5 at 26 years. This far exceeds the incidence of neoplasia in cryptorchid testes found in all other intersex categories.

The question of whether gonadal neoplasia is purely a genetic event remains unanswered. Early age at the time of tumor development and the increased incidence of bilateral tumors have been used to support the concept that a mutant gene is responsible [52]. Certainly, the markedly lessened risk of neoplasia in individuals without a Y chromosome makes the Y chromosome or Y chromosome-directed genetic information suspect as a contributing factor to the development of gonadal neoplasia [53]. Conversely, the neoplastic potential of dysgenetic gonads may be related to an abnormal environment. This concept is supported by the increased incidence of tumors found in abdominal gonads over that found in inguinal gonads, and the increased risk for inguinal over descended gonads. Muller et al. found carcinoma in situ in the gonads of four children with mixed gonadal dysgenesis, further stressing the propensity for neoplasia in these patients [54]. It may be surmised that this tendency is a result of a two-hit mechanism, as proposed by Knudsen at al: an inherent genetic tendency toward neoplasia (the first hit) is accentuated by environmental factors such as an abdominal or inguinal location (the second hit) [55].

Dysgenetic gonads should be identified and removed soon after diagnosis in patients with gonadal dysgenesis and a Y chromosome. Neoplasia in the cryptorchid testes of individuals with other intersex states appears to be related to the risk associated with cryptorchidism in general [56]. Early orchidopexy or extirpation of abdominal and inguinal gonads is appropriate in all cases, with life-long followup [57,58]. The case of testicular feminization, however, appears to be special. The risk of gonadal neoplasia clearly increases significantly after the age of 25 [10]. Most authors recommend elective gonadectomy once normal pubertal development has taken place.

SPECIAL GONADAL TUMORS ASSOCIATED WITH DISORDERS OF SEXUAL DIFFERENTIATION

Gonadoblastoma

Scully first described this rare tumor in 1953 and coined the term gonado-blastoma [59]. In 1970, he reviewed 101 tumors in 74 patients, 80% of whom were phenotypic females. Fifty-eight percent of patients showed evidence of virilization. The remainder were phenotypic males with cryptorchidism and hypospadias, most with evidence of persistent mullerian structures. The karyotype of all patients in whom it was obtained revealed the presence of a Y chromosome [60]. In Scully's series, the tumors originated in gonads of indeterminate nature in most patients, in a streak gonad in 22%, and in a cryptorchid dysgenetic testis in 18%. Subsequent series have confirmed that this tumor occurs almost exclusively in the dysgenetic gonads of individuals with a 46,XY karotype [40,61,62]. Gonadoblastomas may produce androgenic steroids and may give rise to germ cell neoplasm [63]. Histologically, the gonadoblastoma recapitulates the indifferent fetal gonad with germ cells and primitive sex cords [64]. Most gonadoblastomas have been treated with local resection without evidence of recurrence. Teter reported one patient in whom metastatic disease was documented [39].

Dysgerminoma

The dysgerminoma is a germ cell tumor of the ovary and is histologically identical to seminoma [63]. It is the most common neoplasm of the ovary in the adolescent. Ninety percent of dysgerminomas occur in patients under the age of 30. Dysgerminoma may be found together with teratoma and may arise in a gonadoblastoma [52,65]. Localized dysgerminoma is treated surgically, but local recurrence has been noted after spillage of tumor at surgery. Biopsy of the contralateral ovary and pelvic node biopsy are an important part of staging [66]. Ten-year survival for all patients with pure dysgerminoma is 74% [66].

REFERENCES

1. Ford CE: Cytogenetics and sex determination in man and mammals. J Biosoc Sci 2:7, 1970.
2. Eichwald EJ, Silmser CR: Communication. Transpl Bull 2:148, 1955.
3. Bernstein R: The Y chromosome and primary sexual differentiation. JAMA 245:1953, 1981.
4. Wachtel SS, Ohno S, Koo GC et al.: Possible role for H-Y antigen in the primary determination of sex. Nature 257:235, 1975.
5. Winters SJ, Wachtel SS, White BJ: H-Y antigen mosaicism in the gonad of a 46,XX true hermaphrodite. N Engl J Med 300:745, 1979.
6. Bongiovanni AM, Root AW: The adrenogenital syndrome. N Engl J Med 268:1283, 1963.
7. Wilkins L, Jones HW, Holman GH, et al.: Masculinization of the female fetus associated with administration of oral and intramuscular progestins during gestation: Non-adrenal female pseudohermaphrodism. J Clin Endocrinol Metab 18:559, 1958.
8. Simpson JL, Photopulos G: The relationship of neoplasia to disorders of sexual differentiation. Birth Defects 12:15, 1976.
9. New MI, Dupont B, Grumback K, et al.: Congenital adrenal hyperplasia and related conditions. In Stanbury JB, Wyngaarden JB, Wyngaarden JB, Frederickson DS, et al. (eds): Metabolic Basis of Inherited Disease. 5th ed. New York: McGraw Hill, 1983, p 973.
10. Morris JM, Mahesh VB: Further observations on the syndrome, testicular feminization. Am J Obstet Gynecol 87:731, 1963.
11. Lubs HA, Vilar O, Bergenstal DM: Familial male pseudohermaphrodism with labial testes and partial feminization, endocrine studies and genetic aspects. J Clin Endocrinol Metab 19:1110, 1959.
12. Reifenstein EC: Hereditary familial hypognadism. Proc Am Fed Clin Res 3:86, 1947.
13. Gilbert-Dreyfus S, Sebaoun CA, Blaisch J: Etude d'un cos familial d'androgroidisme avec hypospadias grave, gynecomastie, et hyperestrogenie. Ann Endocrinol Paris 18:93, 1957.
14. Sloan WR, Walsh PC: Familial persistent Mullerian duct syndrome. J Urol 115:459, 1976.
15. Simpson JL, New M, Peterson RE, German J: Pseudovaginal periscrotal hypospadias. Clin Genet 3:1, 1972.
16. Morris, JM: The syndrome of testicular feminization in male pseudohermaphrodites. Am J Obstet Gynecol 65:1192, 1953.
17. Grumbach MM, Conte FA: Disorders of sex differentiation. In William RH (ed): Textbook of Endocrinology. New York: WB Saunders, 1981, p 423.
18. O'Leary JA: Comparative studies of the gonad in testicular feminization and cryptorchidism. Fertil Steril 16:813, 1965.
19. Griffin JE, Wilson JD: Studies in the pathogenesis of the incomplete forms of androgen resistance in man. J Clin Endocrinol Metab 45:1137, 1977.
20. Snow BW, Rowland RG, Seal GM, et al.: Testicular tumor in a patient with persistent Mullerian duct syndrome. Urology 26:495, 1985.
21. Imperato-McGinley JL, Guerrero L, Gauteir T, et al.: Steroid 5-alpha reductase deficiency in man: An inherited form of male pseudohermaphrodism. Science 186:1213, 1974.

22. Imperato-McGinley JL, Peterson RE: Male pseudohermaphrodism. The complexities of male phenotypic development. Am J Med 61:251, 1976.
23. van Niekerk WA, Retief AE: The gonads of true hermaphrodites. Hum Genet 58:117, 1981.
24. van Niekerk WA: True hermaphrodism. An analytical review with a report of 3 new cases. Am J Obstet Gynecol 126:890, 1976.
25. Szokol M, Knodrai G, Papp Z: Gonadal malignancy and 46,XY karyotype in a true hermaphrodite. Obstet Gynecol 49:358, 1977.
26. Nichter LS: Seminoma in a 46,XX true hermaphrodite with positive H-Y antigen. Cancer 53:1181, 1984.
27. Radhakrishnan S, Sivaraman L, Natarajan PS: True hermaphrodite with multiple gonadal neoplasms. Cancer 42:2726, 1978.
28. Schwartz IS, Cohen CJ, Deligdisch L: Dysgerminoma of the ovary associated with true hermaphrodism. Obstet Gynecol 56:102, 1980.
29. Kaisary AV, Williams G: A case of bilateral intra-abdominal testes and seminomas in a previously recognized hermaphrodite. Br J Urol 54:323, 1982.
30. Talerman A, Jarabek J, Amarose AP: Gonadoblastoma and dysgerminoma in a true hermaphrodite with a 46,XX karyotype. Am J Obstet Gynecol 140:475, 1981.
31. Decker JP, Lerner JH, Schwartz I: Breast carcinoma in a 46,XX true hermaphrodite. Cancer 49:1481, 1982.
32. Froland A: Klinefelter's syndrome: Clinical, endocrinological and cytogenetic studies. Dan Med Bull 16(suppl 6):1, 1969.
33. Sogge MR, McDonald SD, Cofold PB: The malignant potential of the dysgenetic germ cell in Klinefelter's syndrome. Am J Med 66:515, 1979.
34. Harnden DG, Maclean N, Langlands AO: Carcinoma of the breast and Klinefelter's syndrome. J Med Genet 8:460, 1971.
35. Cuenca CR, Becker KL: Klinefelter's syndrome and cancer of the breast. Arch Int Med 121:159, 1968.
36. Scheike O, Visfeld J, Peterson B: Male breast cancer. III. Breast carcinoma in association with the Klinefelter syndrome. Acta Pathol Microbiol Scand 81:352, 1973.
37. Simpson JL: Gonadal dysgenesis and abnormalities of the human sex chromosomes: Current status of phenotypic-karyotypic correlations. Birth Defects 11:23, 1975.
38. Wertlecki W, Fraumeni JF, Mulvihill JJ: Nongonadal neoplasia in Turner's syndrome. Cancer 26:485, 1970.
39. Teter J: Prognosis, malignancy, and curability of the germ cell tumor occurring in dysgenetic gonads. Am J Obstet Gynecol 108:894, 1970.
40. Schellhas HF: Malignant potential of the dysgenetic gonad, Part I. Obstet Gynecol 44:298, 1974.
41. Schellhas HF: Malignant potential of the dysgenetic gonad, Part II. Obstet Gynecol 44:455, 1974.
42. Isurugi K, Aso Y, Ishida H, et al.: Prepubertal XY gonadal dysgenesis. Pediatrics 59:569, 1977.
43. Sohval AR: "Mixed" gonadal dysgenesis, a variety of hermaphroditism. Am J Hum Genet 15:155, 1963.
44. Davidoff F, Federman DD: Mixed gonadal dysgenesis. Pediatrics 52:725, 1973.
45. Allen TD: Disorders of sexual differentiation. Urology 7(suppl):1, 1976.
46. Pendergrass TW: Congential anomalies in children with Wilms' tumor. Cancer 37:403, 1976.

47. Drash A, Sherman F, Hartmann WH, et al.: A syndrome of pseudohermaphrodism, Wilms' tumor, hypertension, and degenerative renal disease. J Pediatr 76:585, 1970.
48. Barakat AY, Papadopoulou ZL, Chandra RS, et al.: Pseudohermaphroditism, nephron disorder and Wilms' tumor: A unifying concept. Pediatrics 54:366, 1974.
49. Rajfer J: Association between Wilms' tumor and gonadal dysgenesis. J Urol 125:388, 1981.
50. Beheshti M, Mancer JF, Hardy BE, et al.: External genital abnormalities associated with Wilms' tumor. Urology 24:130, 1984.
51. Manual M, Katayama KP, Jones HW: The age of occurrence of gonadal tumors in intersex patients with a Y chromosome. Am J Obstet Gynecol 124:293, 1976.
52. Simpson JL, Photopulos G: Hereditary aspects of ovarian and testicular neoplasia. Birth Defects 12:51, 1976.
53. Khalid BA, Bond AG, Ennis G, et al.: Dysgerminoma-gonadoblastoma and familial 46,XY pure gonadal dysgenesis: Case report and review of the genetics and pathophysiology of gonadal dysgenesis and H-Y antigen. Aust NZ J Obstet Gynaecol 22:175, 1982.
54. Muller, J. Skakkebaek NE, Ritzen M, et al.: Carcinoma in situ of the testis in children with 45,X/46,XY gonadal dysgenesis. J Pediatr 106:431, 1985.
55. Knudsen AG Jr, Strong LC, Anderson DE: Heredity and cancer in man. Prog Med Genet 9:113, 1973.
56. Batata MA, Whitmore WF, Jr., Chu FC, et al.: Cryptorchidism and testicular cancer. J Urol 124:382, 1980.
57. Levitt SB, Kogan SJ, Engel RM, et al.: The impalpable testis: A rational approach to management. J Urol 120:515, 1978.
58. Farrer JH, Walker AH, Rajfer J: Management of the postpubertal cryptorchid testis: A statistical review. J Urol 135:1071, 1985.
59. Scully RE: Gonadoblastoma. A gonadal tumor related tumor related to the dysgerminoma (seminoma) and capable of sex-hormone production. Cancer 6:445, 1953.
60. Scully RE: Gonadoblastoma, a review of 74 cases. Cancer 25:1340, 1970.
61. Melicow MM, Uson AC: Dysgenetic gonadomas and other gonadal neoplasms in intersexes. Cancer 12:552, 1959.
62. Melicow MM: Tumors of dysgenetic gonads in intersexes: Case reports and discussion regarding their place in gonadal oncology. Bull NY Acad Med 42:3, 1966.
63. Hart WH, Burkons DM: Germ cell neoplasms arising in gonadoblastomas. Cancer 43:669, 1979.
64. Telium G: Special Tumors of the Ovary and Testis and Related Extragonadal Lesions Philadelphia: Lippincott, 1976.
65. Warner BA, Monsaert RP, Stumpf PG: 45,XY gonadal dysgenesis: Is oncogenesis related to H-Y phenotype or breast development? Hum Genet 69:79, 1985.
66. Gordon A, Lipton D, Woodruff JD: Dysgerminoma: A review of 158 cases from the Emil Novak Ovarian Tumor Registry. Obstet Gynecol 58:497, 1981.

Chapter 15
Genetics of Pediatric Genitourinary Tumors

Vincent M. Riccardi

Tumors of the urinary tract, particularly the kidney, are not rare in child-hood. As a matter of fact they represent a relatively common indication for consulting a pediatric urologist, and one of the most common and well-studied tumors of childhood is Wilms' tumor (WT). This paper will review pediatric urology tumors in general, emphasizing, however, WT, renal cell carcinoma, von Hippel-Lindau disease, tuberous sclerosis, and neuro-fibromatosis.

WILMS' TUMOR

WT, also known as nephroblastoma, is one of the most common childhood solid tumors [1–6], accounting for about 10% of the malignant tumors seen in that age-group. In the majority of instances it is unilateral, representing a sporadic event, without any significant heritable contribution. Occasionally (about 10% of the time), WT may be bilateral [7–9]. In all patients with bilateral tumors and as many as one-third of patients with unilateral tumors, WT may represent an autosomal dominant trait with reduced penetrance [10], though some of the data are incomplete or subject to alternative interpreta-tions [11]. In a subset of patients with WT, the genetic contribution is more clear-cut, involving a deletion of the short arm of chromosome 11 [12–15]. Although the number of patients with WT who have del(11p) is small, these patients have been instructive about the pathogenesis and origin of this tumor and about pediatric embryonal tumors in general.

Pediatric Tumors of the Genitourinary Tract, pages 241–261

In the vast majority of instances, WT occurs in the kidney, but extrarenal sites are well-known [16–19].

Clinical Settings Associated With WT

WT is predominantly a disorder of childhood, although adult cases are well-known [20–23]. The tumor may become apparent in an infant or child at any age, but the peak age is 3–4 years [24]. By age 10 years, the risk has decreased to much nearer the background risk.

For a child with WT, there are five specific points for considering the long-term significance of the tumor, both for the child and his or her family: Are there associated anomalies or developmental delay/mental retardation? Is there a chromosome anomaly? Is the tumor unilateral or bilateral? Is the histology favorable? Is there any other family member known or thought to have a WT or other type of childhood cancer?

The most common histology is that of typical nephroblastoma [24]. This "favorable histology" ordinarily signifies the absence of anaplasia and the expectation of a salutary response to medical, surgical, and radiation treatment. On the other hand, there may be varying degrees of anaplasia and/or the presence of other cell types, including elements of rhabdomyosarcomas, neuroblastomas, or combinations thereof [25–36]. Each histologic type can occur in a variety of clinical and genetic settings, though, as indicated above, the favorable-histology variety is the most common for each setting.

Most often, WT develops within an otherwise apparently normal kidney. However, there is also a well-known association of WT with renal cysts [37,38], nephroblastomatosis [39–45], and nodular renal blastema [46], including that occurring in trisomy 18 [47].

Most of the time, WT occurs in "otherwise normal" children, is unilateral, and is an isolated occurrence in a family [48]. However, in individual instances, the burden of proof is on the clinician to establish that, indeed, the child is otherwise normal. This ordinarily means, at the least, a careful physical examination from a dysmorphology perspective [49,50], with special attention to the eyes, the genitalia, and the limbs. Specific features or combinations thereof that are of particular concern can be ascertained from the discussions of the various conditions and syndrome in subsequent sections.

The key issue is whether there is a possible or probable diagnosis of a chromosome anomaly. If the child is old enough for a clinician to document the absence of developmental delay or mental retardation, the likelihood of chromosome abnormality becomes increasingly remote. However, all infants and young children with a WT should have a chromosome analysis as part of the determination that the WT has occurred in the context of an otherwise normal child. Ultimately, a chromosome analysis is highly desirable and generally recommended for children with WT in all age-groups, though for at least some of these, collaboration with a clinical cytogenetics research group might help defray costs and ensure the utilization of the most appro priate techniques. If the family history is negative for other instances of WT, there is no apparent need to study other family members beyond history-taking, unless the child's constitutional chromosomes are abnormal and the parents must have their chromosomes analyzed to rule out a carrier state [51,52].

Having established that the child has no dysmorphic features or a chromosome abnormality, and presuming favorable histology, the next concern is whether the tumor is unilateral or bilateral. A vigorous search, radiographically and at the time of surgery, for bilateral involvement is incumbent upon the involved clinicians. A unilateral tumor in an otherwise normal child is most often a sporadic event, with a relatively low likelihood of recurrence among other siblings and other relatives, except perhaps offspring (see below). However, at best this is a guess that represents the considerations averaged from a combination of high-risk and low-risk families [10]. Moreover, given the higher empiric risk for recurrence among family members of patients with bilateral WT and the possibility that apparent unilaterality merely represents failure of one side's tumor to become obvious, premature or overzealous discounting of some significant recurrence risk must be avoided.

For an otherwise normal child with sporadic (i.e., negative family history) unilateral WT, the recurrence risk among siblings is considered to be less than 1%, and among offspring as high as 10–15%. If the family history is positive for one or more other persons with a WT or another embryonal tumor, generalizations are not possible, and individualized determinations of recurrence risks will be necessary. For an otherwise normal child with sporadic bilateral WT, the recurrence risk among siblings is at least 3–10%, significantly higher than when the tumor is unilateral. The recurrence risk for siblings begins to approach 50% if the WT is not sporadic and there is an affected parent, but the risk is somewhat less than 50% if the additional affected person is more removed in relationship. The recurrence risk for the offspring of a patient with sporadic unilateral WT is relatively uncertain [53], but it is increased compared to the general population, with a magnitude of about 10–15%. The recurrence risk for the offspring of a patient with familial bilateral WT is certainly at or near 50%. The recurrence risks for the offspring of patients with WT who have intermediate situations (e.g., unilateral case with positive family history, bilateral case with a negative family history) are increased, but the quantitation must be individualized. The reasons for vagueness include both somewhat incomplete epidemiologic and genetic data and respect for the notion of decreased penetrance. A fully penetrant mutant gene expresses itself in 100% of the individuals in whom it occurs. A mutant gene with reduced penetrance is expressed (i.e., is obvious) in only a portion of individuals in whom it occurs, whether as a de novo mutation or one transmitted from a parent. If the mutant gene is expressed in 60% of those who bear it, the mutant gene is said to have a penetrance of 60%. Variable, that is decreased, penetrance appears to be characteristic of the mutant genes contributing to the origin of unilateral or bilateral WT. Thus, in recurrence risk calculations for WT, distinctions must be made between the likelihood of transmitting a mutant gene and the likelihood of the tumor occurring in a more distant relative [54].

The possibility of a second malignancy developing at some later time should always be kept in mind for survivors of WT. However, a high risk for this complication has not been established, as it has for patients surviving retinoblastomas.

Syndromic Associations With WT

AGR triad—aniridia, genitourinary anomalies, and retardation—and del(11p). In the time period 1973–1976, this investigator had the opportunity to study a series of three patients with the combination of bilateral aniridia, genitourinary anomalies (i.e., ambiguous genitalia, including pseudovaginal perineoscrotal hypospadias), and various degrees of retarded mental development, referred to as the AGR triad. All three of these youngsters turned out to have overlapping deletions of the short arm of chromosome 11. (It may be of some interest that each had previously been said to have normal karyotypes.) When one of them developed a WT, all the pieces fell into place, and a chromosomal basis for at least some instances of WT was established [12]. Once the relationship of del (11p) to the AGR triad and WT became apparent and several important genes were assigned to the short arm of chromosome 11 (see below), a great deal of interest developed around the AGR triad and WT, both in the patients themselves and in in vitro experimental systems [13–15,55–69]. At times, the tumor developing in the context of aniridia and del(11p) may be a gonadoblastoma [70,71].

Aniridia denotes total absence of the iris and as a clinical label it may be somewhat of a misnomer. Literal aniridia is only one end of the spectrum of the iris dysplasia discussed below as "autosomal dominant aniridia." Both true aniridia and less severe iris dysplasia have been seen in association with WT [72]. For the sake of brevity, and respecting previous usage, the term aniridia will be used in this paper to designate both literal aniridia and the full spectrum of related iris dysplasias.

Aniridia usually occurs as an isolated anomaly, and as such it is ordinarily heritable as an autosomal dominant trait [73,74]. Tentative assignment of at least one autosomal dominant aniridia gene to the long arm of chromosome 2 has been made [75]. Aniridia associated with absent patellae may also represent an autosomal dominant trait [76]. Aniridia appears to occur as an autosomal recessive trait when other features, such as mental retardation or cerebellar ataxia, are present [74]. The occurrence of apparently sporadic aniridia in association with other birth defects, particularly ambiguous genitalia, has been known for some time [49]. The association of aniridia with WT has been known for almost equally as long [49,77].

All newborns, infants, and children with aniridia (including less severe iris dysplasia of the same type) must be considered at high risk for developing a WT, and each of them should have at least one good quality high resolution chromosome analysis. All associated constitutional chromosomal aberrations have involved chromosome arm 11p, either as unbalanced deletions [12,13,15] or as a balanced translocation [78]. The finding of either requires followup parental chromosome analyses. And both types of chromosome aberration should alert the clinician to a dramatically increased risk for WT, that is well established for the deletion at least. Given the finding of normal chromosomes in a child with inherited or sporadic aniridia, the risk for development of a WT is certainly less than 1%, but significantly higher than for the general population [72]. If a del(11p) is found, the risk for a WT is between 30 and 50%. In either event—that is, aniridia with or without a del(11p)—close followup and periodic monitoring for the development of such a tumor is mandatory.

Parenthetically, it may be of some interest that anterior chamber ocular defects may also occur with deletions of the long arm of chromosome 11 [79] or chromosome 11 pericentric inversions [80], and at least one instance of craniopharyngioma has accompanied autosomal dominant aniridia [81]. In addition, aniridia has been noted with familial pheochromocytoma [82].

Perineoscrotal hypospadias. As indicated above, pseudovaginal perineoscrotal hypospadias can be a component of the AGR triad when the sex chromosome complement of the patient is XY. There are also reports of patients with this type of distorted anatomy (including ambiguous genitalia and male pseudohermaphroditism) and/or gonadal dysgenesis having a WT [83–87]. WT with bladder exstrophy has also been reported [88].

Beckwith-Wiedemann syndrome. The Beckwith-Wiedemann syndrome (BWS) is the prototype of overgrowth (e.g., segmental hypertrophy) disorders. The full-blown syndrome includes hemihypertrophy, macroglossia, and an omphalocele, and is associated with a relatively high risk (30-40%) [89] for an embryonal tumor, particularly WT, neuroblastoma, adrenocortical carcinoma, hepatoblastoma, hepatocellular carcinoma, or cerebellar hemangioblastoma.

Segmental or regional overgrowth, including hemihypertrophy, has a well-established association with WT [90]; at least several percentages of patients with BWS manifest this tumor [89]. Moreover, a significant number of those who develop WT do not have the complete syndrome, but rather only a more limited segmental hypertrophy [91–94]. Thus, all children with segmental hypertrophy of any sort need to be considered at increased risk for WT, and appropriate followup measures should be taken (see below). In addition, all children for whom the diagnosis of BWS is entertained or established must have a chromosome analysis. A significant, though yet unspecified portion of these youngsters will have triplication 11p [95] or a pericentric inversion of chromosome 11 [96]. It is intriguing that two quite distinct syndromes associated with WT also have aberrations of chromosome 11, though at different sites. This type of finding emphasizes the need to perform a chromosome analysis for all children with WT and other embryonal tumors. It should also be noted that other types of segmental overgrowth disorders, such as the Klippel-Trenaunay-Weber syndrome [97], may be associated with WT.

Other chromosome aberrations. Constitutional trisomy 8 [98] has been associated with at least two cases of WT [99,100]. Wilms' tumor has occurred in at least two cases of trisomy 18 [47] and in one case with a balanced 7;13 translocation [101].

Perlman syndrome. The Perlman syndrome [102] is an autosomal recessive gigantism syndrome that is associated with a very significant risk for WT. This disorder has recently been reviewed by Greenberg and associates [103]. Chromosomal analyses have been normal, but in the patient reported by Greenberg et al., there was apparent mosaicism for del(11p) in the cells cultured from the surgically removed WT (VM Riccardi, unpublished data).

Neurofibromatosis. Neurofibromatosis (NF) is another Mendelian condition well-known to be associated with WT [104–106], although the pathogenetic mechanism or mechanisms underlying the association remain uncertain. While the NF-WT association is clear, the actual frequency of the two in combination is uncertain. Nonetheless, all children with NF must be considered at increased risk for WT, and, conversely, all children with WT should be examined for café-au-lait spots and other stigmata of NF. This investigator has previously hypothesized that the neurocristopathy nature of

NF and the neural crest origin of the iris indicate WT ultimately to be of neural crest origin. From a totally different vantage point, Masson [107] has derived a similar conclusion.

In utero hydantoin exposure. A series of reports have emerged indicating what appears to be an excess of embryonal tumors among infants exposed in utero to hydantoin anticonvulsants [108,109]. Included among these reports have been at least two patients with WT. This set of facts is especially interesting in view of the neural crest hypothesis noted above, since hydantoin compounds appear to have at least some of their teratogenic effects explained in terms of disturbed neural crest cell migration.

Drash syndrome. The Drash syndrome is the combination of the nephrotic syndrome, diffuse glomerulonephritis, and WT [86,110,111]. The pathogenetic interrelationship between the glomerulonephritis and WT is obscure [83]. In infants and small children, the two appear to be concomitant, in contrast to some older survivors of WT who develop glomerulonephritis somewhat later [112,113]. Chromosome analyses in these patients have been normal, and, based on this investigator's experience, none of the del(11p) patients have developed glomerulonephritis, regardless of whether they have had a WT.

Health Care and Management Considerations

For the average child, the risk of WT is sufficiently remote that screening efforts for early detection of WT are inappropriate. However, for the child with a first- or second-degree relative with WT [54] or with one of the syndromic diagnoses discussed above, specific efforts should be made to screen the child initially and periodically thereafter [114]. At the initial evaluation, the following are recommended: history-taking (abdominal protuberance or mass, unexplained fever, gross hematuria, etc.) abdominal palpation, routine urinalysis (looking specifically for hematuria), renal ultrasound, and an intravenous pyelogram [115].

Followup evaluations should take place at 3–4-month intervals through about age 6 years and then at least at 6–9-month intervals through age 10 years. Although presumably there is still some increased risk beyond that age, the benefit of frequent, structured followup evaluations then is problematic. The followup evaluation should include the history-taking, abdominal palpation, routine urinalysis, and renal ultrasound. If there is any suspicion of a tumor, more definitive studies, including an IVP and/or a CT scan or nuclear magnetic resonance imaging [6,116–119] should be utilized. In addition, the parents should be encouraged to learn how to palpate the child's abdomen so that they may be able to identify the development of a mass in a timely manner. And, of course, they should be alerted to the importance of gross hematuria.

Research Considerations

It has become overwhelmingly clear that the importance of WT goes far beyond the affected patients themselves. As with retinoblastomas [120], WT holds a key to understanding the intracellular genetic mechanisms that appear to underlie the origin of cancers in general. In order to clarify this point and emphasize the critical need for all patients with WT to be included in various research projects, it is necessary to provide some background information.

Chromosome 11 gene localizations. As noted above, a series of genes have been localized to the short arm of chromosome 11 [121–126]. These include insulin, the beta-globin (or non-alpha-globin) gene cluster, LDH-A, parathormone, the Harvey-ras (Ha-ras) proto-oncogene, calcitonin-1, at least two antibody-defined cell surface antigens (MIC1 and MIC4), acid phosphatase-2, follicle stimulating hormone B (FSHB), and catalase. The latter two, FSHB and catalase, appear to be located in band 11p13, where a putative gene for the Wilms' tumor-AGR (WAGR) complex is thought to be, on the basis of analysis of 11p breakpoints among patients with WAGR. Direct DNA probes, utilizing endonuclease restriction fragment length polymorphisms (RFLP), for many of these genes can be used to define the specific gene forms (alleles) that are present on each of the two chromosome 11 homologues, both in normal tissues and tumor specimens from patients with WT.

Genetic linkage. Through the use of polymorphic gene products or RFLPs, families with heritable WT can be studied to determine whether the "WT gene" is located on (that is, co-segregates with) chromosome arm 11p. This will afford both more accurate genetic counseling and prenatal diagnosis (as has already been done for retinoblastoma [120]) and allow for the identification of the gene itself at the DNA level. To date, the use of red blood cell levels of catalase as an indicator of a risk for WT has not been fruitful, even though it has been assigned to 11p13 [127].

In addition, the respective number 11 chromosomes from a sporadic WT patient (with or without other clinical findings) and his/her parents can be studied for their 11p alleles. Such data suggest that the parental origin of the 11p appears to contribute specifically to the development of the tumor. This approach, combined with direct tumor studies described below, would allow for the direct testing of the previous suggestion that paternal environmental exposures may be contributory to the risk for an offspring's WT [128,129].

In vitro tumor studies. Numerous studies have documented both the frequent loss of chromosome 11 or portions thereof in WTs studied in vitro

[130–135] and the presence of other chromosome anomalies as well, especially those involving chromosomes 1 and 16 [131,132,134–136].

RFLP analysis of 11p genes in DNA prepared directly from WT and normal tissue specimens from the same patient have already demonstrated that one of the 11p homologues is preferentially lost in the tumor [135,137–147]. The retained 11p is presumed to have been structurally altered (microscopically or submicroscopically) and is present in single doses. This can be shown when one or more of the 11p genes is present in two forms (alleles), that is, when the person is heterozygous for the gene in question. When the heterozygosity is lost (i.e., when one of the alleles is lost) in the tumor, the inference is that the tumor cells have become homozygous or hemizygous for the critical gene or genes on the remaining 11p [135].

Such findings make it obvious to students of oncology that one schema for the development of at least certain types of cancers is as follows: a genetic alteration (e.g., point mutation, chromosomal deletion) occurs at a specific chromosomal site, but that change is "recessive" in terms of its expression (i.e., it will not be expressed as long as the normal homologous site is present); the normal homologous site then undergoes a similar mutation or is lost through a variety of cytogenetic mechanisms (e.g., deletion, loss of the chromosome); the alteration of the critical site is then expressed, the phenotype being the cancer. This schema is emphasized in order to demonstrate how studies directed at WT have begun to have impact far beyond that tumor itself, and to suggest that there is even more to be learned. But the key is collaboration between the clinicians caring for these young children with the researchers in the laboratory. To facilitate collaboration in the future, readers are encouraged to contact the author.

RHABDOMYOSARCOMA

Rhabdomyosarcoma (RMS) occurs in five forms [148]: 1) the embryonal tumor that is the primary focus of this discussion; 2) the alveolar form that has a distinctive pseudoalveolar pattern as well as rhabdomyoblastic elements, although strict histologic differentiation of alveolar and embryonal RMS can not always be established [149]; 3) botryoid RMS; 4) pleomorphic RMS; and 5) mixed RMS, showing combinations of any of the preceding histologic patterns.

In embryonal RMS the tumor cells are elongated and spindle-shaped, and arranged in parallel arrays. At least a portion of the cells manifest histologic and/or biochemical features of muscle tissue (e.g., expression of creatine phosphokinase M). It occurs mainly in children, with two peak ages of presentation, 2–6 years and the mid-teens [150]. It can develop in many different sites and many different tissues, even those that do not ordinarily contain muscle cells, such as the meninges [151]. It is not uncommon at various sites along the genitourinary tract, from the ureters to the vagina to the prostate [152–156]. RMS is rarely familial, and no clear evidence has been garnered to suggest an autosomal dominant mutant gene as appears with WT and RB. Likewise, no consistent chromosomal aberration has been identified, although its occurrence as part of trisomy 8 has been sited [98]. Nonetheless, for all instances of RMS, a careful family history should be obtained and cytogenetic analyses carried out, both on peripheral blood cells and tumor specimens themselves.

RMS is generally underrepresented in the investigative efforts being applied to childhood cancer, and every attempt should be made to effect collaborations, after the manner described above for WT. Many WT investigators would be more than willing to work with RMS material for a variety of reasons, including the fact that some WTs include RMS elements [36] and, by analogy, a comparable chromosomal locus should be identifiable with a modicum of effort.

RENAL CELL CARCINOMA

Renal cell carcinoma (RCC) is also known as a hypernephroma. Most often it occurs sporadically, but it can be familial and/or a component of von Hippel-Lindau disease (see below). When it occurs sporadically, it is usually unilateral, though bilateral cases are known [157,158]. The age of onset extends from childhood to later adult years, with a preponderance in the sixth and seventh decades. It accounts for 85–90% of all renal cancers in adults and has a clear male predominance (3:1).

In at least one instance, a familial form of RCC has been associated with a translocation between chromosomes 3 and 8 [t(3;8)(p21;q24)] [159], although an alternative 3p breakpoint (3p14.2) has been suggested [160], and the concordance between the chromosomal aberration and the tumor has not been absolute. Moreover, other families with segregating RCC have not shown the t(3p;8q) aberration [161]. A significant relationship between the chromosome aberration and the tumor is still likely, however, in view of the finding of a comparable chromosome rearrangement in cells cultured from RCCs [162,163].

VON HIPPEL-LINDAU DISEASE

RCC is a critical element of von Hippel-Lindau disease (VHLD), one of the so-called phakomatoses, which, along with neurofibromatosis and tuberous sclerosis, are considered to be neuroscristopathies as well [164]. RCC occurs in at least 5% of VHLD patients [118,157,165–171]. This means, at the least, that every patient with RCC must have a family history and personal history-taking and physical examination to consider the possibility that he or she has VHLD. And, conversely, every VHLD patient must be considered at risk to manifest RCC, and should be studied and followed-up accordingly [167,169,172]. In VHLD the RCC is usually unilateral, but bilateral involvement is known [157], and a second lesion in the contralateral kidney must always be a consideration. Some authors urge a very conservative surgical management approach to this tumor in the context of VHLD [165].

It is not at all clear as to the pathogenetic relationship of RCC to the remainder of the individual tissue abnormalities that are part of VHLD. Moreover, the likelihood of developing RCC as part of that syndrome seems to be independent of its other features.

Pheochromocytomas, which not infrequently manifest as a suprarenal mass, also occur with significant frequency in VHLD [173,174] and must be considered in the differential diagnosis of renal masses associated with that disorder. On the other hand, pheochromocytomas in any setting are distinctly unusual in the pediatric population.

Cystadenomas of the epididymis are also occasionally seen as part of the urologic tumor manifestations of VHLD [175–177].

TUBEROUS SCLEROSIS

As indicated above, tuberous sclerosis (TS) is one of the neural crest-derived phakomatoses, with a wide variety of manifestations in the skin, nervous system, lungs, and kidneys [178]. The renal manifestations are primarily an unusual type of hamartomatous tumor, angiomyolipomas [179–181]. The occurrence of the renal tumors is apparently unrelated to the presence or absence of other TS features, and the pathogenetic relationship of the renal angiomyolipomas to these other features is totally obscure. Renal angiomyolipomas occur in at least several percentages of patients with TS, if all ages are taken into account; in any event they are not rare components of TS. They are almost always bilateral, but the timing of their onset is variable. They may grow progressively and eventually lead to compromise of renal function and even lead to renal failure and death. In keeping with the types of recommendations made for previously discussed disorders, any patient with TS must be evaluated, both at presentation and periodically thereafter, for the presence of renal angiomyolipomas. And, conversely, any patient with such tumors must have a personal and family evaluation to consider the possibility of underlying TS.

NEUROFIBROMATOSIS

Neurofibromatosis (NF), the most common form of which is von Reckling-hausen's disease (VRNF) [104,182], is characterized by two types of urologic tumors. First, but least frequent, is the WT that occurs in a small number of VRNF patients [105], as discussed above in the section on WT. Second, and relatively common, is the occurrence of neurofibromas at various sites along the urinary tract, including the external genitalia and perineum.

Neurofibromas in and about the renal hilum, often associated with reno-vascular hypertension may occur in upwards of 1% of VRNF patients. Neurofibromas may also develop as intramural lesions along the lengths of the ureters, and/or the latter might be compressed by an adjacent retroperi-toneal neurofibroma. The most frequent urologic site of neurofibromatous involvement in VRNF is the urinary bladder. Neurofibromas may develop in the bladder wall itself or there may be external compression by pelvic retroperitoneal tumors; such problems may occur in as many as 1–2% of patients with VRNF. Diffuse plexiform neurofibromas arising in or near the perineum may, with progressive growth, come to distort the external genitalia of young girls (e.g., clitoromegaly) sufficiently to suggest sexual differentia-tion abnormalities. All patients with NF who have evidence of abdominal, retroperitoneal, and perineal neurofibromas must be evaluated by a urologist to define the extent and nature of impingement on the urinary tract and appropriate treatment and/or followup plans made.

SUMMARY

Tumors of the urinary tract that occur in children may be isolated, non-familial findings, or they may represent a distinctive heritable tumor disorder (e.g., WT), or they may be part of a more pleiotropic disorder (e.g., VHLD, TS, NF). This means that all pediatric patients with urologic tumors should be considered at risk for having additional personal or family-related risks. And further, patients with each of the syndromes and disorders considered above should be considered to be at risk for the development of urologic tumors. The consequences of research investigation of the tumors discussed in this paper has proved invaluable, both for gleaning facts about the disorder itself and for gaining new insights into oncogenesis in general. We are just beginning to make progress, but to continue we must assure timely access to tumor specimens. The basis for and benefits of collaboration between the clinician and basic researcher are clear.

ACKNOWLEDGMENTS

Support for this project was provided by the Texas NF Foundation and NCI grant CA 25597. Thanks to Ms. Gail Barnard for expert assistance with manuscript preparation.

REFERENCES

1. Lemerle J, Tournade M-F, Gerard-Marchant R, et al.: Wilms' tumor: Natural history and prognostic factors. A retrospective study of 248 cases treated at the Institut Gustave-Roussy 1952–1967. Cancer 37:2557, 1976.
2. Lennox EL, Stiller CA, Jones PHM, et al.: Nephroblastoma: Treatment during 1970–3 and the effect on survival of inclusion in the first MRC trial. Br Med J 2:567, 1979.
3. D'Angio G, Beckwith JB, Breslow NE, et al.: Wilms' tumor: An update. Cancer 45:1791, 1980.
4. Jaffe MH, White SJ, Silver TM, et al.: Wilms tumor: Ultrasonic features, pathologic correlation, and diagnostic pitfalls. Radiology 140:147, 1981.
5. Küss R, Murphy GP, Khoury S, et al. (eds): Renal Tumors: Proceedings of the First International Symposium on Kidney Tumors. Progress in Clinical and Biological Research, vol. 100. New York: Alan R. Liss, 1982.
6. Jaffe N (ed): Oncology Overview. Selected Abstracts on Diagnosis and Treatment of Wilms' Tumor. National Cancer Institute/International Cancer Research Data Bank Program. Bethesda, Md.: U.S. Dept. of Health and Human Services, 1983.
7. Bond JV: Bilateral Wilms' tumour. Age at diagnosis, associated congenital anomalies, and possible pattern of inheritance. Lancet 2:482, 1975.
8. Garrett RA, Donohue JP: Bilateral Wilms tumors. J Urol 120:586, 1978.
9. Casale AJ, Flanigan RC, Moore PJ, et al.: Survival in bilateral metachronous (asynchronous) Wilms tumors. J Urol 128:766, 1982.
10. Knudson AG, Jr., Strong LC: Mutation and cancer: A model for Wilms' tumor of the kidney. JNCI 48:313, 1972.
11. Matsunaga E: Cancer susceptibility: Family studies of retinoblastoma and Wilms tumor. Prog Clin Biol Res 103:241, 1982.
12. Riccardi VM, Sujansky E, Smith AC, et al.: Chromosomal imbalance in the aniridia-Wilms' tumor association: 110 interstitial deletion. Pediatrics 61:604, 1978.
13. Narahara K, Kikkawa K, Kimira S, et al.: Regional mapping of catalase and Wilms tumor—aniridia, genitourinary abnormalities, and mental retardation triad loci to the chromosome segment 11p1305→p1306. Hum Genet 66:181, 1984.
14. Turleau C, de Grouchy J, Nihoul-Fekete C, et al.: Del11p13/nephroblastoma without aniridia. Hum Genet 67:455, 1984.
15. Turleau C, de Grouchy J, Tournade M-F, et al.: Del11p/aniridia complex. Report of three patients and review of 37 observations from the literature. Clin Genet 26:356, 1984.
16. Akhtar M, Kott E, Brooks B: Extrarenal Wilms' tumor. Cancer 40:3087, 1977.
17. Madanat F, Osborne B, Cangir A, Sutow WW: Extrarenal Wilms tumor. J Pediatr 93:439, 1978.
18. Alterman K, Grantmyre E, Gillis DA: Extrarenal Wilms' tumor: A review and case report. Invest Cell Pathol 2:309, 1979.

19. McCauley RGK, Safaii H, Crowley CA, et al.: Extrarenal Wilms' tumor. Am J Dis Child 133:1174, 1979.
20. Bard RH, Greenwald ES, Kalnicki S, et al.: Adult Wilms tumor treated with radiotherapy and chemotherapy: A case report. J Urol 121:679, 1979.
21. Kilton L, Matthews MJ, Cohen MH: Adult Wilms tumor: A report of prolonged survival and review of literature. J Urol 124:1, 1980.
22. Hara T, Fujime M, Kawabe K, et al.: Adult Wilms tumor and bilateral germ cell tumors of testes: A case report. J Urol 128:1296, 1982.
23. Hartman DS, Davis CJ, Jr., Madewell JE, et al.: Primary malignant renal tumors in the second decade of life: Wilms tumor versus renal cell carcinoma. J Urol 127:888, 1982.
24. Bove KE, McAdams AJ: Nephroblastomatosis complex and Wilms' tumor: A clinicopathologic treatise. Perspect Pediatr Pathol 3:185, 1976.
25. Lawler W, Marsden HB, Palmer MK: Wilms' tumor—histologic variation and prognosis. Cancer 36:1122, 1975.
26. Kuo T-T: Observation of nervous tissue in a Wilms' tumor: Its histogenetic significance. Cancer 39:1105, 1977.
27. Kurtz SM: A unique ultrastructural variant of Wilms' tumor. Its possible histogenetic implications. Am J Surg Pathol 3:257, 1979.
28. Harms D, Gutjahr P, Hohenfellner R, et al.: Fetal rhabdomyomatous nephroblastoma. Pathologic histology and special clinical and biologic features. Eur J Pediatr 133:167, 1980.
29. Llombart-Bosch A,: Peydro-Olaya A, Cerda-Nicolas M: Presence of ganglion cells in Wilm's tumours: A review of the possible neuroepithelial origin of nephroblastoma. Histopathology 4:321, 1980.
30. Giagaspero F, Zanetti G, Mancini A, et al.: Sarcomatous variant of Wilms' tumor. A light and immunohistochemical study of four cases. Tumori 67:367, 1981.
31. Grimes MM, Wolff M, Wolff JA, et al.: Ganglion cells in metastatic Wilms' tumor. Review of a histogenetic controversy. Am J Surg Pathol 6:565, 1982.
32. Kawano N, Morii S, Kenzoh Y, et al.: Contiguous malignant astrocytoma and Wilms'-like tumor in the brain. Cancer 49:2505, 1982.
33. Leblanc A, Caillaud JM, Hartmann O, et al.: Hypercalcemia preferentially occurs in unusual forms of childhood non-Hodgkin's lymphoma, rhabdomyosarcoma, and Wilms' tumor. A study of 11 cases. Cancer 54:2132, 1984.
34. Mayes LC, Kasselberg AG, Roloff JS, et al.: Hypercalcemia associated with immunoreactive parathyroid hormone in a malignant rhabdoid tumor of the kidney (rhabdoid Wilms' tumor). Cancer 54:882, 1984.
35. Sens MA, Garvin AJ, Drew CD, et al.: Skeletal muscle differentiation in Wilms' tumor. Antibody identification and explant culture. Arch Pathol Lab Med 108:58, 1984.
36. Weinberg AG, Currarino G, Hurt GE, Jr.: Botryoid Wilms' tumor of the renal pelvis. Arch Pathol Lab Med 108:147, 1984.
37. Havers W, Stambolis C: Benign cystic nephroblastoma. Eur J Pediatr 131:119, 1979.
38. Andrews MJ, Askin FB, Fried A, et al.: Cystic partially differentiated nephroblastoma and polycystic Wilms tumor: A spectrum of related clinical and pathologic entities. J Urol 129:577, 1983.
39. de Chadarevian JP, Fletcher BD, Chatten J, et al.: Massive infantile nephroblastomatosis. Cancer 39:2294, 1977.
40. Bove KE, McAdams AJ: Multifocal nephroblastic neoplasia. JNCI 61:285, 1978.
41. Machin GA: Nephroblastomatosis and multiple bilateral nephroblastomata—histologic, therapeutic and theoretical aspects. Arch Pathol Lab Med 102:639, 1978.

42. Kulkarni R, Bailie MD, Bernstein J, et al.: Progression of nephroblastomatosis to Wilms tumor. J Pediatr 96:178, 1980.
43. Rosenfield NS, Shimkin P, Berdon W: Wilms tumor arising from spontaneously regressing nephroblastomatosis. AJR 135:381, 1980.
44. Franken EA, Jr., Yiu-Chiu V, Smith WL, et al.: Nephroblastomatosis: Clinicopathologic significance and imaging characteristics. AJR 138:950, 1982.
45. Machin GA, McCaughey WT: A new precursor lesion of Wilms' tumour (nephroblastoma): Intralobar multifocal nephroblastomatosis. Histopathology 8:35, 1984.
46. Cromie WJ, Engelstein MS, Duckett JW: Nodular renal blastema, renal dysplasia and duplicated collecting systems. J Urol 123:100, 1980.
47. Karayalcin G, Shanske A, Honigman R: Wilms' tumor in a 13-year-old girl with trisomy 18. Am J Dis Child 135:665, 1981.
48. Breslow NE, Beckwith JB: Epidemiological features of Wilms' tumor: Results of the National Wilms' Tumor Study. JNCI 68:429, 1982.
49. Miller RW, Fraumeni JF, Manning MD: Association of Wilms' tumor with aniridia, hemihypertrophy and other congenital malformations. N Engl J Med 270:922, 1964.
50. Pendergrass TW: Congenital anomalies in children with Wilms' tumor. A new survey. Cancer 37:403, 1976.
51. Hittner HM, Riccardi VM, Francke U: Aniridia caused by a heritable chromosome 11 deletion. Ophthalmology 86:1173, 1979.
52. Yunis JJ, Ramsay NKC: Familial occurrence of the aniridia-Wilms tumor syndrome with deletion 11p13-14.1. J Pediatr 96:1027, 1980.
53. Green DM, Fine WE, Li FP: Offspring of patients treated for unilateral Wilms' tumor in childhood. Cancer 49:2285, 1982.
54. Cordero JF, Li FP, Holmes LB, et al.: Wilms tumor in five cousins. Pediatrics 66:716, 1980.
55. Bader JL, Li FP, Gerald PS, et al.: 11p chromosome deletion in four patients with aniridia and Wilms' tumor. Am Assoc Cancer Res (abstracts) 20:210, 1979.
56. Francke U, Holmes LB, Atkins L, et al.: Aniridia-Wilms' tumor association: Evidence for specific deletion of 11p13. Cytogenet Cell Genet 24:185, 1979.
57. Junien C, Turleau C, de Grouchy J, et al.: Regional assignment of catalase (CAT) gene to band 11p13. Association with the aniridia-Wilms' tumor-gonadoblastoma (WAGR) complex. Ann Genet 23:165, 1980.
58. Riccardi VM, Hittner HM, Francke U, et al.: The aniridia- Wilms tumor association: The critical role of chromosome band 11p13. Cancer Genet Cytogenet 2:131, 1980.
59. Strobel RJ, Riccardi VM, Ledbetter DH, et al.: Duplication 11p11.3-14.1 to meiotic crossing-over. Am J Med Genet 7:15, 1980.
60. Warburg M, Mikkelsen M, Andersen SR, et al.: Aniridia and interstitial deletion of the short arm of chromosome 11. Met Pediatr Ophthalmol 4:97, 1980.
61. Dufier JL, Phug LH, Schmelck P, et al.: Intercalary deletion of the short arm of chromosome 11: Aniridia, glaucoma, growth and mental retardation, sexual ambiguity, gonadoblastoma, and catalase deficiency. Bull Soc Ophthalmol Fr 81:747, 1981.
62. Fryns JP, Beirinckx J, DeSutter E, et al.: Aniridia-Wilms tumor association and 11p interstitial deletion. Eur J Pediatr 136:91, 1981.
63. Godde-Salz E, Behnke H: Aniridia, mental retardation and an unbalanced reciprocal translocation of chromosomes 8 and 11, with an interstitial deletion ot 11p. Eur J Pediatr 136:93, 1981.
64. Gilgenkrantz S, Vigneron C, Gregoire MF, et al.: Association of del(11)(p15.1p12), aniridia, catalase deficiency, and cardiomyopathy. Am J Med Genet 13:39, 1982.

65. Niikawa N, Fukushima Y, Taniguchi N, et al.: Chromosome abnormalities involving 11p13 and low erythrocyte catalase activity. Hum Genet 60:373, 1982.

66. Shannon RS, Mann JR, Harnden DG, et al.: Wilms's tumour and aniridia: Clinical and cytogenetic features. Arch Dis Childhood 57:85, 1982.

67. Waziri M, Patil SR, Hanson JW: Chromosomal and clinical findings in aniridia patients. Am J Hum Genet 34:125a, 1982.

68. Nakagome Y, Ise T, Sakurai M, et al.: High-resolution studies in patients with aniridia-Wilms tumor association, Wilms tumor or related congential abnormalities. Hum Genet 67: 245, 1984.

69. Barletta C, Castello MA, Ferrante E, et al.: 11p13 deletion and reduced RBC catalase in a patient with aniridia, glaucoma and bilateral Wilms' tumor. Tumori 71:119, 1985.

70. Andersen SR, Geertinger P, Larsen H-W, et al.: Aniridia, cataract and gonadoblastoma in a mentally retarded girl with deletion of chromosome 11. A clinicopathological case report. Ophthalmologica 176:171, 1978.

71. Junien C, Turleau C, Lenoir GM, et al.: Catalase determination in various etiologic forms of Wilms' tumor and gonadoblastoma. Cancer Genet Cytogenet 10:51, 1983.

72. Riccardi VM, Hittner HM, Strong LC, et al.: Wilms tumor with aniridia/iris dysplasia and apparently normal chromosomes. J Pediatr 100:574, 1982.

73. Hittner HM, Riccardi VM, Ferrell RE, et al.: Variable expressivity in autosomal dominant aniridia by clinical, electrophysiologic and angiographic criteria. Am J Ophthalmol 89:531, 1980.

74. Nelson LB, Spaeth GL, Nowinski TS, et al.: Aniridia. A review. Surv Ophthalmol 28:261, 1984.

75. Ferrell RE, Chakravarti A, Hittner HM, et al.: Autosomal dominant aniridia: Probable linkage to acid phosphatase-1 on chromosome 2. Proc Natl Acad Sci USA 77:1580, 1980.

76. Mirkinson AE, Mirkinson NK: A familial syndrome of aniridia and absence of the patella. Birth Defects 11(5):129, 1975.

77. Fraumeni JF, Jr., Glass AG: Wilms' tumor and congenital aniridia. JAMA 206:825, 1968.

78. Simola KOJ, Knuutila S, Kaitila I, et al.: Familial aniridia and translocation t(4;11)(q22;p13) without Wilms' tumor. Hum Genet 63:158, 1983.

79. Bateman JB, Maumenee I, Sparkes RS: Peters' anomaly associated with partial deletion of the long arm of chromosome 11. Am J Ophthalmol 97:11, 1984.

80. Broughton WL, Rosenbaum KN, Beauchamp GR: Congenital glaucoma and other ocular abnormalities associated with pericentric inversion of chromosome 11. Arch Ophthalmol 101:594, 1983.

81. Blethen SL, Taysi K: Autosomal dominant aniridia in association with craniopharyngioma. Am J Dis Child 135:575, 1981.

82. Ohno F, Yamano T, Kataoka K: A case of congenital aniridia and familial pheochromocytoma—with special reference to aniridia-Wilms' tumor syndrome. Jpn J Hum Genet 27:335, 1982.

83. Barakat AY, Papadopoulou ZL, Chandra RS, et al.: Pseudohermaphroditism, nephron disorder and Wilms' tumor: A unifying concept. Pediatrics 54:366, 1974.

84. Bond JV: Wilms's tumour, hypospadias, and cryptorchidism in twins. Arch Dis Childhood 52:243, 1977.

85. Rajfer J: Association between Wilms tumor and gonadal dysgenesis. J Urol 125:388, 1981.

86. McCoy FE, Franklin WA, Aronson AJ, et al.: Glomerulonephritis associated with male pseudohermaphroditism and nephroblastoma. Am J Surg Pathol 7:387, 1983.
87. Beheshti M, Mancer JFK, Hardy BF, et al.: External genital abnormalities associated with Wilms tumor. Urology 24:130, 1984.
88. Candia A, Zegel HG: The occurrence of Wilms tumor in 2 patients with exstrophy of the bladder. J Urol 128:589, 1982.
89. Wiedemann HR: Tumours and hemihypertrophy associated with Wiedemann-Beckwith syndrome. Eur J Pediatr 141:129, 1983.
90. Fraumeni JF, Jr., Geiser CF, Manning MD: Wilms' tumor and congenital hemihypertrophy: Report of five new cases and review of literature. Pediatrics 40:886, 1967.
91. Sotelo-Avila C, Gonzalez-Crussi F, Fowler JW: Complete and incomplete forms of Beckwith-Wiedemann syndrome: Their oncogenic potential. J Pediatr 95:47, 1980.
92. Sotelo-Avila C, Gonzalez-Crussi F, Starling KA: Wilms' tumor in a patient with an incomplete form of Beckwith-Wiedemann syndrome. Pediatrics 66:121, 1980.
93. Tolchin D, Koenigsberg M, Santorineou M: Early detection of Wilms' tumor in a child with hemihypertrophy and ovarian cysts. Pediatrics 70:135, 1982.
94. Olshan AF: Wilms' tumor, overgrowth, and fetal growth factors: A hypothesis. Cancer Genet Cytogenet 21:303, 1986.
95. Turleau C, de Grouchy J, Chavin-Colin F, et al.: Trisomy 11p15 and Beckwith-Wiedemann syndrome. A report of two cases. Hum Genet 67:219, 1984.
96. Waziri M, Patil SR, Hanson JW, et al.: Abnormality of chromosome 11 in patients with features of Beckwith-Wiedemann syndrome. J Pediatr 102:873, 1983.
97. Ehrich JHH, Ostertag H, Flatz S, et al.: Bilateral Wilms' tumour in Klippel-Trenaunay syndrome. Arch Dis Childhood 54:405, 1979.
98. Riccardi VM: Trisomy 8: An international study of 70 patients. Birth Defects 13(3c):171, 1977.
99. Niss R, Passarge E: Trisomy 8 restricted to cultured fibroblasts. J Med Genet 13:229, 1976.
100. Nakamura Y, Nakashima H, Fukuda S, et al.: Bilateral cystic nephroblastomas and multiple malformations with trisomy 8 mosaicism. Hum Pathol 16:754, 1985.
101. Bernard JL, Baeteman MA, Mattei JF, et al.: Wilms' tumor, malformative syndrome, mental retardation and de novo constitutional translocation, t(7;13)(q36;q13). Eur J Pediatr 141:175, 1984.
102. Perlman M, Levin M, Wittels B: Syndrome of fetal gigantism, renal hamartomas, and nephroblastomatosis with Wilms' tumor. Cancer 35:1212, 1975.
103. Greenberg F, Stein F, Gresik MV, et al.: The Perlman familial nephroblastomatosis syndrome. Am J Med Genet 24:101, 1986.
104. Riccardi VM: Von Recklinghausen neurofibromatosis. N Engl J Med 305:1016, 1981.
105. Hope DG, Mulvihill JJ: Malignancy in neurofibromatosis. Adv Neurol 29:33, 1981.
106. Chu J-Y, O'Connor DM, Danis RK: Neurofibrosarcoma at irradiation site in a patient with neurofibromatosis and Wilms' tumor. Cancer 31:333, 1981.
107. Masson P: The role of the neural crests in the embryonal adenosarcomas of the kidney. Am J Cancer 33:1, 1938.
108. Allen RW, Ogden B, Bentley FL, et al.: Fetal hydantoin syndrome, neuroblastoma, and hemorrhagic disease in a neonate. JAMA 244:1464, 1980.
109. Taylor WF, Myers M, Taylor WR: Extrarenal Wilms' tumour in an infant exposed to intrauterine phenytoin. Lancet 2:481, 1980.
110. Goldman SM, Garfinkel DJ, Oh KS, et al.: The Drash syndrome: Male pseudohermaphroditism, nephritis, and Wilms tumor. Radiology 141:87, 1981.

111. Eddy AA, Mauer SM: Pseudohermaphroditism, glomerulopathy, and Wilms tumor (Drash syndrome): Frequency in end-stage renal failure. J Pediatr 106:584, 1985.

112. Thorner P, McGraw M, Weitzman S, et al.: Wilms' tumor and glomerular disease. Arch Pathol Lab Med 108:141, 1984.

113. Welch TR, McAdams AJ: Focal glomerulosclerosis as a late sequela of Wilms Tumor. J Pediatr 108:105, 1986.

114. Green DM: The diagnosis and management of Wilms' tumor. Pediatr Clin North Am 32:735, 1985.

115. Cohen MD, Siddiqui A, Weetman R, et al.: A rational approach to the radiologic evaluation of children with Wilms' tumor. Cancer 50:887, 1982.

116. Cohen MD, Weber T, Smith JA, et al.: The role of computerized tomography in the diagnosis and management of patients with bilateral Wilms tumor. J Urol 130:1160, 1983.

117. Zimmer WD, Williamson B, Hartman GW, et al.: Changing the patterns in the evaluation of renal masses: Economic implications. AJR 143:285, 1984.

118. Levine E: Computed tomography of renal masses. CRC Crit Rev Diagn Imaging 24:91, 1985.

119. Peretz GS, Lam AH: Distinguishing neuroblastoma from Wilms tumor by computed tomography. J Comp Assist Tomogr 9:889, 1985.

120. Cavenee WK, Murphree AL, Shull MM, et al.: Prediction of familial predisposition to retinoblastoma. N Engl J Med 317:1201, 1986.

121. Ferrell RE, Riccardi VM: Catalase levels in patients with aniridia and/or Wilms' tumor: Utility and limitations. Cytogenet Cell Genet 31:120, 1981.

122. Cowell JK: Tracking the cancer genes in paediatric predisposition syndromes: Opportunity for prenatal diagnosis. Cancer Surveys 3:573, 1984.

123. Fisher JH, Miller YE, Sparkes RS, et al.: Wilms' tumor-aniridia association: Segregation of affected chromosome in somatic cell hybrids, identification of cell surface antigen associated with deleted area, and regional mapping of c-Ha-ras-1 oncogene, insulin gene, and beta-globin gene. Somatic Cell Mol Genet 10:455, 1984.

124. Lewis WH, Goguen JM, Powers VE, et al.: Gene order on the short arm of human chromosome 11: Regional assignment of the LDH A gene distal to catalase in two translocations. Hum Genet 71:249, 1985.

125. Scoggin CH, Fisher JH, Shoemaker SA, et al.: The E7-associated cell surface antigen: A marker for the 11p134 chromosomal deletion associated with aniridia-Wilms tumor. Am J Hum Genet 37:883, 1985.

126. van Heyningen V, Porteus DJ: Mapping a chromosome to find a gene. Trends Genet 2:4, 1986.

127. Punnett HH, Marshall LS, Qureshi AR, et al.: Deletion 11p13 with normal catalase activity. Pediatr Res 17:217A, 1983.

128. Wilkins JR, Sinks TH, Jr.: Paternal occupation and Wilms tumour in offspring. J Epidemiol Commun Health 38:7, 1984.

129. Wilkins JR, III, Sinks TH, Jr.: Occupational exposures among fathers of children with Wilms' tumor. J Occup Med 26:427, 1984.

130. Kaneko Y, Egues MC, Rowley JD: Interstitial deletion of short arm of chromosome 11 limited to Wilms' tumor cells in a patient without aniridia. Cancer Res 41:4577, 1981.

131. Slater RM, de Kraker J, Voute PA, et al.: A cytogenetic study of Wilms' tumor. Cancer Genet Cytogenet 14:95, 1985.

132. Kaneko Y, Kondo K, Rowley JD, et al.: Further chromosome studies on Wilms' tumor cells of patients without aniridia. Cancer Genet Cytogenet 10:191, 1983.

133. De Blois MC, Philip T, Lenoir GM, et al.: Etude cytogenetique en prometaphase de 13 cas de tumeur de Wilms sans aniridie. J Genet Hum 31:25, 1983.

134. Kondo K, Chilcote RR, Maurer HS, et al.: Chromosome abnormalities in tumor cells from patients with sporadic Wilms' tumor. Cancer Res 44:5376, 1984.

135. Slater RM: The cytogenetics of Wilms' tumor. Cancer Genet Cytogenet 19:37, 1986.

136. Douglass EC, Green AA, Hayes FA, et al.: Chromosome 1 abnormalities: A common feature of pediatric solid tumors. JNCI 75:51, 1985.

137. Gardner RJM, Grindley RM, Chewings WE, et al.: Wilms' tumour with somatic rearrangement of chromosome 11 at band p13. Proc Univ Otago Med Sch 61.32, 1983.

138. Huerre C, Despoisse S, Gilgenkrantz S, et al.: c-Ha-ras1 is not deleted in aniridia-Wilms' tumour association. Nature 305:638, 1983.

139. Eccles MR, Millow LJ, Wilkins RJ, et al.: Harvey-ras allele deletion detected by in situ hybridization to Wilms' tumor chromosomes. Hum Genet 67:190, 1984.

140. Fearon ER, Vogelstein B, Feinberg AP: Somatic deletion and duplication of genes on chromosome 11 in Wilms' tumours. Nature 309:176, 1984.

141. Koufos A, Hansen MF, Lampkin BC, et al.: Loss of alleles at loci on human chromosome 11 during genesis of Wilms' tumour. Nature 309:170, 1984.

142. Orkin SH, Goldman DS, Sallan SE: Development of homozygosity for chromosome 11p markers in Wilms' tumour. Nature 309:172, 1984.

143. Reeve AE, Housiaux PJ, Gardner RJM, et al: Loss of a Harvey ras allele in sporadic Wilms' tumour. Nature 309:174, 1984.

144. Dao DD, Schroeder WT, Chao LY, et al.:Genetic mechanisms of tumor-specific loss of 11p DNA sequences in Wilms' Tumor. Am J Hum Genet 41:202, 1987.

145. Michalopoulos EE, Bevilacqua PJ, Stokoe N, et al.: Molecular analysis of gene deletion in aniridia-Wilms tumor association. Hum Genet 70:157, 1985.

146. Schroeder WT, Chao LY, Dao DD, et al.: Nonrandom loss of maternal chromosome 11 alleles in Wilms' Tumors. Am J Hum Genet 40:413, 1987.

147. van Kessel AG, Nusse R, Slater R, et al.: Localization of the oncogene c-Ha-ras1 outside the aniridia-Wilms' tumor-associated deletion of chromosome 11(del 11p13) using somatic cell hybrids. Cancer Genet Cytogenet 15:49, 1985.

148. Gonzalez-Crussi F, Black-Schaffer S: Rhabdomyosarcoma of infancy and childhood: Problems of morphologic classification. Am J Surg Pathol 3:157, 1979.

149. Seidal T, Mark J, Hagmar B, et al.: Alveolar rhabdomyosarcoma: A cytogenetic and correlated cytological and histological study. Acta Pathol Microbiol Immunol Scand (Sect A) 90:345, 1982.

150. Young J, Miller RW: Incidence of malignant tumors in U.S. children. J Pediatr 86:254, 1975.

151. Smith MT, Armbrustmacher VW, Violett TW: Diffuse meningeal rhabdomyosarcoma. Cancer 47:2081, 1981.

152. Rogers PCJ, Howards SS, Komp DM: Urogenital rhabdomyosarcoma in childhood. J Urol 115:738, 1976.

153. King DG, Finney RP: Embryonal rhabdomyosarcoma of the prostate. J Urol 117:88, 1977.

154. Kotecha NM: Embryonal rhabdomyosarcoma of the kidney. J Urol 118:325, 1977.

155. Flamant F, Chassagne D, Cosset JM, et al.: Embryonal rhabdomyosarcoma of the vagina in children: Conservative treatment with curietherapy and chemotherapy. Eur J Cancer 15:527, 1979.

156. Kaplan WE, Firlit CF, Berger RM: Genitourinary rhabdomyosarcoma. J Urol 130:116, 1983.

157. Das S, Egan RM, Amar AD: Von Hipple-Lindau syndrome with bilateral synchronous renal cell carcinoma. Urology 18:599, 1981.

158. Yashiro N, Itai Y, Iio M: Bilateral synchronous renal cancer. Radiat Med 2:123, 1984.

159. Li FP, Marchetto DJ, Brown RS: Familial renal cell carcinoma. Cancer Genet Cytogenet 7:271, 1982.

160. Wang N, Perkins KL: Involvement of band 3p14 in t(3;8) hereditary renal cell carcinoma. Cancer Genet Cytogenet 11:479, 1984.

161. Marchetto D, Li FP, Henson DE: Familial carcinoma of ureters and other genitourinary organs. J Urol 130:772, 1983.

162. Pathek S, Goodacre A: Chromosome anomalies and predisposition to human breast, renal cell, and colorectal carcinoma. Cancer Genet Cytogenet 19:29, 1986.

163. Yoshida MA, Ohyashiki K, Ochi H, et al.: Rearrangement of chromosome 3 in renal cell carcinoma. Cancer Genet Cytogenet 19:351, 1986.

164. Hardwig P, Robertson DM: Von Hippel-Lindau disease: A familial, often lethal, multisystem phakomatosis. Ophthalmology 91:263, 1984.

165. Pearson JC, Weiss J, Tanagho EA: A plea for conservation of kidney in renal adenocarcinoma associated with von Hippel-Lindau disease. J Urol 124:910, 1980.

166. Selli C, Hinshaw WM, Woodard BH, et al.: Stratification of risk factors in renal cell carcinoma. Cancer 52:899, 1983.

167. Levine E, Collins DL, Horton WA, et al.: CT screening of the abdomen in von Hippel-Lindau disease. AJR 139:505, 1982.

168. Christenson PJ, Craig JP, Bibro MC, et al.: Cysts containing renal cell carcinoma in Von Hippel-Lindau disease. J Urol 128:798, 1982.

169. Levine E, Weigel JW, Collins DL: Diagnosis and management of asymptomatic renal cell carcinomas in von Hippel-Lindau syndrome. Urology 21:146, 1983.

170. Outzen HC, Maguire HC, Jr.: The etiology of renal-cell carcinoma. Semin Oncol 10:378, 1983.

171. Nagendran V, Dimond AH: Renal carcinoma in Lindau's disease. Postgrad Med J 60:624, 1984.

172. Pyhtinen J, Suramo I, Lohela P, et al.: Abdominal ultrasonography and computed tomography in von Hippel-Lindau disease. Ann Clin Res 14:172, 1982.

173. Hoffman RW, Gardner DW, Mitchell FL: Intrathoracic and multiple abdominal pheochromocytomas in von Hippel-Lindau disease. Arch Int Med 142:1962, 1982.

174. Mulshine JL, Tubbs R, Sheeler LR, et al.: Clinical significance of the association of the von Hippel-Lindau disease with pheochromocytoma and pancreatic apudoma. Am J Med Sci 288:212, 1984.

175. Kallie NR, Fisher GF, Harker JR: Papillary cystadenoma of the epididymis. Can J Surg 26.174, 1983.

176. de Sousa-Andrade J, Bmbirra EA, Bichalo OJ, et al.: Bilateral papillary cystadenoma of the epididymis as a component of von Hippel-Lindau's syndrome: Report of a case presenting as infertility. J Urol 133:288, 1985.

177. Witten FR, O'Brien DP III, Sewell CW, et al.: Bilateral clear cell papillary cystadenoma of the epididymis presenting as infertility: An early manifestation of von Hippel-Lindau's syndrome. J Urol 133:1062, 1985.

178. Gomez MR: Tuberous Sclerosis. New York: Raven Press, 1979.

179. Shapiro RA, Skinner DG, Stanley P, et al.: Renal tumors associated with tuberous sclerosis: The case for aggressive surgical management. J Urol 132:1170, 1984.

180. Pode D, Meretik S, Shapiro A, et al.: Diagnosis and management of renal angiomyolipoma. Urology 25:461, 1985.
181. Yu DT, Sheth KJ: Cystic renal involvement in tuberous sclerosis. Clin Pediatr 24:36, 1985.
182. Riccardi VM, Eichner JE: Neurofibromatosis: Phenotype, Natural History and Pathogenesis. Baltimore: Johns Hopkins University Press, 1986.

Chapter 16
Radiotherapy of Pediatric Genitourinary Tumors

P.N. Plowman

WILMS' TUMOR

The use of multimodal therapy for Wilms' tumor (combinations of radical nephrectomy with or without radiotherapy to the tumor bed and chemotherapy with actinomycin D, vincristine, and adriamycin) has led to improved survival rates (Fig. 16-1). The National Wilms' Tumor Study Group (NWTS) has been instrumental in improving the survival for Wilms' tumor as well as adjusting therapy to achieve the optimal quality of life without affecting survival. Data from both the NWTS and United Kingdom trials, however, are valuable in arriving at the optimal management recommendations for each stage of the disease.

NWTS derived a grouping system (later amended to the staging system) based on the extent of tumor presentation [1–3] (Table 16-1). It is important to note that this grouping is based on clinical stage and not on surgical stage as in some other studies. It is relevant to note that with progressively more accurate and meticulous radiographic surgical and pathological staging over the last decade, there has been a skew towards lower-extent disease in all stages. This tends to improve the prognosis of the individual stages but not of overall survival. It is important to remember that while early NWTS findings clearly demonstrated that the staging system related to overall prognosis, now that more aggressive and considerably lighter treatment strategies are being applied to high and low stage disease, respectively, it is not surprising that the prognostic impact of staging might be blunted in the more recent trials.

Pediatric Tumors of the Genitourinary Tract, pages 263–281
© 1988 Alan R. Liss, Inc.

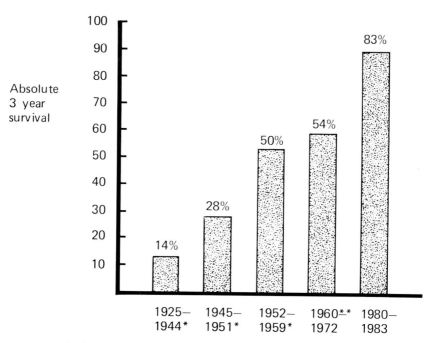

Fig. 16-1. Absolute 3-year survival of children with Wilms' tumor presenting to the Hospital for Sick Children, Great Ormond Street. *Data from D.I. Williams (1964).**Data from J.V. Bond (1976).

In the first NWTS trial (NWTS-1), postoperative radiotherapy and adjuvant chemotherapy were analyzed in a systematic fashion [1]. In children aged less than 2 years who had group 1 (Stage I) tumors and who received 15 months of adjuvant single agent actinomycin D, the use of postoperative radiotherapy did not significantly add to local recurrence-free or overall survival. In group 1 patients over the age of 2 years, there were five intraabdominal relapses in the 41 non-irradiated patients (three being in the original tumor bed) versus one (in the contralateral kidney and questionably a second primary) among 39 irradiated patients. This was a non-significant trend favoring radiotherapy in 1976, but later became a significant survival advantage to radiotherapy patients.

In groups 2 and 3 (stages II and III), patients treated by radical nephrectomy and postoperative radiotherapy, adjuvant double agent (actinomycin D and vincristine) chemotherapy proved superior to single agent therapy (either actinomycin D or vincristine). Thus, approximately 80% of patients treated

TABLE 16-1. Staging System for Wilms' Tumor (NWTS System)

Stage I
>   Tumor limited to kidney and completely excised.
>
> The surface of the renal capsule is intact. The tumor was not ruptured before or during
>   removal. There is no microscopic evidence of tumor at resection margins.

Stage II
>   Tumor extends beyond the kidney but is completely excised.
>
> There is local extension of the tumor, i.e., penetration beyond the pseudocapsule into the
>   perirenal soft tissues. The renal vessels outside the kidney substance are infiltrated or
>   contain tumor thrombus. There is no residual tumor apparent at the resection margins
>   microscopically.
>
> Local flank spillage at operation is allowable within stage II.
>
> (Biopsy-positive lymph nodes place the patient in stage III.)

Stage III
>   Residual non-hematogenous tumor confined to the abdomen (i.e., incomplete
>   resection).
>
> This stage includes microscopic tumor at operative resection specimen margins, all
>   positive lymph cases, and all patients in whom there was operative tumor spillage
>   throughout the abdomen.

Stage IV
>   Hematogenous metastases including liver.

Stage V
>   Bilateral renal involvement.

with combination chemotherapy were disease-free at 2 years versus approximately 55% for those receiving vincristine alone [1].

Other data arising from NWTS-1 allowed other conclusions to be reached with regard to histopathologic, radiotherapeutic, and surgical assessment and practice. Beckwith and Palmer demonstrated that Wilms' tumors with anaplastic or sarcomatous variants were "poor prognosis" tumors [4]. These unfavorable histological patterns proved to be the most important single determinant of patient outcome in NWTS-1 [5] Although comprising only 11.5% of tumors studied, the unfavorable histology tumors accounted for 52% of the deaths. The radiotherapy recommendations in the NWTS-1 study differed from the current ones, and their discussion here is merited by the insight it gives into the evolution of present recommendations. The radiation dose recommendation ranged from 18–24 Gy in children over 40 months by parallel opposed megavoltage photon portals with daily treatments of up to 2 Gy. For group 1–2 patients (stage I–II but excluding "flank spillage" cases and including resected paraaortic node positive cases), the portal irradiated came across the midline medially to encompass the whole width of the vertebral bodies but not the surviving kidney. Superiorly, inferiorly, and laterally the field borders were to encompass the site of the kidney and associated tumor as visualized on the preoperative intravenous urogram (Fig. 16-2).

Initially, group 3 patients (stage III excluding resected positive paraaortic node cases) were treated by whole abdominal radiation from the domes of the diaphragm to the pelvic floor and to the lateral peritoneal reflections. The recommended doses of 25 Gy in 3 weeks to children less than 4 years and 35 Gy in 4 weeks to children over 4 years were delivered in 1.5-Gy daily fractions with shielding of the contralateral kidney and liver so they received no more than a total of 15 Gy and 30 Gy, respectively. In analyzing the NWTS-1 radiation data, Tefft et al. concluded that whole abdominal radiotherapy was unnecessary when tumor spillage was confined to the flank [6]. In group 3 patients, there was an intraabdominal recurrence rate of 8/58 cases (12%) that included two Wilms' tumors in the contralateral kidney, most likely second primaries. Tefft et al. considered that radiotherapy had been effective in producing this low recurrence rate [6]. In a later analysis of NWTS radiotherapy data up to that time, D'Angio et al. could demonstrate no statistically significant differences in the relapse patterns locally or distantly regardless of radiation dose [7]. This later influenced recommended radiotherapy doses.

An analysis of the surgical management of NWTS-1 patients is also instructive. Leape et al. did not find any statistically significant difference in

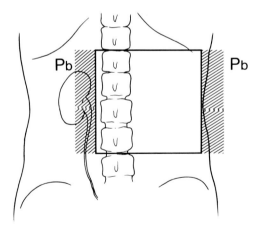

Fig. 16-2. Typical megavoltage photon (linear accelerator) radiation portal for postoperative renal bed radiotherapy in Wilms' tumor. Note that the portal extends across the midline to encompass both vertebral growth epiphyses but none of the contralateral kidney. A tangential body wall shield is shown and usually recommended.

relapse-free survival in comparable treatment groups whether the tumor was diffusely distributed throughout the kidney or localized to one pole, whether it was unicentric or multicentric, or whether it was nodular or smooth [8]. Soft tumors were associated with a higher incidence of preoperative rupture and operative spillage than hard tumors. While operative spillage was found to be associated with a significantly higher incidence of abdominal recurrence and consequent higher mortality, it was found that preoperative rupture did not lead to a significantly higher abdominal relapse rate. Whether the wider field, higher dose radiotherapy protocol in NWTS-1 contributed to this lack of significance is not answered and probably no longer a vital issue.

Older patients had larger tumors in NWTS-1 and larger tumors tended to be associated with more advanced disease stage. Positive lymph nodes, hepatic invasion, and capsular infiltration led to a lower survival rate, but the finding of tumor in the renal vein did not. Leape et al. thus recommended a transabdominal approach to the tumor to allow careful inspection of the opposite kidney, early ligation of the renal vascular pedicule, and radical nephrectomy [8]. Whether the incision was vertical, transverse, or thoracoabdominal made no difference with regard to spillage rates, but flank incisions were to be avoided.

NWTS-2 was built on the findings of NWTS-1. Having established that actinomycin D and vincristine were superior to single agents, radiotherapy was removed from the postoperative management of all group 1 patients in favor of two-drug adjuvant therapy for either 6 or 15 months. More advanced group/stage patients all received radiotherapy and either two drugs as above or the addition of a third drug (adriamycin). The radiation dosage remained the same as in the first study [3].

The important conclusions from NWTS-2 were that the omission of radiotherapy in the treatment of all group 1 patients appeared safe, and the 6-month adjuvant double agent chemotherapy was as effective as longer chemotherapy for this subset of patients. Overall, the survival of group 1 patients was better than NWTS-1, but patients with unfavorable histology tumors were still considerably more likely to relapse (locally and distantly) after this treatment program than those with favorable histology tumors. Group 2–4 patients receiving the third drug (adriamycin) in the adjuvant chemotherapy regimen had a superior survival rate to those patients receiving two drugs. This difference was most marked in the survival of unfavorable histology patients and not apparent in group 2 or 3 (stage II and III) favorable histology patients.

NWTS-3 was the logical sequel to NWTS-2. Considering the approximate 90% survival of stage I patients in NWTS-2, NWTS-3 sought to examine whether double agent adjuvant chemotherapy for even less than 6 months was equally curative. The results of NWTS-3 now demonstrate that 10 weeks of such therapy are sufficient. For higher stage patients (II or III) in whom there was concern regarding the cardiotoxicity of anthracyclines, there was stratification to compare more intensive double agent actinomycin D and vincristine versus triple agent chemotherapy. At the same time they elected to compare 10-Gy radiotherapy to the renal bed versus 20-Gy for stage III favorable histology patients and radiotherapy (20 Gy) versus no radiotherapy in stage II favorable histology patients. The results of NWTS-3 demonstrate a better survival rate for stage III favorable histology cases given three-drug chemotherapy. This is largely accounted for by nine infradiaphragmatic relapses (excluding liver and contralateral kidney) in the children having the reduced radiotherapy dose and double agent chemotherapy. Thus, it would seem unwise to reduce both the radiotherapy below 20 Gy and to stay with double agent chemotherapy. It also seems likely that stage II favorable histology disease may be safely managed without radiotherapy and adriamycin, as NWTS-3 does not appear to show an advantage for stage II favorable histology irradiated patients. Now that operative spillage is allowable within stage II and bearing in mind the findings of Leape et al. [8], the need for radiotherapy in some stage II cases must still be appraised in each trial. In NWTS-4, adriamycin has been retained, but radiotherapy to the renal bed has been reduced (10 Gy) in stage III favorable histology patients.

The NWTS trials have established the dominant treatment patterns for stage I–III Wilms' tumor, but can we learn from other series? The United Kingdom Children's Cancer Study Group trial differs in that single agent vincristine (1.5 mg/m^2 weekly × 10, then three weekly for a further five doses) was the only adjuvant therapy given to stage I favorable histology cases. This policy avoids intercalating agent administration to young children but runs counter to modern curative oncologic practices of using drug combinations. The 2-year survival figures for favorable histology stage I cases in the United Kingdom Children's Cancer Study Group trial is 98%.

The United Kingdom Children's Cancer Study Group has yet to be fully analyzed but two firm conclusions on prognostic factors are already apparent. First, the recognition of and the more aggressive treatment regimens employed for unfavorable histology cases of all stages have substantially increased survival over the previous UK (MRC) trial. Second, among stage III cases, the survival of children who were stage III by virtue of residual disease or positive aortic lymph nodes was significantly better than among children who were stage III because of both these factors. In other respects, the United Kingdom Children's Cancer Study Group corroborates the NWTS data.

Flank spillage and difficulty in initial operation has been a major concern to the European group International Society of Pediatric Oncology. This led the International Society of Pediatric Oncology to a different therapeutic strategy for non-metastatic Wilms' tumor, employing preoperative therapy [9]. The NWTS staging system was used. The first group of patients was randomized to 20 Gy preoperatively followed by 0–15 Gy postoperatively (depending on operative stage). The second group of patients received only postoperative radiotherapy. The analysis demonstrated a much lower rate of tumor rupture in the preoperative radiotherapy group. Although at first this appeared to be associated with a lower rate of distant metastases, the long-term survival of both groups has proved similar. The adjuvant chemotherapy given was single agent actinomycin D and the recurrence-free survival results are inferior to NWTS, although the overall survival is good: 91% for stage I, 76% for stage II, and 84% for stage III. This is due presumably to effective salvage chemotherapy. It is worth noting the arguments against preoperative radiotherapy. First, the diagnosis and staging of Wilms' tumor is best assessed at the time of primary radical nephrectomy when there is no perturbation of disease extent or alteration of histology by therapy. Second, the radiation portal will be substantially larger to encompass the unoperated growth. When the tumor crosses the midline, it may be necessary to encompass part of the contralateral kidney, leave some tumor unirradiated, or use a radiation plan other than a parallel opposed portals technique (all of which may be complex and unsatisfactory, especially in young children). In favor of preoperative radiotherpy, however, is the reduced incidence of tumor rupture at operation and the reduced postoperative radiation volume in those who would have had tumor spill. Lemerle et al. therefore recommended preoperative radiotherapy for all Wilms' tumors other than those with small stage I [9,10].

Later International Society of Pediatric Oncology trials have examined preoperative double-agent (actinomycin D and vincristine) chemotherapy versus preoperative radiotherapy and have found no differences in disease-free or overall survival rates [11,12]. Not unexpectedly the proportion of early stage growths at operation is considerably higher than in other series, and these authors claim that unfavorable histology is still perceptible after pretreatment. In the more recent International Society of Pediatric Oncology trials, preoperative actinomycin D and vincristine therapy has influenced the aggressiveness of postoperative chemotherapy that is based on the amount of disease persisting at operation. This argument is possibly weakened by an earlier finding from the Gustave Roussay Institute (a major contributor to the International Society of Pediatric Oncology studies) that cases in which preoperative radiotherapy resulted in complete destruction of tumor cells were a very unfavorable prognostic group [10]. In conclusion, the UK and American groups are not convinced that preoperative therapy is indicated or useful for stage I–III disease. The one exception to this is the patient with massive abdominal growth with inferior vena cava invasion or diaphragmatic infiltration. In such situations, preoperative chemotherapy is favored.

In stage IV disease, preoperative therapy is more logical, although a pathological diagnosis is certainly first indicated by biopsy of the primary tumor. In NWTS-1 the use of preoperative vincristine to group 4 patients in addition to postoperative radiotherapy (to the primary tumor bed and all metastatic sites) and chemotherapy (actinomycin D and vincristine) did not improve results. In NWTS-2, no preoperative therapy was given, but the addition of adriamycin to the other two postoperative drugs appeared to improve results. In NWTS-3, again no preoperative therapy was given but a fourth drug (cyclophosphamide) was introduced. This was not found to improve survival and did add to toxicity.

In United Kingdom Children's Cancer Study group 1, initial surgery was indicated if the tumor in the abdomen was thought to be resectable. In other cases, preoperative aggressive chemotherapy commenced the program with delayed nephrectomy. The survival results of stage IV United Kingdom Children's Cancer Study Group patients at present appear inferior to NWTS figures. This is not attributed to any difference in indications for initial surgery (although this remains possible), but may be due to the lesser use of radiation to metastatic sites. In the United Kingdom series, pulmonary radiation is not used following a chemotherapeutic response in lung secondaries. This is an issue because the dose of radiotherapy that can be given to the whole lung is limited. Thus, the current NWTS protocols for stage IV (pulmonary metastatic) cases call for 1,200 cGy mid-plane in 150 cGy daily fractions (this dose having been reduced from the previously recommended 1,500 cGy due to the radiosensitization effected by actinomycin D and adriamycin). In cases with liver metastases, hepatic radiation is also recommended by NWTS, used primarily after chemotherapy to consolidate the response for metastases in both these sites. In the United Kingdom Children's Cancer Study Group study, radiotherapy to metastatic sites is not part of the initial treatment strategy for any stage IV cases but is reserved for relapsers or incomplete responders. This is currently being reviewed in light of the American stage IV survival figures.

The salvage of Wilms' tumor patients who relapse during or after treament merits further discussion. Lemerle et al. established that despite a relatively low relapse-free survival following single agent adjuvant chemotherapy (actinomycin D), a high overall survival is still obtainable [9]. One infers from their paper that this is from multiple agent chemotherpay. One would expect the salvage rate to be lower in patients relapsing having received multiple drug adjuvant therapy. In general, patients who relapse on therapy fare worse than those who relapse later after therapy has ceased. All workers would now employ actinomycin D, vincristine, adriamycin, and radiotherapy to all sites in salvage programs, and occasionally surgery may be required for single residual masses. The place of alkylating agents is controversial.

In an early study from St. Bartholomew's Hospital, London, 70 patients with Wilms' tumor presented over an 18-year period and seven (10%) had bilateral tumors. Four out of the seven patients died and three survived. Actinomycin D was the only chemotherapeutic agent used [13]. In the modern literature and from larger series, it now appears that bilateral Wilms' tumor accounts for approximately 5% of all cases [14]. Usually, the second tumor is small and discovered only by careful operative inspection of the contralateral kidney at the time of definitive primary radical nephrectomy for clinically diagnosed unilateral Wilms' tumor (Fig. 16-3). The initial operative inspection of the contralateral kidney is always to be advised in the surgical management of Wilms' tumor. If bilateral tumors are found and if there is a chance of preservation of some normal functioning kidney on the side of the larger tumor, then only bilateral biopsies are recommended initially. If the larger tumor has destroyed its kidney of origin as a functioning organ, then radical nephrectomy on this side and biopsy of the incidentally discovered tumor is indicated. It is only recently that radical nephrectomy has been questioned as an essential procedure for Wilms' tumor [15]. Where a heminephrectomy is possible (perhaps only after preoperative therapy), this should be considered. Bishop et al. analyzed 33 NWTS patients with bilateral Wilms' tumor reporting a 2-year survival of 87% [14]. As only four patients had died, it was difficult for these authors to make treatment comparisons but certain features were apparent. Although extirpative surgery was important, leaving microscopically involved margins did not seem to affect survival as long as these second tumors were small and surgery was backed up by adjuvant radiotherapy and chemotherapy. Double agent actinomycin D and vincristine were effective in reducing tumor bulk and might supplant radiotherapy to the surviving kidney. Radiotherapy to the surviving kidney, at least with the few years followup available in this 1977 series, was tolerated to a dose of 1,500 cGy in 150 cGy daily fractions. The present policy in London is 1,000 cGy similarly fractionated. Radiotherapy to the surviving kidney of a young child is a potential worry in the management of these cases, and a greater emphasis on combination chemotherapy, and second

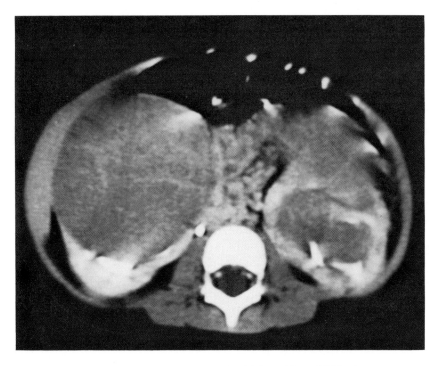

Fig. 16-3. CT scan of abdomen of a child with large bilateral Wilms' tumors.

look surgery followed by lower dose and partial renal radiotherapy, is to be recommended in the future. Certainly, the work of Bishop and associates [14] as well as our own smaller experience [16] are cause for optimism in the management of bilateral cases. More recently, "bench" surgery of awkwardly placed (usually centrally situated) Wilms' tumors has added a new dimension to kidney sparing. Thus, bilateral nephrectomy should only be considered as a last resort.

Wilms' tumor in adults is rare. When it does occur, it tends to present with higher stage of disease but the likelihood of unfavorable histology disease does not seem greater than in children [16,17]. Nevertheless, the prognosis is considerably worse than in the pediatric age range, with the 3-year survival rate being 24% [16]. It would seem advisable to routinely employ postoperative radiotherapy to the tumor bed as well as the most aggressive adjuvant chemotherapy regimen (vincristine, actinomycin, adriamycin).

GENITOURINARY RHABDOMYOSARCOMAS

Genitourinary and intrabdominal rhabdomyosarcomas (RMS) account for approximately one-third of all rhabdomyosarcomas, with pure genitourinary accounting for just under one quarter [18]. There is currently great controversy as to the ideal management program for treating rhabdomyosarcoma as intensive multimodality therapy is now not only effective but has late and undesirable side effects. Within the group of genitourinary rhabdomyosarcomas, there are cases with both a good and bad prognosis. Since the most intensive therapy regimens lead to severe late normal tissue morbidity, a full discussion of the problems and controversies regarding optimal management is necessary. It is important to remember that, in general, rhabdomyosarcoma is a more highly lethal disease than Wilms' tumor and that curative salvage programs for children who relapse through their first treatment regimen are usually unsuccessful.

It must not be forgotten that radical surgery alone and radical radiotherapy alone both have curative potential in this disease. Radical surgery leads to a 70% survival rate in children with bladder rhabdomyosarcoma, and radical radiotherapy leads to a 66% survival rate in orbital rhabdomyosarcoma [19,20]. Since the introduction of systemic combination chemotherapy, not only have the local control rates in the primary site improved but overall survival has also greatly increased. The routine use of pulse VAC (vincristine, actinomycin D, cyclophosphamide) adjuvant chemotherapy for rhabdomyosarcoma was introduced widely in the early 1970s. Since there have been no major advances in rhabdomyosarcoma chemotherapy since that time, several large groups have accumulated more than a decade of experience with similar chemotherapy in the multimodality management of rhabdomyosarcoma. Conventional management of apparently localized rhabdomyosarcoma is 1) radical excision of easily excised tumors followed by radiotherapy and then adjuvant VAC for 1 year plus; 2) initial chemotherapy (2–3 cycles of pulse VAC) followed by surgery or radiotherapy or both, after which pulse VAC is continued for 1 year plus. This second approach is used for larger invasive tumors or those that are not easily resectable at diagnosis.

The Children's Solid Tumor Group (CSTG) comprising a collaborative group from St. Bartholomew's Hospital and the Royal Marsden Hospital, London, reported 73 patients treated according to the above policies [21]. The extent of the local (or distant) disease at presentation was found to be the major prognosticator of outcome. Children with tumors confined to the tissue of origin had a predicted 5-year survival rate of 86%, while this figure was 21% for patients whose tumors extended beyond the tissue of origin. Boys with paratesticular tumors and girls with vaginal tumors had 5-year survival rates of 81 and 67%, respectively, whereas children with primaries at other pelvic sites did much worse with an overall survival at 5 years of 31%. Embryonal histology appeared a more prognostically favorable microscopic diagnosis than alveolar histology. Age at diagnosis did not seem to influence outcome. A later analysis of CTSG data reveals more information. Of 102 children with rhabdomyosarcoma (all sites) presenting to CSTG participants over a 13-year period and with a minimum of 2 years' followup, 54 patients have relapsed. Of the 54 relapsers, the primary site was the first site of relapse in 35 patients (65%), whereas distant metastatic disease was evident in 19 (35%). The relapse rate in the primary site is considerably higher in this CSTG series than in a comparable American Intergroup Rhabdomyosarcoma Study (IRS). It seemed likely that radiotherapy was given less frequently in the CSTG series, being withheld from cases that were deemed to be low risk, despite the infrequent use of radical surgery. Of 35 relapsers at the primary site, 15 cases had received no radiotherapy, two cases less than 20 Cy, a further four cases less than 40 Gy, while the other 14 patients had received over 40 Gy to the primary site. Thus, 64% of patients not receiving radiotherapy to the primary site relapsed, whereas 31% of patients receiving radiotherapy relapsed (Kingston and Plowman, unpublished CSTG data). The local relapse rate in the otherwise comparable IRS trials where radiotherpy (more than 40 Gy) was routinely prescribed, except where early surgical excision had achieved microscopic clear margins, is considerably lower, on the order of 15% (Tefft, personal communication).

Bladder and Prostate Rhabdomyosarcoma

Bladder and prostate primary rhabdomyosarcomas are worthy of separate scrutiny. In an early study from the Hospital for Sick Children, London, Claireux and Williams found eight out of 13 survivors among children with primary bladder rhabdomyosarcoma treated by radical surgery, whereas among nine children with prostate region primaries treated by radical surgery, there was only one survivor [22]. The average age of the latter group was older. Tefft and Jaffe found that half of bladder rhabdomyosarcoma patients presented before the age of 2 years and three-quarters before the age of five years [19], a slightly younger age range than boys presenting with primary prostatic rhabdomyosarcoma. Two-thirds of cases arose in the region of the trigone, eliminating the feasibility of partial cystectomy. Bladder rhabdomyosarcoma usually arises as a pedunculated mass in the submucosa but later develops a broader and then sessile base as it ultimately invades the bladder wall (Fig. 16-4). Nevertheless, for some considerable time the lesion remains intravesical, accounting for the high survival rates following radical

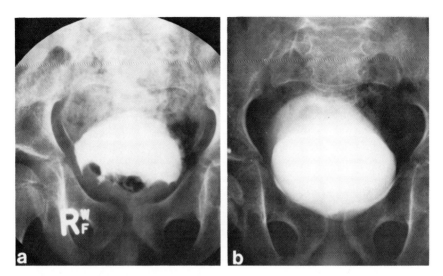

Fig. 16-4. **a**: Presentation cystogram of a child with a bladder rhabdomyosarcoma (demonstrated as the filling defect) prior to treatment by chemo-radiotherapy. **b**: Two years later the bladder remains of good volume and is radiologically (and cystoscopically) free of disease.

resection. Indeed, in their pre-VAC era analysis, Tefft and Jaffe concluded that no patients survived following less than total cystectomy [19]. Of the entire group of 37 patients who had local or segmental resections, all had recurrences. Conversely, they found that of 31 patients undergoing total cystectomy as the minimum primary surgical procedure, 21 patients (70%) were alive and disease-free. Local recurrence was the major problem following the more conservative procedures. In a more modern study, Hays et al. encountered only two out of 11 relapsers in patients with bladder rhabdomyosarcoma where the primary therapy had been pelvic exenteration [23]. These studies have led other clinicians attempting to save children from cystectomy to more routinely employ radiotherapy early in the management of bladder rhabdomyosarcoma.

Prostate rhabdomyosarcoma behaves in a quite different manner. In the pre-VAC era, Claireux and Williams found that prostate rhabdomyosarcoma tends to be more locally invasive and to disseminate earlier [22]. Several authors have reported that radical surgery was, in general, less effective in local control or survival. Tefft and Jaffe found 20/25 (80%) of primary prostatic rhabdomyosarcoma patients had died with both local and distant recurrences [19]. The subsequent IRS data on bladder and prostate rhabdo-

myosarcoma from the VAC era are important. In their first study, IRS-1
patients were treated broadly according to the above cited principles [23].
Nineteen of 64 patients relapsed, but none were in the group of eight patients
with disease localized to the tissue of origin and completely excised. Ten of
the 19 relapses occurred within the pelvis plus one peritoneal and one multiple
site relapse. Thus, 12 of the 19 relapsing patients recurred locally in this
study. These data are echoed by the VAC era CSTG data where eight out of
13 pelvic (not paratesticular, vagina, or corpus uteri) rhabdomyosarcoma
relapsers recurred in the primary site. Hays et al. concluded that pelvic
exenteration (anterior exenteration in most cases), when combined with local
radiotherapy and appropriate chemotherapy, resulted in high rates of survival
[23]. Exenteration may also be successful in the salvage of patients in whom
other surgical (or non-surgical) approaches have failed. The sequelae of
pelvic exenteration, however, makes it desirable to formulate other therapeutic strategies. Partial cystectomy must be complete (i.e., tumor excision
without residual or nodal involvement) to be successful. It if is incomplete,
lethal relapse usually follows. The primary chemotherapy-radiotherapy approach was inferior to pelvic exenteration in respect to overall survival in the
IRS-1 series, but this study did not employ the most aggressive pulse VAC
regimen. Finally, Hays et al. concluded that patients can be salvaged by
exenteration after failure of a primary chemotherapy-radiotherapy regimen if
the decision for surgery is not delayed [23].

It should be noted that radiotherapy to high dose equivalent to the bladder
(plus cyclophosphamide) may lead to late bladder dysfunction, namely hemorrhagic cystitis, that could ultimately necessitate cystectomy. In addition,
occasional radiation enteropathy may occur. In an attempt to avoid radiation
complications, the IRS group initiated a study (IRS-2) of primary chemotherapy in the treatment of bladder-prostate rhabdomyosarcoma [24]. This study
comprising 29 patients represented an attempt to avoid pelvic exenteration
and irradiation to pelvic organs. The results demonstrated that 11 patients
(38%) overall (and 52% of survivors) retained functional bladders and
survived without recurrence. Only two of 29 patients (7%) achieved a
successful outcome without either radiotherapy or tumor excision, and only
3/29 (10%) without radiotherapy or exenteration [24]. An update on a large
number of patients treated by primary chemotherapy for bladder-prostate
primary rhabdomyosarcoma has shown that 90% will require radiotherapy
and that the survival rate of those coming to radiotherapy later rather than
earlier is worse (Tefft, personal communication).

A primary chemotherapy approach was also attempted for 81 children with
rhabdomyosarcoma (arising in all body sites) by a (non-UK) European group

(International Society of Pediatric Oncology). This study used initial pulse VAC chemotherapy. In responders, chemotherapy was continued without local therapy, whereas non-responders moved to radical local therapy. There were 15 poor responders who moved straight to local therapy, with a 33% survival rate. In the good VAC responder group, the survival rate was only 39% (a figure substantially lower than that obtained by CSTG or IRS). The local relapse rate is not documented but these workers state that no patients with bladder or prostate primaries achieved a complete response to chemotherapy alone [25]. Thus, all the current data on bladder-prostate rhabdomyosarcoma lead us to the following conclusions: 1) Primary radical surgery, radiotherapy, and chemotherapy leads to the highest survival figures but with a high morbidity rate. 2) Primary bladder dome tumors that may be completely excised (perhaps after 2–3 cycles of pulse VAC) may be safely managed in some cases by conservation surgery and adjuvant VAC, without radiotherapy. This approach is less commonly possible for trigone, bladder neck, or prostatic primaries. 3) Chemo-radiotherapy as primary treatment is often safe, with surgery as a salvage procedure if necessary. Radiotherapy should be sandwiched early into the chemotherapy program. If salvage surgery is later required, it must be both radical and employed without delay. 4) Primary chemotherapy-only regimens have failed to date and are not to be recommended; the delay to radiotherapy is potentially dangerous to the patient.

The next controversy relates to the radiation dose delivered and the associated morbidity. There is IRS data corroborated by CSTG data that seem to demonstrate that conventionally fractionated doses of 40 Gy plus are more effective than lower doses [26]; however, the early work showing that 50 Gy plus was required to sterilize rhabdomyosarcoma was from a pre-VAC era. It is currently recommended that 40–45 Gy be delivered to younger children and cases with a better prognosis, whereas 45–50 Gy be delivered to others. In the St. Bartholomew's Hospital and Hospital for Sick Children, London, data (all radiotherapy at St. Bartholomew's), the bladder radiation complications have occurred with higher radiation doses or concomitant administration of actinomycin D or cyclophosphamide. With regard to radiation technique, a parallel opposed pair of anterior and posterior pelvic megavoltage photon portals is preferred. This allows the therapist to spare the acetabular and proximal femoral epiphyses. Also, the small separation across the child's pelvis allows good dosimetry that is not greatly improved by a multi-portal approach. Finally, the whole pelvis is not automatically irradiated unless the tumor is that extensive.

Paratesticular Rhabdomyosarcoma

Rhabdomyosarcoma arising within the scrotal contents or in the spermatic cord is a relatively common site of occurrence presenting clinically as a painless mass. Such growths are usually of embryonal histology. Treatment recommendations are radical inguinal orchiectomy followed by radiotherapy and pulse VAC chemotherapy. Treatment differs in the United States as radical orchiectomy is generally followed by retroperitoneal node dissection. Although a node dissection does carry with it the possible morbidity of infertility secondary to either retrograde or no ejaculation, it is justified by the report of Raney et al. in which four of 12 cases with an otherwise negative metastatic workup had positive nodes [27]. The UK attitude is (as for teratoma of testis) entirely different: embryonal rhabdomyosarcoma is not considered a tumor with a preferentially higher likelihood of earlier lymphatic than blood dissemination, and the findings of microscopic tumor in four of 12 cases when over 20 regional nodes were sampled from each case are not considered evidence for such preferential lymphatic spread meriting en bloc node dissection. In a recently analyzed cohort of 14 CSTG paratesticular rhabdomyosarcoma treated in the VAC era, the undissected retroperitoneal lymph nodes do not appear to be a high risk site of regional relapse, and node dissection is not recommended. There is now a trend in America to reserve this operation for lymphogram-positive cases.

A similar difference of opinion occurs between the American attitude towards "hemiscrotectomy" as advocated by some IRS workers and the British approach. In the UK, an initial radical transinguinal orchidectomy with radiotherapy is favored if disease reaches to resection margins or if the disease is locally advanced (e.g., fungating) (initial chemo-radiotherapy). If necessary, the contralateral testis is translocated to the inguinal canal or thigh out of the radiation portal. We do not advocate wide surgical resections of the scrotum but agree that most of the scrotum must lie within the radiation portal. Other workers favor hemiscrotectomy to reduce the need for radiotherapy. In the UK-CSTG data, there were four local relapses in 14 cases of paratesticular rhabdomyosarcoma, and one of these was in a translocated contralateral testis; fortunately, this child has been salvaged. The overall survival rate is 81%. This survival rate is in agreement with the preliminary report of a later American series where the children were similarly managed without node dissection and without hemiscrotectomy. The survival rate was 87% [28]. Thus, paratesticular is considered a relatively good prognostic site for rhabdomyosarcoma where resection of a small bulk primary can be complete. It is therefore reasonable to question the routine use of the alkylating agent (cyclophosphamide) in VAC. American studies have demonstrated equivalent efficacy of VA alone in early rhabdomyosarcoma cases. If cyclophosphamide were omitted, the contralateral testis would be left within an intact seminiferous epithelium provided this lies outside any radiation portal.

Vaginal/Corpus Uteri Rhabdomyosarcomas

Rhabdomyosarcoma of the vagina or corpus uteri accounted for six of 102 consecutive children presenting to CSTG members in London. Hays et al. have recently reported on 37 such patients [29]. The average age at presentation of children with vaginal primaries was 1.6 years as compared to 12.4 years for uterine primaries. There was only one death from disease in 23 patients with primary vaginal rhabdomyosarcoma, but five children out of 14 with uterine primaries succumbed to the disease. Salvage by further surgery was possible after some local relapses and less than exenterative procedures

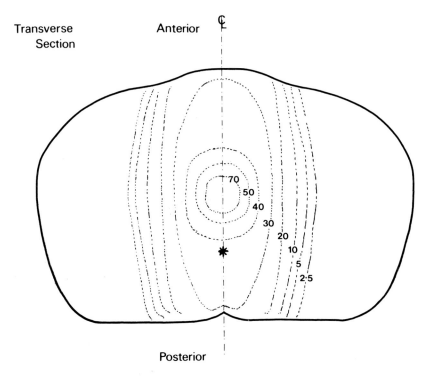

Fig. 16-5. Isodosimetry of mixed external beam and intracavitary radiotherapy to demonstrate the concentration of dose in the region of a primary vaginal rhabdomyosarcoma.

could be curative (e.g., conservative hysterectomy and partial vaginectomy). Adjuvant chemotherapy is routine, and radiotherapy is given when required.

Contact or brachy-radiotherapy may be useful in this situation. Figure 16-5 illustrates a child presenting with primary vaginal rhabdomyosarcoma who had persisting local tumor after initial chemotherapy and limited surgery. The figure demonstrates the composite isodosimetry of low pelvic external beam therapy supplemented by an intracavitary/intravaginal brachytherapy boost. The child is currently disease-free 3 years later. In these tumors, it is now considered safe to attempt to manage without cystectomy and with ovarian preservation. In addition, in good prognostic vaginal cases, the omission of cyclophosphamide from pulse VAC may be safe, and it is in these cases that we are currently transposing the ovaries to the upper abdomen prior to radiotherapy.

REFERENCES

1. D'Angio GJ, Evans AE, Breslow N, et al.: The treatment of Wilms' tumor. Results of the National Wilms' Tumor Study. Cancer 38:633–646, 1976.
2. D'Angio GJ, Beckwith JB, Breslow NE, et al.: Wilms' tumor: An update. Cancer 45:1791–1798, 1980.
3. D'Angio GJ, Evans A, Breslow N, et al.: The treatment of Wilms' tumor: Results of the Second National Wilms' Tumor Study. Cancer 47:2302–2311, 1981.
4. Beckwith JB, Palmer NF: Histopathology and prognosis of Wilms' tumor. Results from the First National Wilms' Tumor Study. Cancer 41:1937–1948, 1978.
5. Breslow NE, Palmer NF, Hill LR, et al.: Wilms' tumor: Prognostic factors for patients without metastases at diagnosis. Cancer 41:1577–1589, 1978.
6. Tefft M, D'Angio GJ, Grant W: Postoperative radiation therapy for residual Wilms' tumor. Review of group III patients in the National Wilms' Tumor Study. Cancer 37:2768–2772, 1976.
7. D'Angio GJ, Tefft M, Breslow N, et al.: Radiation therapy of Wilms' tumor: Results according to dose, field, postoperative timing and histology. Int J Radiat Oncol Biol Phys 4:769–780, 1978.
8. Leape LL, Breslow NE, Bishop HC: The surgical treatment of Wilms' tumor. Results of the National Wilms' Tumor Study. Ann Surg 187:351–356, 1978.
9. Lemerle J, Voute PA, Tournade MF: Preoperative versus postoperative radiotherapy, single versus multiple courses of actinomycin D in the treatment of Wilms' tumor. Cancer 38:647–654, 1976.
10. Lemerle J, Tournade MF, Gerard-Marchant R, et al.: Wilms' tumor: Natural history and prognostic factors. Cancer 37:2557–2566, 1976.
11. Voute PA, Tournade MF, Perry HJM, et al.: Wilms' tumor trials and studies: SIOP no. 1, no. 2, no. 5, and no. 6. Proc XIVth Meeting of the Int Soc Ped Oncol (Bern, Switzerland), 1982. (Abstract 9)
12. Voute PA, Lemerle J, Tournade MF, et al.: Preoperative chemotherapy in Wilms' tumor. Results of clinical trials and studies on nephroblastomas conducted by SIOP. In Raymand E, Clement, Lebreuiz (eds): Pediatric Oncology. Excerpta Medica 1982, pp 272–283.

13. Williams IG: Tumors of Childhood—A Clinical Treatise. London: Heinemann, 1972, pp 103–104.
14. Bishop HC, Tefft M, Evans AE, et al.: Survival in bilateral Wilms' tumor—Review of 30 national Wilms' tumor study group cases. J Pediatr Surg 12:631–638, 1977.
15. Martins AG, Sousinha M, De Sousa IV, et al.: Is total nephrectomy always advisable in the treatment of nephroblastoma? Proc XIVth Meeting of Int Soc Ped Oncol (Abstract 8), Bern, Switzerland, 1982.
16. Bond JV: Prognosis and treatment of Wilms' tumor at Great Ormond Street Hospital for Sick Children 1960–1972. Cancer 36:1202–1207, 1975.
17. Byrd RL, Evans AE, D'Angio GJ: Adult Wilms' tumor: Effect of combined therapy on survival. J Urol 127:648–651, 1982.
18. Biolletot A, Tournade MF, Delemarre JF, et al.: Wilms' tumor in adult patients: SIOP results in 15 patients. Proc 3rd Eur Conf on Clin Oncol, Stockholm (Abstract), p 179, 1985.
19. Tefft M, Jaffe N: Sarcoma of the bladder and prostate in children. Rationale for the role of radiation therapy based on a review of the literature and a report of fourteen additional patients. Cancer 32:1161–1177, 1973.
20. Cassady JR, Sagerman RH, Treffer P, et al.: Radiation therapy for rhabdomyosarcoma. Radiology 91:116–120, 1963.
21. Kingston JE, McElwain TJ, Malpas JS: Childhood rhabdomyosarcoma: Experience of the children's solid tumor group. Br J Cancer 48:195–207, 1983.
22. Claireux AE, Williams DI: Tumors in childhood. In Taylor S (ed): Recent Advances in Surgery. London: J and A Churchill, 1969, pp 48–83.
23. Hays DM, Raney RB, Lawrence W, et al.: Bladder and prostatic tumors in the Intergorup Rhabdomyosarcoma Study (IRS-I). Results of therapy. Cancer 50:1472–1482, 1982.
24. Hays DM, Raney RB, Lawrence W, et al.: Primary chemotherapy in the treatment of children with bladder-prostate tumors in the Intergroup Rhabdomyosarcoma Study (IRS-II). J Pediatr Surg 17:812–819, 1982.
25. Flamant F, Rodary C, Voute PA, Otten J: Primary chemotherapy in the treatment of rhabdomyosarcoma in children: Trial of the International Society of Pediatric Oncology (SIOP): Preliminary results. Radiotherapy Oncol 3:227–236, 1985.
26. Tefft M, Wharram M, Ruymann F, et al.: Radiotherapy for rhabdomyosarcoma in children. A report for the Intergroup Rhabdomyosarcoma Study (IRS-2). Proc Am Soc Clin Oncol 4:234, 1985.
27. Raney RB, Hays DM, Lawrence W, et al.: Paratesticular rhabdomyosarcoma in childhood. Cancer 42:729–736, 1978.
28. Raney RB, Tefft M, Lawrence W, et al.: Treatment results in paratesticular sarcoma of children and adolescents. A report from the Intergroup Rhabdomyosarcoma Studies (IRS-I and IRS-II). Proc Am Assoc Cancer Res 183, 1984.
29. Hays DM, Shimada H, Raney RB, et al.: Vaginal-uterine rhabdomyosarcoma study. Proc Am Assoc Clin Oncol 4:244, 1985.

Chapter 17
Adverse Effects and Sequelae of Pediatric Genitourinary Cancer Therapy

Frederick A. Klein

Multidisciplinary treatment for childhood genitourinary cancer has not only improved survival but also brought about cures from malignant neoplasms that were uniformly fatal in previous decades. These successful outcomes, however, can be affected by the appearance of adverse therapy-related sequelae. Ionizing irradiation is known to produce spinal deformities (kyphosis and scoliosis), renal disease, infertility, pulmonary fibrosis, chest wall deformities, and abnormalities in the skin, subcutaneous tissue, and muscle. Chemotherapy-related complications include hemorrhagic cystitis, gonadal failure, pulmonary fibrosis, cardiomyopathies, and neuropathies. The sequelae of exenterative surgery are immediately obvious and manifested by the presence of bowel and/or urinary stomas and sexual dysfunction. Finally, oncogenic sequelae include both benign and malignant solid neoplasms as well as hematopoietic malignancies. Whether therapy-induced immunosuppression is responsible for secondary malignancies or the development of malignancies in patients is secondary to congenital immunosuppression deficiencies is yet unclear. What needs to be strongly emphasized is that long-term survivors of malignancies are at significant risk for delayed complications. In addition, long-term periodic surveillance and continual research to find the most effective curative therapeutic regimens with the least amount of acute and long-term toxicities are essential.

RADIATION THERAPY

Radiation therapy in the 20th century has been the most commonly used non-surgical therapeutic modality for treating malignancy. As such, radia-

Pediatric Tumors of the Genitourinary Tract, pages 283–298
© 1988 Alan R. Liss, Inc.

tion-induced tissue damage is well documented, particularly with respect to long-term survivors from Wilms' tumor. In a classic manuscript by Neuhauser and associates, the adverse effects of radiation on the vertebral body were described [1]. The degree of abnormality appeared to correlate with the quantity of irradiation; thus the recommendation at the time was to include the entire vertebral body in the treatment portal. Including this report, there have been numerous others describing radiation-induced spine changes with doses ranging anywhere from 1,500 to 6,100 rad [2–8]. Although in general the larger the radiation dose, the more likely a deformity will occur, scoliosis and reduction in sitting height may be observed with doses of less than 2,500 rad [9].

In the study reported by Riseborough and associates of 75 patients treated with orthovoltage irradiation, radiographic bony deformities were divided into four categories [5]. These included early alterations in the architecture of individual vertebral units, alterations in axial alignment, other skeletal alterations, and no alterations. The earliest changes that occurred in the vertebral body included growth arrest lines, end-plate irregularity, altered trabecular pattern, and decreased vertebral body height. Scoliosis was observed in 70.4% of these patients, with the extent of the deformity due to the cumulative effect of the architectural alterations in the individual segments. These patients' ages at the time of irradiation ranged from 1 week to 6 years, with doses varying from 2,631 to 6,160 rad (mean 3,218 rad).

The exact time of appearance of scoliosis has not been reliably determined; however, mild curvatures were generally observed by the age of 8 or 9 years. No deformities of more than 20° were manifested before the age of 10 years. When scoliosis did develop, the curves were reported to become rigid early; however, the most progression occurred concomitantly with growth during adolescence. There was no correlation with age at the time of irradiation. In addition, early loss of vertebral body height was not a reliable predictor of the severity of subsequent scoliosis.

In the same study, kyphosis was observed in 25.9% of patients [5]. Although no correlation could be established between age at the time of irradiation, dose of irradiation, and interval preceding the kyphosis, most deformities of 10° or more also had scoliosis of 25° or more. Worsening of the kyphosis occurred primarily with the onset of the adolescent growth spurt. An example of a patient following irradiation for Wilms' tumor is shown in Figure 17-1.

Other skeletal alterations reported following irradiation include sternal and chest wall abnormalities manifested by hypoplasia, asymmetry, pectus excavatum, and pectus carinatum [10]. When treatment portals include the ilium,

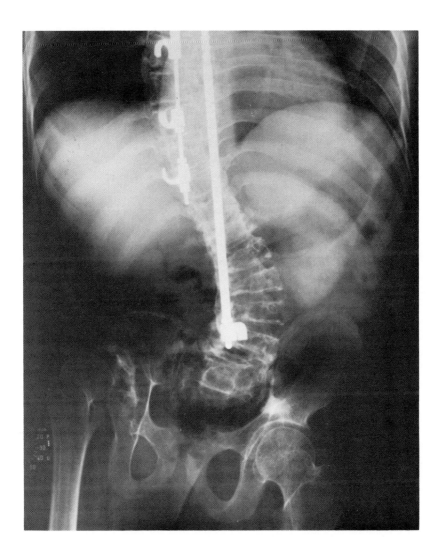

Fig. 17–1. Plain abdominal film of a 23-year-old patient. Radiation therapy was given following radical nephrectomy for Wilms' tumor at age 2. Note the severe osteoporosis and scoliosis requiring placement of Harrington rods.

growth epiphyses are affected resulting in iliac wing hypoplasia in as many as 68% of patients [11]. In addition, when the acetabular fossa and femoral head are included within the treatment portal, acetabular dysplasia, coxa valga, coxa vara, dislocation of the hip, and leg shortening have been reported.

Both the ovaries and testes are sensitive to the effects of irradiation. In a study by Doll and Smith estimated ovarian doses of only 360–720 rad caused menstrual failure in 97% of women [12]. Shalet and associates [13] studied ovarian function in 18 females who received 2,000–3,000 rad abdominal irradiation over 25 to 44 days during childhood for various non-gonadal tumors, predominately Wilms' [1]. Of those who reached pubertal age, abnormalities were manifested by amenorrhea, underdeveloped breasts, inadequate pubic hair development, and elevated levels of serum follicle stimulating hormone and luteinizing hormone. In an autopsy study of children with abdominal tumors, all children treated with radiation therapy either alone or with chemotherapy had severe ovarian damage [14]. There was a marked reduction in the number of small non-growing follicles in all cases. Decreased fertility and/or sterility have been shown to be dependent on age, dose, and regimen used in delivering irradiation [15]. Lushbaugh and Casarett reported that permanent amenorrhea is produced in women over 40 years of age by only 600 rad, whereas 2,000 rad is necessary in girls and young females [15]. Preservation of ovarian function in females requiring pelvic irradiation has been reported in patients where ovaries were surgically relocated so that they would receive only scattered irradiation [16–18].

In males it is documented that fractionated radiation therapy doses are more damaging to testicular function than single therapy doses [9]. Therefore, radiation scatter received during pelvic irradiation is damaging. Sperm counts may drop to aspermic levels anywhere from 1 to 3 months after the initiation of pelvic radiotherapy [19]. Whether adequate function returns over prolonged followup remains unanswered.

Radiation therapy also has adverse effects on other organ systems including the bowel, kidney, liver, lung, skin, and subcutaneous tissue. Radiation enteritis and proctitis may be manifested by diarrhea, abdominal pain, bleeding, and tenesmus. Although most symptoms can be handled conservatively and are not a chronic problem, the incidence and severity of changes may be on the increase with the use of radiation sensitizing chemotherapy agents such as actinomycin D and doxorubicin. Radiation doses as low as 1200–1500 rad may cause renal failure as well as affect the rate of compensatory hypertrophy of the remaining kidney following nephrectomy for Wilms' tumor [11]. When doses of more than 2,000 rad have been administered, progressive renal insufficency has been said to be inevitable. [20–22]. In addition, the appearance of radiation nephritis 20 years following the delivery of 1,400 rad to the kidney has been reported [23] as well as a case of renal artery stenosis causing renin-dependent hypertension 11.5 years postirradiation for Wilms' tumor [24].

The liver has been shown to be quite sensitive to radiotherapy, showing decreased function after doses as low as 1,200–1,500 rad [25,26]. In the National Wilms' Tumor Study number I, 15 patients developed liver abnormalities manifested primarily by transient abnormalities of liver function tests and/or liver isotope scans [26]. Of these, ten developed clinical liver failure manifested by jaundice, hepatosplenomegaly, and ascites. Evidence of damage appeared in all within 2 months of beginning therapy and within 4 weeks in nine patients. Recovery was evident in another 2-4 months in all but three patients. It should be emphasized that these patients also received some form of chemotherapy. The degree of hepatic damage was related to the liver volume radiated and the dose delivered (Table 17-1). Although no definite relation of radiation damage to age was noted, the very young developed liver toxicity even though doses were less than 1,500 rad [25]. It should be pointed out that radiation-associated patches of hepatic fibrosis may be confusing on liver scans because "cold spots" may be seen along with lobar enlargement and be misinterpreted as hepatic metastases rather than fibrosis or hypertrophy [9].

Pulmonary damage from radiation therapy ususally occurs with doses greater than 2,000 rad and is seen most often in patients treated for metastatic Wilms' tumor [9]. In the National Wilms' Tumor Study number I, seven of 24 patients who received lung radiation developed toxicity [26]. Four of these patients received the recommended dose to both lung fields, and three required additional treatment for larger lesions. Three of the four mentioned above recovered without sequelae, one died of pneumocystis infection, and two of those receiving larger doses died. It was felt, however, that additional factors such as high inspiratory oxygen tension, healing Pneumocystis, and necrotizing Klebsiella pneumonia infection may have been of more significance than the radiation effects.

Finally, radiation therapy is known to cause impairment of growth and development of skin, muscle, fat, and other soft tissue, as well as affect the immune system by a prolonged suppression of the number of circulating T cells [9]. These soft tissue effects are primarily manifested by hyperpigmentation, hair loss, telangiectasia, hypoplasia, and atrophy.

CHEMOTHERAPY

The effects of chemotherapy can be divided into acute and chronic toxicities. The most obvious sites of acute toxicity are the hair, skin, and mucous

TABLE 17–1. National Wilms' Tumor Study Number 1: Randomized Patients With Liver Toxicities vs Total Number NWTS Patients

Radiation dose (rad)	Volume of liver rradiated				Age of NWTS patient (yr)			
	Rt. lobe	Lt. lobe	Entire liver	Total	<1	1–4	>4	Total
<1,500	0/1	0/6	2[1]/3 (3[1])	2/10	0/2	1[1]/5 (2[2])	1[1]/2 (1[2])	2/8
1,501–2,400	0/26	1/33	2/10 (4[1])	3/69	2/29	0/31 (2[2])	1/9 (2[2])	3/69
2,401–3,000	1/36 (2[2])	0/34 (1[2])	1/12 (2[1])	2/82	0/1	2/60 (4[2])	0/21 (1[2])	2/82
>3,001	5[2]/29 (1[2])	3[2]/71 (5[2])	2/3	10/103	0/3	3[2]/46 (3[2])	7[2]/54 (3[2])	10/103
Total	6/92	4/143	7/28	17/263	2/35	6/142	9/86	17/263

[1]Each patient had boost to portion of liver >3,000 rad.
[2]One patient each as noted in the above footnote.

membranes. Although this toxicity is probably more a psychological concern with regard to cosmetics, mucous membrane ulceration and local tissue necrosis can be severe and even life-threatening. Table 17-2 lists commonly used chemotherapy agents and their effects on skin, hair, and mucous membranes.

The loss of hair is caused by damage to the dividing cells in the germinal portion of the hair bulb and is manifested by rendering the hair shaft fragile and easily broken by the trauma of brushing or combing. In general, a normal amount and distribution of hair returns with the cessation of chemotherapy. Preventive measures such as ice caps or scalp tourniquets may prevent some loss depending on the drug used and its duration of toxic blood

TABLE 17–2. Effect of Cytotoxic Chemotherapy on Skin, Hair, and Mucous Membranes[1]

Drug		Effect			
Generic name	Brand name	Vesicant	Alopecia	Mucosal ulceration	Other[2]
Cyclophosphamide	Cytoxan	0	4	0	C
Mechlorethamine (nitrogen mustard)	Mustargen	4	1	0	
Melphalan	Alkeran	0[3]	1	0	
Chlorambucil	Leukeran	0[3]	1	0	
Busulfan	Myleran	0[3]	1	0	C
Bleomycin	Blenoxane	0	2	2	A,B,C
Methotrexate	Methotrexate	0	3	4	A,C
5-Fluorouracil	Fluorouracil	0	2	4	A,C
Doxorubicin	Adriamycin	4	4	2	A,B,C
Mitomycin C	Mutamycin	4	2	4	
Mithramycin	Mithracin	3	2	0	
Actinomycin D	Dactinomycin	4	2	3	
Vinblastine	Velban	2	2	0	
Vincristine	Oncovin	2	2	0	
6-Mercaptopurine	Purinethol	0[3]	2	0	C
Procarbazine	Matulane	0[3]	2	0	
Carmustine (BCNU)	BiCNU	3	2	0	
Lomustine (CCNU)	CeeNU	0[3]	2	0	
Dacarbazine	DTIC	2	2	1	
Cis-diamminedichloro-platinum (DDP)	Cis-platinum	0	0	0	
Cytarabine (cytosine arabinoside)	Cytosar	0	2	1	

[1]Grade 1 = mild or none; 2 = moderate; 3 = marked; 4 = severe.
[2]A = Photosensitivity; B = keratosis; C = pigmentation.
[3]Oral drug.

levels. Skin toxicity may be characterized by local reaction at a site of direct exposure to the chemical, a generalized eruption, or changes in pigmentation. Extravasation and local complications can generally be alleviated by careful administration by trained oncology nurses. If a systemic eruption is noted, the drug needs to be discontinued; however, the hypersensitivity reaction should not be confused with other types of skin reactions including Herpes zoster, bacterial or fungal embolic lesions, skin metastases, other allergic or connective tissue disorders, or parasites. Photosensitivity and hyperpigmentation may occur so patients should be counseled to use protective clothing and sun screen when exposed to sunlight. Ulceration of mucous membranes can be a life-threatening complication especially in a leukopenic patient. The drugs that ulcerate the mucous membranes destroy this normal barrier and expose the patient to the possibility of acute overwhelming gram-negative bacteremia. If it occurs, local treatment of mucositis can be carried out by the use of topical antibiotics, antifungals, and good oral hygiene.

The only drug commonly used to treat childhood malignancies that has significant cardiotoxicity in the form of cardiomyopathy is Adriamycin. In addition to dose-related cardiomyopathy, other acute cardiac changes may occur in 25% of patients [27]. These cardiac effects include electrocardiographic abnormalities consisting of non-specific ST segment and T-wave changes which usually resolve by the end of a month or two. Arrhythmias that may occur in some patients generally resolve within minutes to hours. Therefore, if there is a history of arrhythmias, cardiac monitoring during drug administration is recommended. In addition, acute cardiac decompensation manifested by a pericarditis-myocarditis syndrome and acute left ventricular dysfunction has been described in patients with no previous history of cardiac disease and in some patients who have borderline reserve [28,29]. Singer and associates demonstrated a decrease in ejection fraction following therapy using cardiac scans [30]. This decrease resolved after 22 hours in all cases. Congestive heart failure depends on the cumulative dose of Adriamycin, with an incidence of less than 1% in patients receiving less than 500 mg/m^2 ranging from 30 to 40% at doses of greater than 600 mg/m^2 [32–34]. Heart failure may occur anywhere from 9 to 280 days posttherapy, with a mean of 89 days [33,35]. It is generally recommended that doses should not exceed 550 mg/m^2 because of the dose-related incidence of cardiomyopathy and a mortality rate of around 50% in those who are affected. In those patients receiving radiation therapy for pulmonary metastases, the risk of developing cardiac toxicity is also greater; therefore, in these patients the total Adriamycin dose should be reduced to 450 mg/m^2 or less [27].

Lung damage secondary to several chemotherapeutic agents is well documented. Pulmonary infiltrates and alveolar pneumonitis have been associated with methotrexate, bleomycin, and busulfan [35]. More severe pulmonary toxicities have been reported in from 2 to 15% with bleomycin and from 2.5 to 11.5% with busulfan [36]. Busulfan toxicity usually only occurs with long-term use of the drug (longer than 8 months). If diffuse pulmonary fibrosis with infiltrates develops, there is usually progressive respiratory insufficiency leading to death [27].

The primary target of bleomycin toxicity is the lung. The earliest abnormality is inspiratory rales [37]. On pulmonary function studies, restrictive pulmonary disease, arterial hypoxemia, and a decreased diffusion capacity are evident. On radiologic examination, a pattern of diffuse interstitial fibrosis with patch basilar infiltrates is noted, and on lung biopsy, atypical alveolar cells, fibrinous exudate, and hilar membranes are evident in the acute state, with diffuse interstitial and intraalveolar fibrosis noted in the chronic stage [9]. Fibrosis is known to be dose-related and occurs in approximately 5% as long as the dose is kept below 450 mg of drug [32]. If the dose exeeds this, the risk increases to approximately 20% [32]. There is no documentation that patients receiving radiation to the lungs or mediastinum are at any increased risk of developing fibrosis. Although in some cases fibrosis is reversible, progressive respiratory failure occurs in many cases.

The major chemotherapeutic agent in childhood cancer treatment with long-term sequelae of the urinary tract is cyclophosphamide. While cyclophosphamide does not cause renal tubular or glomerular destruction, it may cause severe chemical cystitis and hemorrhage. The incidence is dose-related ranging from less than 10% with 1–3 mg/kg to over 40% with doses of over 60 mg/kg. In addition, the time of onset may be anywhere from 1 month to several years following initiation of treatment [27]. The toxicity is secondary to direct contact of the drug metabolites with the bladder mucosa. Acute changes with administration of the drug include ulceration of the epithelium, edema, and hemorrhage, whereas chronic problems include submucosal telangiectasia and fibrosis, which may result in a chronically contracted bladder, reflux, and hydronephrosis [38–40]. The clinical symptoms and signs of cystitis in addition to hematuria include urgency, frequency, and dysuria. Bleeding may be severe and life-threatening. The most important means of reducing the likelihood of epithelial damage by cyclophosphamide is adequate hydration. A forced diuresis not only keeps the toxic metabolites dilute, but frequent voiding limits exposure of the mucosal surface to the toxic agents. DeFronzo and associates reported that cyclophosphamide has an antidiuretic action that may impede the therapeutic diuresis needed to reduce toxicity [41]. The peak impairment of water excretion occurs from 4 to 12 hours after administration, also the peak time when the urinary concentration is the highest.

Gonadal dysfunction in both males and females has been most frequently associated with cyclophosphamide. In adolescent females amenorrhea or menstrual irregularities have been reported in 50–60% of patients receiving this drug [9]. The primary effect seems to be destruction of oocytes; however, this is not necessarily permanent with short-term administration [42]. In preadolescents the ovary seems to be more resistant to the effects of the drug [43,44]. When cyclophosphamide is administered to the male during puberty, reduced spermatogenesis and an elevation in serum FSH may be noted [45]. This may result in gonadal atrophy and gynecomastia in pubertal boys. Testicular biopsy in men following alkylating agents has shown the absence of germinal cells with resultant azoospermia [46–48]. Sertoli and Leydig cells are preserved. Although the effects of alkylating agents are reversible in some cases, the time to recovery may be as long as 5 years [47,49]. It has recently been shown that the use of GnRH, a synthetic analogue of gonadotropin releasing hormone, administered before using chemotherapy may result in preservation of reproductive function [51]. In addition, this protection may be enhanced by adding testosterone to the GnRH analogue [51].

ONCOGENIC EFFECTS OF THERAPY

There have been numerous reports documenting the association between radiation therapy, chemotherapy, and the development of benign and malignant neoplasms. Since this concern increases as life expectancy increases from the primary tumor, the pediatric population harbors the greatest risk of sequelae from initial treatment modalities. Malignant neoplasms have been reported in nearly all organs and structures included in radiotherapy portals used for the treatment of malignant disease [52]. The etiology of the second malignant neoplasm in 200 children and the association with radiation therapy is shown in Table 17-3. Li and associates reviewed the experience with Wilms' tumor from 1917 to 1981 at the Dana-Farber Cancer Institute and Children's Hospital [53]. Of 487 patients treated, 30 (6%) developed second primary tumors: 11 cancers, 16 benign tumors, and 3 with borderline neoplasms. Of the 11 with second cancers, all received radiation therapy, and nine occurred within the radiation field. In other studies analyzing the carcinogenic risk of radiotherapy for childhood tumors other than Wilms' tumor, a 12–17% cumulative probability of developing a new cancer within

TABLE 17–3. Etiology of Second Malignant Neoplasms in 200 Children[1]

	Radiation-associated	Not radiation-associated
Bone sarcoma	34	9
Soft tissue sarcoma	31	11
Leukemia/lymphoma	21	12
Thyroid carcinoma	15	3
Skin carcinoma	11	11
Brain tumor	5	16
Breast carcinoma	4	2
Other	12	10
Total	133	74

[1]Source: Meadows et al. [53].

TABLE 17–4. Factors That Influence Carcinogenicity Due to Ionizing Radiation

Type of neoplasm induced
Type of irradiation
Volume of tissue irradiated
Specific tissues included in ports and near edge of field
Use of chemotherapy, immunosuppressive therapy, or immunostimulating therapy
Latency period until tumor presentation
Length of patient followup

5 to 25 years was found. This is more than a 15-fold increase over the rate in the general population [53,54].

In general, there are seven factors that are associated with carcinogenicity due to ionizing radiation as reported by Coleman (Table 17-4) [55]. The type of neoplasm may be a leukemia-lymphoma, epithelial carcinoma, or sarcoma. The type of irradiation may be orthovoltage, megavoltage, or interstitial with orthovoltage being the one most commonly associated with radiation-associated neoplasms. The volume of irradiated tissue and what specific tissue is included in the ports and near the edge of the field are important as different tissues are more susceptible to carcinogenic effects than others. Finally, the use of adjuvant chemotherapy and immunosuppression as well as the length of patient followup are additional factors related to the influence of ionizing radiation on carcinogenicity.

Chemotherapy can be carcinogenic whether used to treat cancer or nonmalignant conditions. Sieber [56] and Harris [57] have listed the carcinogenic drugs including alkylating agents and antibiotics. A list of second neoplasms in children treated by chemotherapy alone is shown in Table 17-5. The combination of irradiation and actinomycin D in patients surviving for long periods of time may place these patients at greater risk for the development

TABLE 17–5. Second Malignant Neoplasms in Children Treated by Chemotherapy Alone[1]

Neoplasm 1	Neoplasm 2	Interval (yr)	Drug
Wilms' tumor	Brain tumor	2	Actinomycin D (AMD)
Wilms' tumor	Brain tumor	3	AMD
Wilms' tumor	Basal cell carcinoma	7	AMD
Acute myelogenous leukemia (AML)	Ewing's sarcoma	4	Vincristine (VCR), prednisone, 6-mercaptopurine, methotrexate (MTX), cytosine arabinoside, cyclophosphamide (CPM)
Osteosarcoma	Pancreatic sarcoma	7	AMD, mitomycin C
Hodgkin's disease	AML	10	Mustard, CPM, chlorambucil, vinblastine (VBL), VCR procarbazine, adriamycin (ADR), L-asparaginase
Hodgkin's disease	Osteosarcoma	8 (3)[2]	CPM, VBL, chlorambucil
Hodgkin's disease	Acute myelomonocytic leukemia	3	Cyclophosphamide, Oncovin, prednisone, and procarbazine (COPP), ADR
Hodgkin's disease	AML	5	COPP, ADR, CCNU
Histiocytosis X	Hepatoma	18	MTX
Medulloblastoma	Melanoma	4	CCNU, VCR

[1]Source: Meadows et al. [53].
[2]Eight years from diagnosis, 3 years from chemotherapy.

of adverse effects. In fact, three of the five patients who developed leukemia after treatment for Wilms' tumor reported by Schwartz and associates were treated with this combination [58].

SURGERY

The delayed effects attributable to surgery are secondary to organ removal. Radical procedures primarily for sarcomas involving the bladder, prostate, or female genital organs result in urinary and/or fecal diversion and the resultant complications of chronic urinary tract infections, pyelonephritis, sexual dysfunction, psychosocial disturbances, and the potential for developing carcinoma of the sigmoid colon if ureterosigmoidostomies are used as the form of urinary diversion. Fortunately, the number of patients undergoing exenterative surgery for these lesions is on the decline.

CONCLUSIONS

In recent years significant advancements have been made in the management of children with cancer. These results have been achieved because of improvements in surgery, radiation, and chemotherapy. Each of these modalities of therapy, however, have their own immediate and late effects. In assessing a therapeutic program, the physician and patient must balance the expected benefits of treatment against the anticipated and possibly unexpected side effects. Although the knowledge of delayed effects has led to alterations in therapy to improve quality of life and safety, cure of the primary cancer remains the basis of therapy. Thus, sequelae of some presently used treatment regimens as well as those produced by new and innovative forms of treatment must be accepted. Nevertheless, it should be remembered that patients cured of cancer are still at risk of developing late effects of treatment and that continued, careful surveillance is needed to revise presently used treatment modalities and to devise new alternative forms of management.

REFERENCES

1. Neuhauser EBD, Wittenborg MH, Bergman CZ, et al.: Irradiation effects of roentgen therapy on the growing spine. Radiology 59:637, 1952.
2. Arkin AA, Pack GT, Ransohoff NS, Simon N: Radiation-induced scoliosis. A case report. J Bone Joint Surg 32:401, 1950.
3. Donaldson WF, Wissinger HA: Axial skeletal changes following tumor dose radiation therapy. Proc Am Orthop Assoc J Bone Joint Surg 49:1469, 1967.
4. Katzman H, Waugh T, Berdon W: Skeletal changes following irradiation of childhood tumors. J Bone Joint Surg 51:835, 1969.
5. Riseborough EJ, Grabias SL, Burton RI, et al.: Skeletal alterations following irradiation for Wilms' tumor: With particular reference to scoliosis and kyphosis. J Bone Joint Surg 58:526, 1976.
6. Whitehouse WM, Lampe I: Osseous damage of irradiation in infancy and childhood. Am J Roentgenol 70:721, 1953.
7. Vaeth JM, Levitt SH, Jones MD, et al.: Effects of radiation therapy in survivors of Wilms' tumor. Radiology 79:560, 1962.
8. Rubin P, Duthie RB, Young LW: The significance of scoliosis in post-irradiated Wilms' tumor and neuroblastoma. Radiology 79:739, 1962.
9. Karayalcin G: Late effects of cancer treatment. In Lanzkowsky P (ed): Pediatric Oncology. New York: McGraw-Hill, 1983, p 477.

10. Jaffe N: Late side effects of treatment: Skeletal genetic, central nervous system and organic. Pediatr Clin North Am 23:233, 1977.
11. Jaffe N, Paed D, McNeese M, et al.: Childhood urologic cancer therapy related sequelae and their impact on management. Cancer 45:1815, 1980.
12. Doll R, Smith PG: The long term effects of x-irradiation in patients treated for metropathia hamemorrhagica. Br J Radiol 41:362, 1968.
13. Shalet SM, Beardwell CG, Jones PHM, et al.: Ovarian failure following abdominal irradiation in childhood. Br J Cancer 33:655, 1976.
14. Himelstein-Braw R, Peters H, Faber M: Influence of irradiation and chemotherapy on the ovaries of children with abdominal tumors. Br J Cancer 36:269, 1977.
15. Lushbaugh CC, Casarett GW: The effects of gonadal irradiation in clinical radiation therapy: A review. Cancer 37:1111, 1976.
16. Ray GR, Trueblood HW, Enright LP, et al.: Oophoropexy: A means of preserving function following pelvic megavoltage radiotherapy for Hodgkin's disease. Radiology 96:175, 1970.
17. Lewis JL: Surgical transposition of the ovaries as part of staging laparotomy for Hodgkin's disease. In Lacher M (ed): Hodgkin's Disease. New York: John Wiley, 1976, p 111.
18. Tan C, Tan R, Jones W, et al.: Ovarian transposition in childhood Hodgkin's disease. Proc Am Assoc Clin Oncol 17:300, 1976.
19. Slanina J, Musshoff K, Rahner T, et al.: Long term effects in irradiated patients with Hodgkin's disease. Int J Radiat Oncol Biol Phys 2:1, 1977.
20. Arneil GC, Harris F, Emmanuel IG, et al.: Nephritis in two children after irradiation and chemotherapy for nephroblastoma. Lancet 1:960, 1974.
21. Jereb B, Asperia A, Berg U, et al.: Renal function in long term survivors after treatment for nephroblastoma Acta Paediatr Scand 62:577, 1973.
22. Mitus A, Tefft M, Fellers FX: Long-term follow-up of renal functions of 108 children who underwent nephrectomy for malignant disease. Pediatrics 44:912, 1969.
23. O'Malley B, D'Angio GJ, Vawter GF: Late effects of roentgen therapy given in infancy. Am J Roentgenol 89:1067, 1963.
24. Gerlock AJ, Jr, Goncharenko VA, Ekelund L: Radiationosis of the renal artery causing hypertension: Case report. J Urol 118:1064, 1977.
25. Tefft M, Mitus A, Dask L, et al.: Irradiation of the liver in children: Review of experience in the acute and chronic phases, and in the intact normal and partially resected. Am J Roentgenol 108:365, 1970.
26. Tefft M: Radiation related toxicities in National Wilms' Tumor Study number 1. Int J Radiat Oncol Biol Phys 2:455, 1977.
27. Lenhard RE, Jr., Saral R: Acute complications of chemotherapy. In Abeloff MD (ed): Complications of Cancer Diagnosis and Management. Baltimore: Johns Hopkins University Press, 1979, p 357.
28. Kehoe R, Singer OH, Trapani A: Adriamycin-induced cardiac dysrhythmias in an experimental dog model. Cancer Treat Rep 62:963, 1978.
29. Bristow MR, Mason JW, Billingham ME, Daniels JR: Clinical spectrum of anthracycline antibiotic cardiotoxicity. Cancer Treat Rep 62:873, 1978.
30. Singer JW, Narahara KA, Ritchie JL, et al.: Time and dose dependent changes in ejection fraction determined by radionuclide angiography after anthracycline therapy. Cancer Treat Rep 62:945, 1978.
31. Rinehart JJ, Lewis RP, Balcerzak SP: Adriamycin cardiotoxicity in man. Ann Intern Med 81:475, 1974.

32. Blum RH, Carter SK: Adriamycin: A new anticancer drug with significant clinical activity. Ann Intern Med 80:249, 1974.
33. Minow RA, Benjamin RS, Gottlieb JA: Adriamycin (NSC-123127) cardiomyopathy: An overview with determination of risk factors. Cancer Chemother Rep 6:195, 1975.
34. Von Hoff DD, Rozencweig M, Layard M, et al.. Daunomycin-induced cardiotoxicity in children and adults: A review of 110 cases. Am J Med 62:200, 1977.
35. Von Hoff DD: Time relationship between last dose of daunorubicin and congestive heart failure. Cancer Treat Rep 61:1411, 1977.
36. Sostman HD, Malthay RA, Putman CE: Cytotoxic drug-induced lung disease. Am J Med 62:608, 1977.
37. DeLena M, Guzzon A, Monfardini S, et al.: Clinical, radiologic and histopathologic studies on pulmonary toxicity induced by treatment with bleomycin. Cancer Chemother Rep 56:343, 1972.
38. Anderson EE, Cobb OE, Glenn JF: Cyclophosphamide hemorrhagic cystitis. J Urol 97:857, 1967.
39. Riggenbach R, Barrett O, Shawn T: Hemorrhagic cystitis due to cyclophosphamide. South Med J 61:139, 1968.
40. Johnson WW, Meadows DC: Urinary-bladder fibrosis and telangiectasia associated with long-term cyclophosphamide therapy. N Engl J Med 284:290, 1971.
41. DeFronzo RA, Braine H, Colvin OM, et al.: Water intoxication in man after cyclophosphamide therapy: Time course and relation to drug activation. Ann Intern Med 78:861, 1973.
42. Warne GL, Fairley KF, Hobbs LB, et al.: Cyclophosphamide-induced ovarian failure. N Engl Med 289:1159, 1973.
43. Pennisi AJ, Grushkin CM, Lieberman E: Gonadal function in children with nephrosis treated with cyclophosphamide. Am J Dis Child 129:315, 1975.
44. Penso J, Lippe B, Ehrlich R, Smith FE: Testicular function in prepubertal and pubertal male patients treated with cyc;pphosphamide for nephrotic syndrome. J Pediatr 84:1831–1836, 1974.
45. Richter P: Effect of chlorambucil on spermatogenesis in the human with malignant lymphoma. Cancer 25:1026, 1970.
46. Fairley KF, Barrie JV, Johnson W: Sterility and testicular atrophy related to cyclophosphamide therapy. Lancet 1:568, 1972.
47. Cheviakolff S: Recovery of spermatogenesis in patients with lymphoma after treatment with chlorombucil. J Reprod Fertil 33:155, 1973.
48. George CRP, Evans RA: Cyclophosphamide and infertility. Lancet 1:840, 1972.
49. Buchanan JD, Fairley KF, Barrier JU: Return of spermatogenesis after stopping cyclophosphamide therapy. Cancer 2:156, 1975.
50. Globe LM, Robinson J, Gould SF: Protection from cyclophosphamide-induced testicular damage with an analogue of gonadotropin-releasing hormone. Lancet 1:1132, 1981.
51. Heber D, Swendloff RS: Male contraception: Synergism of gonadotrophin-releasing hormone analog and testosterone in suppressing gonadotropin. Science 209:936, 1980.
52. Meadows AT, Kregmas NL, Belasco JB: The medical cost of cure: Sequelae in survivors of childhood cancer. In Van Eys J, Sullivan MP (eds): Status of Curability of Childhood Cancers. New York: Raven Press, 1980, p 270.
53. Li FP, Cai-jie Van J, Sallan S, et al.: Second neoplasms after Wilms' tumor in childhood. JNCI 6:1205, 1983.
54. Li FP, Cassady JR, Jaffe N: Risk of second tumors in survivors of childhood cancer. Cancer 35:1230, 1975.

55. Coleman CN: Adverse effects of cancer therapy. Am J Pediatr Hematol Oncol 4:103, 1982.
56. Sieber SM: The action of antitumor agents: A double-edged sword? Med Pediatr Oncol 3:123, 1977.
57. Harris CC: The carcinogenicity of anticancer drugs: A hazard of man. Cancer 37:1090, 1976.
58. Schwartz AD, Lee H, Baum ES: Leukemia in children with Wilms' tumor. J Pediatr 83:374, 1975.

Chapter 18
Coping With Cancer in Childhood: Support for the Family Unit

Martha Blechar Gibbons

When a child is diagnosed with cancer, the illness reverberates throughout the entire family system. Hospitalization of a child creates maximal stress on the family unit. Parents who may never have cared for a sick child must adapt to caring for one who is chronically, perhaps even critically ill.

The American Cancer Society estimates that 6,000 cases of cancer occur in children under 15 years of age in the United States each year, with approximately 1,600 deaths annually [1]. Though cancer in childhood is rare, it remains the leading cause of death due to disease in children between the ages of 3 and 14 years [1].

In the 1980s, more children are surviving cancer than at any time in the past. However, there is growing recognition that both chemotherapy and radiotherapy may have adverse effects on normal body tissue that may be manifested months or even years after completion of treatment. Such late effects are both physiologic and psychologic, ranging in severity from scanty hair growth to the life-threatening complications of a second malignancy. [2].

The family of the child with cancer is frequently displaced from home to hospital. In the hospital setting, parents and children often have difficulty articulating their needs. Lack of communication can result in frustration and solitude; some families withdraw from staff. Intense involvement with the management of the child's care can be an isolating experience in itself, a test of endurance that can plague the family system.

Pediatric Tumors of the Genitourinary Tract, pages 299-321

Parenthood implies the responsibility of protecting the child from harm. The diagnosis of cancer in childhood robs parents of the ability to maintain this integral aspect of their role. Parents experience anxiety and acute disappointment if the child relapses or fails to respond to treatment. Such experiences lead to parental self-doubt. Feelings of helplessness and worthlessness are frequently expressed by families of a child with cancer [3].

The stress of parenting a child with cancer is intensified when the disease process is not well understood by family members. Confusion regarding the treatment plan may result in parental apprehension and sleep deprivation. When the child is hospitalized for an extended period of time, the family may become overwhelmed and ineffective in providing support, often at a time when the child needs them most.

Awareness of periods in which families may experience particular difficulty in adapting to the demands resulting from the child's illness will enable staff to intervene more therapeutically. A significant relationship has been found between the degree of support parents receive and their psychosocial adjustment to their child's illness [4].

Crisis points in the course of cancer and its treatment that represent times of increased stress for patients and their families have been identified. These include: 1) diagnosis; 2) induction of treatment; 3) negative physical reactions to treatment and to treatment side effects; 4) termination of the treatment protocol; 5) reentry into school, family, and social life; 6) recurrence or metastasis of the disease; 7) initiation of research treatment, 8) termination of active treatment and terminal illness [5]; 9) anniversary phenomena; 10) symptom consciousness; 11) developmental marker events; 12) societal prejudices; and 13) the period several months after the death of a pediatric cancer patient [6].

These crisis points and appropriate supportive interventions will be discussed within the framework of the disease process as experienced from diagnosis through bereavement.

DIAGNOSIS

Initial reactions of parents on hearing their child's cancer diagnosis for the first time have universally been described with such terms as shock, disbelief, numbness, and feeling stunned [7]. Parents react this way even when they have suspicions about the nature of the child's illness before diagnosis. Parents are often unable to hear anything that is said in the initial conference after the word "cancer" is introduced. For this reason, it is essential to repeat the same information shared at this time 2 to 3 days later, when the family has had more time to absorb the shock.

Observations have been made which document a variety of later reactions, ranging from fairly rapid mobilization by parents to act on their child's behalf to denial. Some research suggests that parents progress from initial numbness to a split between emotional acceptance of the diagnosis and prognosis and intellectual acceptance of the reality [7].

The cancer diagnosis represents immediate losses to parents. Future goals must be postponed and sometimes given up entirely. Families express anxiety, sadness, depression, and concern for the child. In the initial phase, many families are too occupied with the beginning of treatment to have opportunity to reflect on what is happening to them. Anger and somatic concerns and complaints may come later, when the family has had time to settle into a routine of treatment. Vacillation of mood may often be observed in family members.

In the initial stages, there may be a cognitive but not emotional acceptance of the illness [5]. What is actually discussed—the amount of illness-related communication—varies from family to family.

When the child is initially hospitalized with cancer, many parents relate feeling a "loss of control." Some express that they "never really know what is going on" [3]. Parents must deal with the stress of the initial diagnosis and then attempt to "regain a new equilibrium in a family and that both encompasses the illness and yet attempts to achieve a new normalcy" [3].

Parents who have been interviewed after the period of diagnosis state that there are certain helpful interventions in the initial stages. Some have shared that it is important that they have conferences alone with the staff first, including the child later. This allows them time to absorb the information and to prepare the child. Parents who have been given information related to diagnosis at the same time as the child state that it is impossible to conceal their shock. They believe this hinders their ability to effectively support the child and to problem-solve as a family unit [3].

Families report that it is important not to dwell on the illness. Many have said that as soon as they are able to acknowledge the facts, it is most helpful to attempt to return to as normal a schedule as possible in order to preserve family unity [3].

Parenting a child with a malignant disease may lead to emotional stress in a variety of ways, some resulting in psychological problems. Parents respond to the diagnosis of cancer with denial, guilt, overprotectiveness, and marital conflict. One study reported that in more than half of the families observed, at least one member required psychiatric hospitalization after the diagnosis of cancer in childhood was made [8].

Communication problems may develop in the family. Both parents and child may understand the severity of the illness, but not communicate fears and apprehensions to each other. The child may want to "protect the parents" from realizing what he or she knows. The parents may believe the child does not know the diagnosis and its implications and hesitate to discuss the illness. At a time when the need for mutual support is most crucial, family members often cope separately, in silence.

COPING PATTERNS

Coping is defined as the cognitive and behavioral efforts made to master, tolerate, or reduce external and internal demands [9]. Coping is a shifting process in which a person must, at certain times, rely more heavily on one form, such as defensive strategies, and at other times on another, such as problem-solving strategies, as the status of the situation changes. The way that a person copes depends to a great extent on the resources available and the constraints that inhibit use of these resources in the context of a specific encounter. Important resources include social support, positive beliefs about oneself, health and energy, problem-solving skills, social skills, and monetary resources. Constraints which might limit the availability of such resources might arise from personal values and beliefs which prohibit action or feeling. In addition, constraints exist in the environment, such as competing demands for the same resources, which may be finite in supply [9].

For the parent of the child with cancer, such factors greatly affect the way in which the illness is interpreted and the individual's management of the disease as it progresses. For example, a family with strong social support, such as consistent, nurturing friendships, may draw upon this resource in crucial times of need throughout the child's illness. A family with monetary resources has easier and more effective access to legal, medical, financial, and other professional assistance. Simply having money may reduce the person's vulnerability to threat and in this way facilitate effective coping [9]. In contrast, a divorced, isolated, single parent who cannot identify sources of social support and who does not have monetary resources may be particularly vulnerable following the diagnosis of cancer and may be ineffective in providing support for the child.

In families coping with cancer in childhood it is important to identify and understand the coping strategies of each member, for each person is affected by the other. Not only will the child with cancer experience his illness, but each member of the family unit will interpret the diagnosis and prognosis and deal with it in his or her unique manner. If family members lose their common objective, become less mutually cooperative, fail to coordinate functions, or lack consensus of emotional attitudes, the family will not be able to provide social support for its members. Family disorganization may ensue, with potential disintegration of the family system [10]. It is unlikely that family members will cope effectively unless active communication is maintained among members of the family unit.

PARENTS OF THE CHILD WITH CANCER

Studies of parents of fatally ill children have reported a number of common behaviors and responses. Strategies used to cope with the illness and to gain psychological protection from overwhelming anxiety include: increased motor activity, denying the diagnosis, seeking explanations for the development of the disease in order to avoid guilt, investing trust in the primary physician and other staff members, avoiding visits to the child, avoiding discussions of death, and reacting with hostility toward the staff [11].

Coping behaviors manifested by parents in attempts to gain mastery or control over the situation include: making practical arrangements for care and transportation, participating in the child's medical care, seeking medical information about the disease in an attempt to master it intellectually, allowing oneself to feel and express sorrow, grieving, giving and accepting emotional support, and openly discussing the illness [11].

It has been stated that the universal use of denial as a coping mechanism seems to aid in long-term adjustment to cancer in childhood [4]. Denial serves an adaptive function by helping the individual to escape from matters over which he or she has no control. Some patients and families who are unable to invoke such defenses effectively may become depressed. Chronic anxiety may result, leading to a loss of future orientation, hypochondriases, or avoidance of hospitals and medical staff. This pattern may result in compliance problems, failure to provide self-care, or failure to continue medical followup [2]. Interventions assisting the child and family to regain a sense of control are important at this particular time.

An opposing view considers denial or avoidance in the context of illness ineffective because the person fails to engage in appropriate problem-solving efforts that would decrease the actual danger or damage of illness [9]. People who defend themselves by avoiding whatever could be threatening must remain forever on guard and may experience depleted energy as a result [13].

Denial may be less damaging and more effective in the early rather than the late stages of a crisis, such as in the diagnosis of cancer, when the situation cannot yet be faced in its entirety. Some studies have shown that denial-like coping processes have proved helpful while the patient was still in the hospital, but seemed to have negative consequences when used after leaving the hospital environment [9].

Some authorities caution that no coping strategy should be labeled as good or bad, for the context must be taken into account for each individual and the particular situation [14].

HIGH RISK FAMILIES

Certain families are particularly high risk for psychological problems when a child is seriously ill. Families whose native language is not English or whose cultural background is significantly different often have major difficulties coping when the child is diagnosed with a disease such as cancer. Factors such as poverty, intellectual limitations, pre-existing psychological maladjustment in a family member, or incongruity of coping styles among family members will negatively affect the child's own ability to cope [5].

Marriages that might previously have been stable are at risk for tension and discord when the child has cancer. The family experiences increased financial pressures, stress resulting from time lost from work, concerns related to the ill child's siblings, and myriad other problems associated with the cancer diagnosis. Differences in parents' coping styles, in addition to these stresses, may exacerbate any pre-existing marital tension and generate friction where none may have previously existed [8].

EFFECTS ON RELATIONSHIPS

Some parents share the fact that the disease has united them as a stronger family unit. They state their values change; some who were materialistic begin to view each day with their child as the most important thing to them.

Friendships may be affected by the child's illness. Those who "don't know what to say" may be so uncomfortable that, not only do they fail to support the family, but they are unsuccessful in coping with their own emotions related to the child's diagnosis. Long silences may ensue, and friendships may end.

New friends are often made who are sharing the same experience. A common bond unites parents who experience the crisis of having a child with cancer. As one mother expressed it, "You (the professional) can't understand what I feel. Only another parent in the same situation can" [15].

Each member of the family adjusts to the disease differently and at an individual pace. This fact emphasizes the importance of family communication. Questions like, "Am I the only one who feels this way? Am I being too extreme?" must be shared and addressed. Not all members of the family will reach the same point emotionally at the same time. When communication within a family unit is poor before the illness is diagnosed, the stress of cancer can result in more severe family dysfunction [16]. All members of the family of a child with cancer are at risk for psychosocial difficulties. The period of risk begins at diagnosis and continues throughout the treatment process. For some families, emotional problems linger long after the death of the child [16].

THERAPEUTIC INTERVENTIONS

One of the most important interventions in providing support for the child with cancer is facilitating consistent communication among the child, family, and those providing care. Family members may need to feel sanction to express ambivalent feelings about the sick child. At some level, there is always resentment at the disruption in their lives, which is complicated by feelings of guilt and anger at the perceived potential loss.

It is important to acknowledge that, even though parents are often aware of their right to be informed of the treatment plan, they may feel uncomfortable asking for further explanation and clarification. Encouraging this type of verbalization—perhaps even identifying someone who can assist them in formulating questions—will help decrease anxiety. If one becomes an astute observer of the family's behavior, much information can be obtained as to how they are coping with the illness. Communication is enhanced by careful, attentive listening, focusing on what family members are sharing, clarifying it to avoid misconceptions, and assisting them to integrate informatioin shared in discussions.

Whenever the patient is a child, the treatment approach should focus on the entire family. Family members will experience psychologic changes as a result of having a child who is seriously ill. A depressed or anxious parent will be unable to conceal feelngs from the child and will be less available to support the child emotionally. In some families, the need for psychosocial intervention may focus on the symptomatic parent or sibling rather than the child [12].

Parents are at risk of losing confidence in their parenting skills when the child is hospitalized for treatment. Confused and bewildered by the diagnosis and treatments, perhaps themselves not having recognized the symptoms or feeling that in some other way they have failed, parents wait helplessly for the outcome. It is crucial to assist parents to regain a sense of confidence in themselves as care givers for their children.

Once past the initial shock, it is imperative to help the family to move from a fear of death to a life focus. A useful technique for facilitating this movement is to enlist the child and family in predicting how they will cope, identifying strengths as well as areas with which they may need assistance, and inquiring how this help may best be provided by the staff providing care. Such exploration gives permission for and models a self-monitoring process [5].

A family that is coping well during the early stage following diagnosis will probably make visible progress by the end of the first week in dealing realistically with the information provided [5]. The family should have begun the process of planning and making appropriate modifications in their lives to begin to prepare for the next stage, the induction of treatment. At this point, the family that is coping effectively will realistically review and evaluate plans they made before the child's diagnosis [5].

THE CHILD WITH CANCER

When a child has cancer, the goals are to: 1) eradicate the disease, 2) return to as normal a life as possible, and 3) live as well as possible [17].

Studies of children with cancer during treatment have noted regression and immature behavior, alterations in self-concept, and increased worry and apprehension [18]. Some children react by living each day to the fullest; they are able to look forward to the future and not dwell on the illness. Others are angry, even hostile, and some withdraw from family and friends.

The chronically ill child must learn to live with various degrees of constant or frequent life disruption and to develop heightened stress tolerance. Many children learn to live with their disability and to develop effective coping mechanisms. Children may ask specific questions beyond what is explained (i.e., as in bone marrow aspirations) in an attempt to cope more effectively. Posing questions may be an example of assertiveness behavior that serves to mediate anxiety and may be related to the child's personality or to a previous pattern of reinforcement or curiosity. Children who express inquisitiveness about procedures tend to exhibit fewer anxious behaviors than children who do not ask questions [19].

Questioning by the school-age child and adolescent can be an indication that positive defenses, such as intellectualization, are being mobilized. This can be encouraged by providing appropriate information at the time it is requested [20]. Patients and family members who actively question various aspects of the treatment and who demonstrate an ability to follow through with instructions are considered in general to be adapting well [5].

SIBLINGS

Siblings of patients with cancer may demonstrate a variety of difficulties. School problems are common. Exaggerated sibling rivalry and jealousy may occur. Siblings who are not allowed to participate in the knowledge and treatment of the child's disease may interpret such "protective treatment" as reinforcement of their irrational fantasies related to the disease. Many siblings experience guilt, believing that they have in some way caused the child's illness. Some are embarrassed by how their sibling appears to others. There may be anger and jealousy of the attention focused on the ill child [21].

Siblings may be neglected while the focus is on the sick child. While some of their problems may be readily apparent, feelings that they experience such as guilt related to the child's diagnosis may surface many months, even years, later [21].

It is important to assist the parents in understanding and interpreting siblings' behavior as symptoms of their stress rather than as an additional annoying burden. The importance of parental communication with siblings of the child with cancer cannot be underestimated. It is now recognized that siblings must be provided with direct factual information at the time of diagnosis and during therapy to ameliorate or prevent adjustment problems [22]. The sibling should be acknowledged as an integral part of the family approach to treatment [23,24]. Psychosocial intervention with siblings, as with other family members, should focus on facilitation of their involvement and participation throughout all stages of the disease.

THE ADOLESCENT WITH CANCER

One of the major goals for the adolescent with cancer is to mitigate the side effects of treatment with medical and behavioral therapy. This is a worthy endeavor, considering the fact that the treatment may be viewed by the adolescent as worse than the disease itself [26].

At a time when the child normally rebels against parents, the adolescent with cancer must be dependent on them. Even the adolescent with a positive self-image suffers greatly with the dramatic change in body image resulting from cancer treatments. Chemotherapy, radiation therapy, and surgery may significantly alter the child that "once was." Rejection by friends and social isolation may follow such treatments.

Cancer is one of the most emotion-laden diagnoses that an adolescent and his or her family can experience. The word itself (which can become a label) can traumatize the family acutely and disrupt previous interactional patterns. The major distresses experienced by adolescents are related to the treatment of the disease process [26].

Adolescence is a period during which multiple and rapid changes are experienced; therefore, additional change due to disease can be particularly anxiety-provoking [20]. Normal teenage concerns include body image, sexuality, and self-esteem. The malignant tumor affects all of these things. The adolescent is in the process of trying to develop control; the diagnosis of cancer halts this developmental process. It is not uncommon for a teenager to say, "I'd rather die than lose my hair." This statement reflects how the adolescent sincerely feels during this period. Loss of hair is one of the greatest concerns expressed by teenagers afflicted with a malignant disease, reported by some to be more difficult than the loss of a limb [27].

Physical changes may affect some female adolescents with cancer more than males. Females tend to believe that physical attributes are strongly related to social acceptance. Males tend to believe they may gain approval from other attributes, such as physical strength and mechanical abilities [26]. Through medical management of the disease, there is often interference with the adolescent's ability to develop sexually, which affects emotional development. Teenagers hesitate to engage in relationships with others for fear others will discover their cancer and reject them. Patients may limit themselves due to lack of confidence resulting from hair loss, weight loss or weight gain, and other alterations in body image. Such self-induced limitations may include dating and any contact potentially leading to intimacy; an important and helpful suggestion is to double date with other teenagers who have cancer, who understand the concerns related to nausea from chemotherapy and hair loss.

Chronically ill adolescents who are under medical surveillance for serious diseases may tend to underplay any but the most major illness as a disruption. This de-emphasis of illness may lead to denial of the disease [26]. Even seriously ill adolescents may be able to deny their disease in order to function adaptively and with hope. Denial is often considered maladaptive, yet the helpful nature of denial should not be overlooked [28].

Severely ill adolescents may displace their anger regarding their illness onto their treatments; decisions to enter or continue with treatments are viewed as potentially controllable [27]. Displaced anger may be a factor in problems of non-compliance, which are common in adolescent patients [26].

Parents are often the ones interfering most in the adolescent's normal growth and development. They assume that because their child has cancer, the child cannot continue to engage in activities shared by well children. This is a common reaction that must be dealt with by the staff as soon as possible. It is essential to assist the parents to understand the concept that it is normal for a child to be sick [29]. It is important to help them to sort out what is best for the child and what is done to alleviate their own anxiety. Home, school, clinic, and hospital environment must be such that a child can live a full life, not one that primarily focuses on disease and treatment [30].

It is crucial in dealing with teenagers to acknowledge their important role in the treatment plan. The adolescent must be provided with knowledge about the disease and therapy. Some treatment centers achieve this by allowing their patients to read their own medical records [28].

Teenagers are risk-takers. This fact should be considered when encouraging them to become actively involved in their own treatment plan. When adolescents are treated as passive recipients, they will not readily cooperate. When explanation is provided as to why therapy is valuable and what the risks are, there is better chance of involvement. It is often effective to encourage the adolescent's natural sense of humor to stimulate his involvement. Some teenagers will find creative ways to cope with treatment, such as painting a flower on an abdominal scar, starting a "trend" [27]. Ill adolescents must develop coping strategies such as forming a hospital or clinic peer group and making arrangements with friends for hospital and home visits during school absences.

It is helpful for staff to address concerns that might not be voiced voluntarily by the adolescent but which do, nevertheless, exist. Topics such as vaginitis, impotence, and ulcerations can be introduced in a manner that normalizes such subjects. This can be done effectively while performing a physical exam, providing the opportunity for the adolescent to share feelings related to the side effects of treatment and to realize that others share similar concerns.

GROUP INTERACTION AS SUPPORTIVE INTERVENTION

It is important to consider that for many children, the diagnosis of cancer may be the first time they experience a serious illness. This diagnosis results in major changes in daily living, altering patterns that previously have been a source of security for the child.

For the very young child, support may be offered by providing the opportunity to play with real equipment that is ordinarily seen as threatening. The child can master anxiety regarding stressful situations by hands-on experiences with tools and supplies, gradually becoming familiar with these objects and viewing them as less "toxic." Such supervised play may take place in sessions with other children or alone, as the need indicates.

Children with cancer experience altered relationships with peers. Obvious changes in body image may be frightening to other children. There is frequently the myth that cancer is contagious. Some children isolate themselves due to fear of peer rejection. Family and friends may refrain from visiting or, alternately, over-indulge the child, both of which are confusing to him.

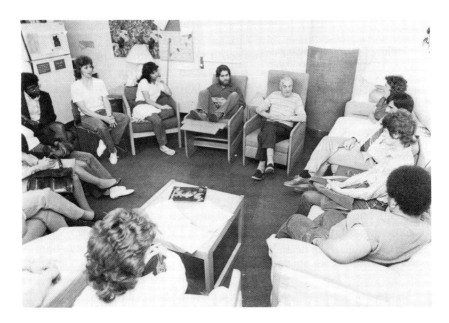

Fig. 18–1. The Parents' Group. Families who have children with cancer collectively pool their knowledge and become resources for each other.

[34]. Many parents are more aware and troubled than their children by the potential terminal nature of the illness. Believing that death is likely or inevitable, with the lengthening of remission, they become increasingly hopeful of a cure. Yet the threat of relapse is an ever-present reality. Many parents continue to have difficulty discussing the illness with each other and with their children during this period. Some continue to have periods of anguish, depression, and intense need for support from family and friends [35].

It has been observed that with the prolongation of remission, at some point there is an attenuation in the process of parental detachment and anticipatory mourning. The mother may display feelings and attitudes that suggest alternately increasing attachment and loosening of ties [35]. In remission there is often a search for meaning, to understand how the child's illness fits into a broader perspective of the family's life. Hope that the remission may be permanent continues. As the remission lengthens, the family moves toward reinvestment in life. Yet the threat of relapse is always present.

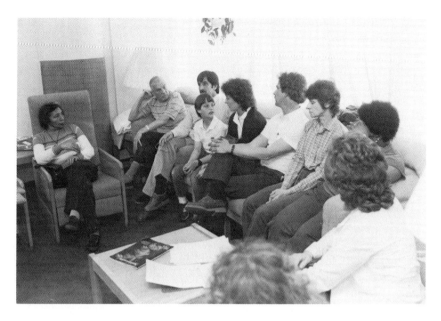

Fig. 18–2. A child in remission joins the Parents' Group to discuss his experiences following diagnosis and treatment.

TERMINATION OF THE TREATMENT PROTOCOL

Long-time survivors of childhood cancer recall the termination of treatment as a time of particular stress. There is relief that treatment is completed, but there is concern of being "unprotected" and of separation from medical and nursing staff [7]. It is helpful at this time to provide a review of the course of treatment, emphasizing the normal feelings of ambivalence experienced regarding the loss of consistent professional monitoring [5]. During the discussion, ways in which the family has succeeded in coping with earlier stress points can be acknowledged and affirmed, encouraging the formulation of new goals for the future. When families can begin to become involved in long-range planning, there is indication that they are effectively managing the treatment termination phase [5].

REENTRY INTO SCHOOL, FAMILY, AND SOCIAL LIFE

The preparation for reentry into school, family, and community life should be completed by the time treatment is terminated. The process of reentry occurs not once, but each time there is a remission [5].

Children with cancer have not lost the potential for growth and development. While in school, they have the opportunity to grow, to develop, and to prepare for the future, as do their healthy classmates [30]. If the health care team places priority on the psychological, social, and educational preparation of patients for cure, then school attendance is particularly significant as a normalizing factor [29]. It has been demonstrated that chronically and even seriously ill children derive much satisfaction from school [36].

Patients and families who are particularly vulnerable during this phase include: 1) those of low socioeconomic status, implying less accommodating schools for children with disabilities; 2) those with a passive attitude; 3) those with a tendency to withdraw; 4) those demonstrating cultural differences with school personnel, which often results in poorer communication; and 5) those with closed communication patterns, limiting their ability to resolve conflicting feelings [5].

Interventions designed to support the child and family at this point require involvement with school personnel and other community agencies. It is necessary to provide school personnel with factual information to help them to understand the disease process and the treatment and how this affects the child and family. A knowledge of available community resources for individual family needs such as transportation, financial aid, medical equipment, and support groups can be of valuable assistance.

The health care team must be committed to doing everything possible to assist the child and family in living as normal a life as possible. School is an integral part of a child's life. Parents who perceive that staff share this attitude will interpret the question of school reentry to be not "if" but "when" the child returns to school [30]. When the child or adolescent is able to return to the school, family, or vocational environment with renewed enthusiasm and enjoyment, there is indication of optimal coping [5].

RELAPSE

Relapse confirms the initial diagnosis and shatters illusions, particularly about the extent of the healing powers of the medical team. Many families express the fact that they experience this period as worse than the crisis of diagnosis [5]. There is recapitulation of earlier stress, accompanied with diminished hope for long-term survival. The family is challenged by the task of confronting their despair and helplessness "in the face of the destructive power of the disease" and yet restoring hope for a prolonged remission and reinvesting in a rigorous treatment protocol [5].

Psychosocial intervention at this time should focus on facilitating the family's processing of information and communication about the patient's new situation. The patient and siblings may require more updated, age-appropriate information, since they may have reached different developmental stages from the time of diagnosis. It is important to assist the family in regaining a life focus with a time perspective reflected of the altered prognosis. Parents may express guilt and self-blame, and reaffirmation of family strength and ability to cope with earlier crisis points is essential. There may be practical problems related to reinduction of treatment with which the family may require assistance.

Families vulnerable at this stage are those that are unrealistically optimistic or excessively pessimistic about the disease process, wishing "it were all over." Psychosocial support at this point is essential to avoid withdrawal of the family's involvement with the child [5]. A family coping effectively at this stage is likely to respond emotionally to the change in prognosis, but be able to reinvest in the next treatment and future plans.

INITIATION OF RESEARCH TREATMENT

The need for research treatment indicates that the disease is uncontrolled. This is a particular stressful time for families. Home life may become chaotic, and the child's condition may require frequent and unpredictable hospitalization.

Facilitation of the communication among the child, family, and the staff providing care is even more critical at this time. Mental health personnel may need to intervene to prevent or minimize alienation between parents and staff. Staff may feel out of control, helpless, and even guilty regarding the failure of the previous treatment. The family may displace their own anger and guilt onto the staff.

Families that have coped well during other crisis points may begin to experience difficulties. Problems may result from the stress experienced in relation to the rapid changes in the child's condition, which negate efforts to maintain a normal schedule.

It is important at this point to provide respite care for the family and to provide them with opportunities to vent their feelings, rather than to blame others. It is likely that families are coping effectively when they can articulate their feelings and can tolerate behavioral changes in the staff, interpreting this as a reflection of the staff's sensitivity to the situation [5].

STRESS POINTS

There are additional crisis or stress points related to the psychological aspects of surviving childhood cancer. These include events that trigger reminders of the residual risks, and therefore precipitate recurring concerns about the illness [6]. Examples are anniversaries, such as in the case of the child whose cancer was diagnosed at the start of the school year. The child may become increasingly anxious each September, without consciously realizing why.

The return of symptoms similar to those that preceded the diagnosis of cancer, "symptom consciousness," is a crisis point. This may generate intense anxiety, which may persist despite the reassurance that such symptoms are not a sign of malignancy [6].

Developmental marker events constitute another stress point. These are social or achievement events that emphasize progress or growth, reminding the patient and family of the future and recalling feelings of uncertainty [6].

Patients diagnosed with cancer encounter societal prejudices, another crisis point. These include the wide range of reactions displayed when others learn that someone has cancer. Non-supportive reactions include avoidance, fantasies of contagion, ostracism, or actual denial of employment to a childhood cancer survivor reaching healthy adulthood [6].

Another event that can trigger anxiety for the child and family is the recent diagnosis of someone known to them with cancer. In addition, media coverge of cancer reminds these children that they are different from others; they have something to worry about. This voids the use of adaptive denial as a defense [12].

It is essential that staff working with the child and family be sensitive to these events and issues as potential stressors of adverse emotional reactions. It is helpful to assist the patient and family to anticipate the stress that may be experienced in relation to these occurrences in order to decrease their anxiety. In addition, it is often effective to assist the child and family in identifying the particular stressor responsible for such apprehension. In these discussions, it is possible to normalize the family's reactions to these stressors.

TERMINATION OF TREATMENT

It is easier for the family if the decision to terminate active treatment is initiated by the medical staff. For all families, guilt needs to be relieved by helping them to see that they have done everything possible. It is essential to assist them to recognize that it is the *treatment* that has failed and not the patient, parent, or hospital staff [5].

COMMUNICATION

Early knowledge of the cancer diagnosis is related to positive psychosocial adjustment among long-term survivors of childhood cancer. Many parents who initially did not share the diagnosis with their child identify this lack of candor as a source of stress both during and after treatment [37].

Children often have fears related to the illness and treatment, which when identified can be addressed. The child who is afraid of a bone marrow aspiration may be greatly relieved when encouraged to express *what* the fears are. An intervention such as suggesting that the parent accompany the child to the procedure may not only lessen the child's fears, but involve the parents, returning some of the sense of control they believe has been robbed by nursing and medical staff.

THE CHILD'S AWARENESS OF DEATH

One of the dilemmas most frequently encountered by parents and staff is how to communicate with the terminally ill child. Should the prognosis be shared with the child, and, if not, does the child sense that he or she is seriously ill, even when this is not explained?

It has been found that, even when the family does not discuss death, children display death anxiety. Childhood affects associated with death are often unhappiness, loneliness, or sadness, suggesting reference to earlier life stages when fears of separation and abandonment are paramount [35].

Studies have demonstrated that a child's conception of death matures developmentally. Children under 5 years of age appear to view death as something reversible such as departure or separation. Death is conceptualized from approximately ages 6 to 10 years as an inevitable, external process often resulting from the actions of others or purposeful forces. God is viewed as such a force. Death is interpreted by children at this age as punishment for evil thoughts or deeds. Past the age of 10, children begin to conceptualize death as an internal process and universal to all forms of life [38].

It is generally accepted that the older children with a fatal prognosis, especially an adolescent, can be aware of the seriousness of the illness. Yet some authorities contend that the fatally ill child under 10 lacks the intellectual capacity to formulate a concept of death and is therefore not aware of his or her prognosis. They theorize that if the adult does not discuss the illness and prognosis with the child, the child will experience little or no anxiety related to this subject [39,40]. Others contest this approach favoring open communication with the dying child and the family. They maintain that the normal development of the ability to conceptualize death is accelerated when the child is terminally ill at an early age. They state that the awareness of impending death becomes stronger as the child progresses through terminal illness [41,42]. Several authorities have stated that "telling" the child is not the most important issue. What should be emphasized is providing a climate of openness and support for the child in dealing with his or her concerns [3,10,41].

The theory of communication referred to as the "open approach" provides an environment that is supportive of the child's questions and concerns from diagnosis on, as the illness progresses [10,42].

If staff does not acknowledge that the child's illness is serious, the child may perceive this as an obvious contradiction to the fact that another child may have died on the same ward, with a similar diagnosis. Such denial may not lend credibility to further statements made by care-givers. Acknowledgement that the illness is serious does not mean eliminating hope, which for many becomes a lifeline throughout the progression of the disease [43].

When cure and remission are beyond the capacity of the available treatment, intervention focuses on paliative care. The goals at this point are to achieve a state in which the patient is as symptom-free as possible, alert, comfortable, and free

Psychosocial interventions at this point should focus on assisting the family to anticipate what lies ahead, exploring with them their desires for their child and alternate methods of achieving these goals [5]. Taking the needs of the patient and all family members into consideration, the parents must decide whether the child should die at home, in the hospital, or in hospice care.

Period of Bereavement

A final crisis point is the period several months after the death of a pediatric cancer patient. Support is often well provided to the family in the first weeks after the child death. Yet often by 5 or 6 months such support is withdrawn when friends and relatives beyond the immediate family do not understand why there is not "full recovery" from the loss. The deceased's birthday, a family holiday, or some similar event may result in renewed mourning or grief reaction among the survivors [6].

There is a period of critical need when contact with former advocates for the family (nurses, physicians, psychosocial staff) might be most helpful; however, this is the time when such support is often unavailable. The inclusion of a plan of followup during the period of bereavement, especially throughout the first year following the child's death, is an essential component of any treatment program. An additionally important time for outreach to the family by the oncology team is at the 1-year anniversary of the child's death [6].

SUMMARY

When a child has cancer, the disease is experienced in some way by all members of the family. Knowledge by staff providing care that there are crisis points, particularly stressful periods that are encountered by the patient and family, is vital to effectively provide consistent psychosocial support. An awarness and understanding of the psychologic implications inherent in each stage of the disease process will enable staff to more realistically formulate guidelines for intervention.

REFERENCES

1. American Cancer Society. Cancer Facts and Figures: 1983. New York: American Cancer Society, 1984.
2. McCalla JL: A multidisciplinary approach to identification and remedial intervention for adverse late effects of cancer therapy. Nurs Clin North Am 20:117, 1985.
3. McQuown L: The parents of the child with cancer: a view from those who suffer most. In Spinetta JJ, Deasi-Spinetta, P (eds): Living with Childhood Cancer. St.Louis: C.V. Mosby, 1981.
4. O'Malley JE, Koocher GP, Foster D, et al.: Psychiatric sequelae of surviving childhood cancer. Am J Orthopsychiatry 49:608, 1979.
5. Christ GH, Adams MA: Therapeutic strategies at psychosocial crisis points in the treatment of childhood cancer. In Christ AE, Flomenhaft K (eds): Childhood Cancer. New York: Plenum Press, 1984, p 109.
6. Koocher GP: The crisis of survival. In Christ AF, Flomenhaft K (eds): Childhood Cancer. New York: Plenum Press, 1984, p 129.
7. Koocher GP, O'Malley JE; Implications for patient care. In Koocher GP, O'Malley JE (eds): The Damocles Syndrome. New York: McGraw Hill, 1981, p 164.
8. Binger CML, Ablin AR, Feuerstein RC, et al.: Childhood leukemia: Emotional impact on child and family. N Engl J Med 280:414, 1969.
9. Lazarus RS, Folkman S: Stress, Appraisal, and Coping. New York: Springer, 1984.
10. Spinetta JJ, Deasy-Spinetta P: Talking with children who have a life-threatening illness. In Spinetta JJ and Deasy-Spinetta P (eds): Living with Childhood Cancer. St. Louis: C.V. Mosby, 1981, p 234.
11. Slavin LA: Evolving psychosocial issues in the treatment of childhood cancer: A review. In Koocher GP, O'Malley JE (eds): The Damocles Syndrome. New York: McGraw Hill, 1981, p 1.
12. Koocher GP: Psychosocial care of the child cured of cancer. Pediatr Nurs 11:91, 1985.
13. Fenichel O: The Psychoanalytic Theory of Neurosis. New York: Norton, 1945.
14. Cohen F, Lazarus RS: Coping and adaptation in health and illness. In Mechanic D (ed): Handbook of Health, Health Care, and the Health Professions. New York: The Free Press, 1983.
15. Gibbons MB, Boren H: Stress reduction: A spectrum of strategies in pediatric oncology nursing. Nursing Clin North Am 20:83, 1985.
16. Kaplan DM, Smith A, Grobstein R, et al.: Family mediation of stress. Social Work 18:60, 1973.

17. van Eyes J: The truly Cured Child: The New Challenge in Pediatric Cancer Care. Baltimore: University Park Press, 1977.
18. Spinetta JJ, Rigler D, Karon M: Anxiety in the dying child. Pediatrics 52:841, 1973.
19. Katz ER, Kellerman J, Siegel S: Behavioral distress in children undergoing medical procedures: Developmental considerations. Consult Clin Psycho 48:356, 1980.
20. Kellerman J, Ellenberg L, Rigler D: Psychological effects of illness in adolescence. I. Anxiety, self-esteem, and perception of control. Pediatr 97:126, 1980.
21. Koocher GP: Coping with survivorship in childhood cancer: Family problems. In Christ AE, Flomenhaft K (eds): Childhood Cancer. New York: Plenum Press, 1984, p 203.
22. Gogan JG, Koocher GP, Foster DJ, et al.: Impact of childhood cancer on siblings. Health Soc Work 2:42, 1977.
23. Lavigne JV: The siblings of childhood cancer patients: Psychosocial aspects. In Schulman JL, Kupst MJ (eds): The Child with Cancer. Springfield: Charles C Thomas, 1980, p 37.
24. Gogal JL, Slavin LA: Interview with brother and sisters. In Koocher GP, O'Malley JE (eds): The Damocles Syndrome. New York: McGraw Hill, 1981, p. 101.
25. Sourkes BM: Siblings of the pediatric cancer patient. In Kellerman J (ed): Psychological Aspects of Childhood Cancer. Springfield: Charles C Thomas, 1980, p 47.
26. Zeltzer L, Ellenberg L, Rigler D: Psychologic effects of illness in adolescence. II. Impact of illness in adolescents; crucial issues and coping styles. J. Pediatr 97:132, 1980.
27. Wilbur J: Sexual development and body image in the teenager with cancer. Front Radiat Ther Oncol 14:108, 1980.
28. Zeltzer L: The adolescent with cancer. In Kellerman J (ed): Psychological Aspects of Childhood Cancer. Springfield: Charles C Thomas, 1980, p 70.
29. van Eyes J: The Normally Sick Child. Baltimore: University Park Press, 1979.
30. Deasy-Spinetta P: The school and the child with cancer. In Spinetta JJ, Deasy-Spinetta P (eds): Living with Childhood Cancer. St. Louis: C.V. Mosby, 1981, p 153.
31. McEvoy M, Duchon D, Schafer D: Therapeutic play groups for patients and siblings in a pediatric oncology ambulatory care unit. Top Clin Nurs 7:10, 1985.
32. Adams MA: A hospital play program: Helping children with serious illness. Am J Orthopsychiatry 46:416, 1976.
33. Mattsson A: Long-term physical illness in childhood: A challenge to psychosocial adaptation. In Garfield GA (ed): Stress and Survival: The Emotional Realities of Life-Threatening Illness. St. Louis: C.V. Mosby, 1979, p 194.
34. Stolberg AL, Cunningham JG: Support groups for parents of leukemic children: Evaluation of current programs and enumeration of participants' emotional needs. In Schulman JL, Kupst MJ (eds): The Child with Cancer. Springfield: Charles C Thomas, 1980.
35. Obetz SW, Swenson WM, McCarthy CA, et al.: Children who survive malignant disease: Emotional adaptation of the children and their families. In Schulman JL, Kupst MJ (eds): The Child with Cancer. Springfield: Charles C Thomas, 1980, p 194.
36. Kaplan DM, Smith A, Grobstein R: School management of the seriously ill child. J Sch Health 44:250, 1974.
37. Koocher GP, O'Malley JE: The special problems of the survivors. In Koocher GP, O'Malley JE (eds): The Damocles Syndrome. New York: McGraw Hill, 1981, p 112.
38. Gartley W, Bernasconi M: The concept of death in children. J Genet Psychol 105:283, 1964.
39. Debuskey M: Orchestration of care. In Debuskey M (ed): The Chronically Ill Child. Springfield: Charles C Thomas, 1970, p 3.
40. Ingalls AJ, Salermo MC: Maternal and Child Health. St. Louis: C.V. Mosby, 1971.

41. Waechter EH: Children's awarness of fatal illness. Am J Nurs 71:1168, 1971.
42. Bluebond-Langner M: Meanings of death to children. In Feifel H (ed): New Meanings of Death. New York: McGraw Hill, 1977, p 97.
43. Gibbons MB: When the dying patient is a child: A challenge for the living. In Hockenberry MJ, Coody DK (eds): Pediatric Oncology and Hematology St. Louis: C.V. Mosby, 1986, p 493.
44. The International Work Group on Death, Dying, and Bereavement: Assumptions and principles underlying standards for terminal care. Am J Nurs 79:296, 1979.

Index